Irritable Bowel Syndrome

AF665723

Takeshi Kamiya • Shin Fukudo
Editors

Irritable Bowel Syndrome

Springer

Editors
Takeshi Kamiya
Department of Medical Innovation
Nagoya City University Graduate School
Medical Sciences
Nagoya, Aichi, Japan

Shin Fukudo
Department of Behavioral Medicine
Tohoku University Graduate School of
Medicine
Sendai, Miyagi, Japan

ISBN 978-981-97-8412-7 ISBN 978-981-97-8410-3 (eBook)
https://doi.org/10.1007/978-981-97-8410-3

© The Editor(s) (if applicable) and The Author(s), under exclusive license to Springer Nature Singapore Pte Ltd. 2024
This work is subject to copyright. All rights are solely and exclusively licensed by the Publisher, whether the whole or part of the material is concerned, specifically the rights of translation, reprinting, reuse of illustrations, recitation, broadcasting, reproduction on microfilms or in any other physical way, and transmission or information storage and retrieval, electronic adaptation, computer software, or by similar or dissimilar methodology now known or hereafter developed.
The use of general descriptive names, registered names, trademarks, service marks, etc. in this publication does not imply, even in the absence of a specific statement, that such names are exempt from the relevant protective laws and regulations and therefore free for general use.
The publisher, the authors and the editors are safe to assume that the advice and information in this book are believed to be true and accurate at the date of publication. Neither the publisher nor the authors or the editors give a warranty, expressed or implied, with respect to the material contained herein or for any errors or omissions that may have been made. The publisher remains neutral with regard to jurisdictional claims in published maps and institutional affiliations.

This Springer imprint is published by the registered company Springer Nature Singapore Pte Ltd.
The registered company address is: 152 Beach Road, #21-01/04 Gateway East, Singapore 189721, Singapore

If disposing of this product, please recycle the paper.

Preface

It is my great pleasure to publish this book *Irritable Bowel Syndrome* with Springer Nature, alongside my colleague, Professor Takeshi Kamiya, and the other authors. Irritable bowel syndrome (IBS) is recognized as a representative gastrointestinal disorder. IBS is not only a prevalent medical illness but also a common medical condition. Anxiety, depression, somatization, and infectious gastroenteritis are high-risk factors for developing IBS. Reciprocally functional gastrointestinal disorders, including IBS, are high-risk factors for anxiety disorders or depressive disorders. IBS is also a risk factor for dementia. IBS patients have a high co-morbidity with functional dyspepsia, gastrointestinal reflux disease, or other functional somatic syndromes. There appears to be a link between IBS and inflammatory conditions, such as inflammatory bowel disease.

Research in IBS focuses on how gut micro-organisms, increased mucosal permeability, mucosal inflammation, and changes in neuroplasticity relate to each other. Many molecules including ion channels, G-protein coupled receptors, toll-like receptors, transporters, tight junction proteins, proteases, chemokines, cytokines, hormones, and neurotransmitters are involved in the pathophysiology and/or pathogenesis of IBS. Moreover, heredity, susceptible genes, and the epigenome are explored in IBS. How the signals originating from the gut conducted to the brain via the autonomic afferent neurons and lamina I neurons in the dorsal horn of the spinal cord has been a subject of research in sensory neurobiology, which has progressed. The research frontier lies in intracerebral connectivity among brain regions including the insula, amygdala, hypothalamus, anterior cingulate cortex, and prefrontal cortex at rest and under gut stimulation, particularly in patients with IBS and their changes. One of great changes in diagnosis is Rome IV criteria as well as coming Rome V criteria instead of Rome III criteria.

Many new treatments have also been developed for IBS. There are many reports on modification of the gut microbiota using probiotics, prebiotics, antibiotics, and fecal microbiota transplantation. Low fermentable oligosaccharides, disaccharides, monosaccharides, and polyols diet therapy is tried to alleviate IBS symptoms. Intestinal secretagogues (gut epithelium modifiers) and agents that modify bile acid are being developed. Agents that modify serotonin, noradrenaline, opioid, histamine, and acetylcholine neurotransmission and receptors provide their efficacy for IBS. Neuroleptics often represented by antidepressants are one of the standard treatments for IBS, but further evidence is being explored. Psychotherapy, e.g., cognitive behavioral therapy or hypnotherapy, is also raising its level of evidence.

Based on these backgrounds, solving IBS as a hub medical condition will give a broad impact on the whole medical science. It is very timely to publish this book by many specialists in Japan. All authors are members of the clinical practice guidelines for irritable bowel syndrome or functional dyspepsia by the Japanese Society of Gastroenterology. Therefore, this book well summarized the deep knowledge on IBS through the contents of each chapter. Japan has the ability to develop new pharmacotherapy for IBS, like United States or European Union. The contents of this book will provide important insights into the new education, clinical practice, and research of IBS worldwide.

Sendai, Japan Shin Fukudo

Contents

Part I
Etiology

Chapter 1
Definition of Irritable Bowel Syndrome

Takeshi Kamiya and Michiko Shikano

Abstract Irritable bowel syndrome (IBS) is a highly prevalent functional bowel disorder. There have been a number of definitions and classifications of IBS, and the diagnostic criteria have changed over the years. The Manning criteria were developed as the first global symptom- based IBS diagnostic criteria in 1978, followed by Rome I in 1992, Rome II in 1999, and Rome III in 2006. After 10 years, in 2016, the latest version of the Rome IV criteria was published and has been used in clinical practice worldwide. Presently, the Rome IV criteria provide valuable resources to investigators, trainers and clinicians for research, education, and management of IBS.

Keywords Irritable bowel syndrome · Definition · Diagnostic criteria · Rome IV

1.1 Introduction

Irritable bowel syndrome (IBS) is one of the common disorders of gut-brain interaction (DGBI), previously called functional gastrointestinal disorders, characterized by chronic and recurrent abdominal pain related to bowel habits of diarrhea or constipation despite the absence of organic disease [1–3]. Although IBS can be diagnosed at any age, younger people are more likely to be affected than those older than age 50 years [1, 4]. IBS was conventionally considered secondary to a neurotic disorder, and several names had been proposed for it: neurogenic mucus colitis [5], colonic neurosis [6], irritable colon, and chronic nonspecific enteropathy. Presently, the Rome criteria proposed by the working expert groups of the Rome Foundation [2, 3] have been most widely accepted globally. This article summarizes changes in the definition of IBS, with particular focus on the latest updated version, Rome IV [1] criteria for IBS.

T. Kamiya (✉) · M. Shikano
Department of Medical Innovation, Nagoya City University Graduate School of Medical Sciences, Nagoya, Japan
e-mail: kamitake@med.nagoya-cu.ac.jp; m_shikano@jg7.so-net.ne.jp

© The Editor(s) (if applicable) and The Author(s), under exclusive license to Springer Nature Singapore Pte Ltd. 2024

T. Kamiya, S. Fukudo (eds.), *Irritable Bowel Syndrome*,
https://doi.org/10.1007/978-981-97-8410-3_1

1.2 History in the Definition of IBS

IBS is a chronic functional bowel disorder that has been recognized as an extremely common disease for a long time. Hippocrates reported of a patient who had symptoms of abdominal discomfort, irregular bowel habits, bloating and rectal urgency [7] more than 3000 years ago in ancient Greece. There have been several IBS definitions over the years although none have proved perfect, and a gold standard for the diagnosis and classification of IBS still does not exist. Manning et al. developed the first global symptom-based IBS diagnostic criteria [8] in 1978, which were widely used by both clinicians and researchers. The Manning criteria consist of six symptoms of abdominal pain relief after defecation, loose stools at the onset of pain, increased frequency of bowel movement after the onset of pain, abdominal distension, passage of mucus in stools, and sensation of incomplete evacuation. Ford et al. [9] found that the overall sensitivity and specificity of the diagnostic accuracy of the Manning criteria were 78% and 72%, respectively. Other studies [10, 11] reported the median sensitivity of the Manning criteria to be 67% and specificity to be 69%. The Manning criteria gradually become unfavorable because they appeared to be more specific for women than for men and was difficult to distinguish IBS with constipation from IBS with diarrhea [12].

Kruis et al. [13] created a diagnostic score to differentiate IBS from organic diseases in 1984. It included the positive points for symptoms suggesting IBS and negative points for suggesting organic diseases. However, this score had not been widely used because it was difficult to validate the scores. In 1988, international experts met in Rome and created the Rome Foundation to classify and establish diagnostic criteria for all DGBIs.

The Rome I criteria [14] for IBS were proposed in 1989 by the working teams of the Rome Foundation. They were developed as a global diagnostic standard and incorporated into research studies, although it was proved difficult to apply for many clinicians in their clinical practice due to their complexity. The diagnostic accuracy of the Rome I criteria was reported with sensitivity from 67% to 71% and specificity from 70% to 85% [10, 15, 16]. After several years, the Rome committee reviewed and revised the Rome I criteria based on feedback from clinicians, investigators, and regulatory agencies and gathered new information from the scientific literature. The revised version of the Rome II criteria [17, 18] was introduced in 1999. The Rome II criteria required that symptoms need to be assessed and present for at least 12 weeks of the preceding 12 months, although this time did not have to be consecutive. Moreover, the term of abdominal pain and discomfort were more clearly defined. The Rome II criteria were used in many studies and clinical trials worldwide because the Rome II criteria were simple and practical and published in the high citation journal *GUT*. They had a median sensitivity of 69% and specificity of 66% [10, 11].

The Rome III criteria [19] were published in 2006 after the Rome II criteria were developed. The Rome III criteria were different from the Rome I and II criteria, using more evidence-based data rather than consensus-based data. The most

Type 1	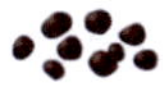	Separate hard lumps, like nuts (hard to pass)
Type 2	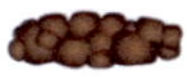	Sausage-shaped but lumpy
Type 3	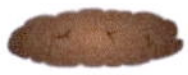	Like a sausage but with cracks on the surface
Type 4	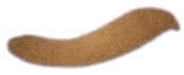	Like a sausage or snake, smooth and soft
Type 5	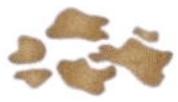	Soft blobs with clear-cut edges
Type 6	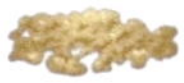	Fluffy pieces with ragged edges, a mushy stool
Type 7	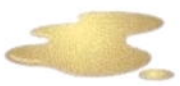	Watery, no solid pieces, entirely liquid

Fig. 1.1 Bristol stool form scale

important change in the Rome III criteria was the definition of the classification of IBS subtypes, including IBS with constipation, IBS with diarrhea, mixed IBS, and unsubtyped IBS. The Rome III committee proposed that researchers and clinicians should use the Bristol Stool Form Scale (BSFS) [1, 20, 21], and patients with IBS could be classified as having constipation or diarrhea bowel pattern using the BSFS (Fig. 1.1). Constipation is defined as hard or lumpy stools and diarrhea as loose or watery stools. Moreover, the duration of symptoms changes from "last 12 months" to "past 6 months." A validation study by Sood et al. [22] reported the sensitivity of the diagnostic accuracy of the Rome III criteria as 69.6% and the specificity as 82.0%. They were published in the highest citation journal *Gastroenterology*. Many creative studies in both basic and clinical sciences had been performed since the publication of the Rome III criteria. These studies provided a better understanding of the pathophysiology that underlies the IBS symptom generation. As the results of these studies, the Rome IV criteria were announced 10 years after the establishment of the Rome III criteria in 2016. They were published in *Gastroenterology*, similar to the Rome III criteria. Therefore, the Rome IV criteria include more addictive information compared to the Rome III criteria in terms of gut microbiota and brain-gut interactions.

1.3 Rome IV Criteria for IBS

The Rome IV criteria [1] for IBS is the most recent definition, and now widely used in diagnosis, treatment, and studies by both researchers and clinicians globally. The Rome IV criteria defined IBS as a functional bowel disorder in which recurrent abdominal pain is associated with defecation or change in bowel habits. Disordered bowel habits are typically present (i.e., constipation, diarrhea, or a combination of constipation and diarrhea), such as symptoms of abdominal bloating/distention. Symptom onset occurs at least 6 months before diagnosis, and symptoms should be present in the last 3 months (Table 1.1).

As shown in Table 1.2, several modifications have been made to the IBS definition from the Rome III to Rome IV criteria [12, 23, 24] (Table 1.2). First, the term "abdominal discomfort" was removed from the definition because the term

Table 1.1 Summary of IBS diagnostic criteria

Criteria
Manning
1. Looser stools at onset of pain
2. More frequent bowel movements at onset of pain
3. Pain eased after bowel movement (often)
4. Visible distension
5. Feeling of distension
6. Mucus per rectum
7. Feeling of incomplete emptying (often)
Rome I
Continuous or recurrent symptoms of the following:
1. Abdominal pain, relieved with defecation, or associated with a change in frequency or consistency of stool
2. Disturbed defecation (two or more of):
(a) altered stool frequency
(b) Altered stool form (hard or loose/watery)
(c) Altered stool passage (straining or urgency, feeling of incomplete evacuation)
(d) Passage of mucus
3. Bloating or feeling of abdominal distension
Rome II
At least 12 weeks, which need not be consecutive, in the preceding 12 months of abdominal discomfort or pain that has two of three features:
1. Relieved with defecation
2. Onset associated with a change in frequency of stool
3. Onset associated with a change in form (appearance) of stool
Rome III
Recurrent abdominal pain or discomfort at least 3 days per month in the last 3 months associated with 2 or more of the following:
1. Improvement with defecation
2. Onset associated with a change in frequency of stool
3. Onset associated with a change in form (appearance) of stool
Rome IV
Recurrent abdominal pain, on average, at least 1 day/week in the last 3 months, associated with two or more of the following criteria:
1. Related to defecation
2. Associated with a change in frequency of stool
3. Associated with a change in appearance of stool

Table 1.2 Rome IV diagnostic criteria for IBS [1]

Recurrent abdominal pain, on average at least 1 day/week in the last 3 months, associated with two or more of the following criteria:
1. Related to defecation
2. Associated with a change in frequency of stool
3. Associated with a change in form (appearance) of stool
Criteria fulfilled for the last 3 months with symptom onset at least 6 months before diagnosis

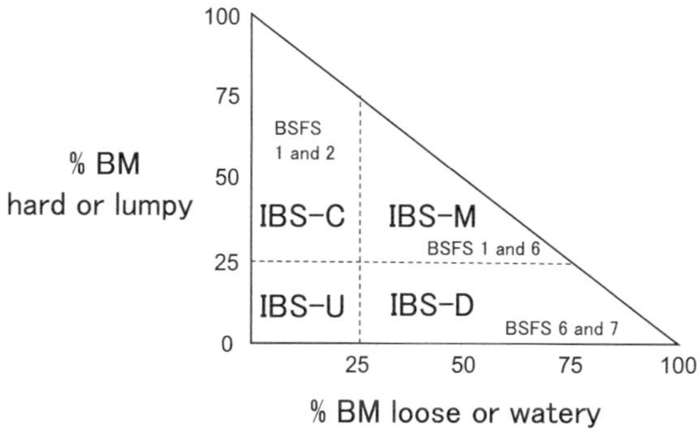

Fig. 1.2 IBS subtypes according to stool consistency. *IBS-C* IBS with predominant constipation, *IBS-D* IBS with predominant diarrhea, *IBS-M* IBS with mixed bowel habits, *IBS-U* IBS unclassified, *BSFS* Bristol Stool Form Scale, *BM* bowel movement

"discomfort" is vague. The difference between pain and discomfort may be unclear for some patients with IBS. Some patients consider the term "discomfort" to be mild pain, while others regard it as bloating. Furthermore, several languages do not have a word for discomfort, or it has a different meaning in various languages. Second, the symptoms of abdominal pain frequency have increased from on average at least 1 day per week in the last 3 months compared to only 3 days per month in the last 3 months in the Rome III criteria. Third, "Improvement of abdominal pain or discomfort after defecation" in the Rome III criteria was replaced with "abdominal pain related to defecation" in the Rome IV criteria. Abdominal pain or discomfort was relieved after defecation in the Rome III criteria, whereas there are some patients who had more pain or no change after defecation in the Rome IV criteria. Finally, the word "onset" was excluded from criteria 2 or 3 in the Rome III criteria. Aziz et al. [25] have described that, overall, 85% of patients that met the Rome III criteria fulfilled the Rome IV criteria for IBS, but 15% did not. The Rome IV criteria was reported to have 62% sensitivity and 97% specificity.

IBS is classified into four subtypes [1, 23] according to the predominant disorder in bowel habits. The term "predominant" was added in the definition of IBS in the Rome IV criteria. Predominant bowel habits are based on stool form by BSFS used to record stool consistency on days with at least one abnormal bowel movement. The three main subtypes are IBS with predominant constipation (IBS-C), IBS with predominant diarrhea (IBS-D), and IBS with mixed bowel habits (IBS-M). The additional subtype is IBS unclassified (IBS-U). The diagnostic criteria for IBS subtypes are as follows (Fig. 1.2):

IBS-C: more than one-fourth (25%) of bowel movements with BSFS types 1 or 2 and less than one-fourth (25%) of bowel movements with BSFS types 6 or 7.
IBS-D: more than one-fourth (25%) of bowel movements with BSFS types 6 or 7 and less than one-fourth (25%) of bowel movements with BSFS types 1 or 2.
IBS-M: more than one-fourth (25%) of bowel movements with BSFS types 1 or 2 and more than one-fourth (25%) of bowel movements with BSFS types 6 or 7.
IBS-U: patients who meet diagnostic criteria for IBS but whose bowel habits cannot be accurately categorized into 1 of the 3 groups above should be categorized as having IBS unclassified. For clinical trials, subtyping based on at least 2 weeks of daily diary data is recommended, using the "25% rule."

The important change from Rome III to Rome IV criteria in subtyping is that the IBS subtype should be based on the patient's reported predominant bowel habit on days with abnormal bowel movements, and not on an average of all days, which might include days with normal bowel habits. IBS is currently considered as not only a functional disease but also a gut-brain axis disorder.

1.4 Asian Consensus on IBS

The first Asian consensus on IBS [26] was published in 2010 by the Asian Neurogastroenterology and Motility Association (ANMA). After the publication of the Rome IV guidelines, ANMA felt that it is timely to examine the literatures from an Asian perspective and to update the Asian IBS consensus. The second Asian consensus on IBS [27] was exhibited in 2019. It consists of 37 statements substantiated by Asian data, and sought to represent current knowledge that will be clinically useful to physicians treating IBS in Asia. The definition of IBS in this Asian consensus is that IBS is a condition characterized by recurrent abdominal pain/discomfort, occurring in association with defecation or change in bowel habits, in the absence of organic causes that are detectable by routine medical tests. The term "discomfort" is still present in this consensus. One global survey indicated that 53.8% patients felt that bloating was the most important feature of IBS, while only 25.6% felt that abdominal pain was. Furthermore, it was reported that 64.6% of IBS patients complained of recurrent abdominal pain and 44.2% with bloating alone in another study from China. This Asian consensus states that patients with IBS may have only abdominal discomfort or bloating as the predominant symptom in clinical practice.

1.5 Japanese Clinical Practice Guidelines for IBS

The Japanese Society of Gastroenterology (JSGE) has proposed to establish clinical guidelines on how to diagnose and treat IBS. Since the symptoms of IBS are influenced by meals, social stress, etc., the formulation of guidelines for Japanese patients was necessary in consideration of geographical differences, such as special medical system, lifestyle, eating habit, and dietary contents compared to Western populations. Furthermore, the Rome criteria were sometimes complex and difficult to apply in daily clinical practice although they were useful for research and clinical trials. Accordingly, the JSGE decided to prepare a draft of these guidelines for IBS. A total of 46 clinical questions were considered by the members of the editorial committee. The evidence-based clinical practice guidelines for IBS, based on the Rome III criteria and the increasing knowledge on the differences between Japan and Western countries, were published in Japanese in 2014 and English in 2015 [28]. IBS is defined as a representative functional gastrointestinal disorder by chronic or recurrent abdominal pain and/or abdominal discomfort associated with abnormal bowel movement in this Japanese clinical guideline. The term "discomfort" was not removed because the JSGE guideline was developed 2 years before the publication of the Rome IV criteria. In addition, internet survey in Japan suggests that abdominal bloating has a great impact on the daily life of the patients with IBS-C.

The JSGE guideline was created to provide assistance in the clinical practice of the management of IBS. Its contents focus on clinical utility and well suited for patients with Japanese IBS. This guideline includes the diagnostic and treatment algorithms of IBS. It makes this disease more widely recognized for general clinicians who are engaged in the primary setting and specialists and researchers. Following the publication of the JSGE-IBS guidelines in 2014/2015, the growing evidence supported by the number of studies using these guidelines and the release of the Rome IV criteria in 2016 led to the need to update the JSGE guidelines. The second version of the JSGE-IBS guidelines [29] were published in 2020. These revised guidelines consist of 41 questions including 12 background questions on epidemiology, pathophysiology, and diagnostic criteria; 26 clinical questions on diagnosis and treatment; and 3 questions on future research. The diagnosis of IBS is in principle based on the Rome IV criteria in these new guidelines. These revised JSGE-IBS guidelines present best practice in the Japanese clinical setting, and the strategies for patients with IBS can be useful for IBS diagnosis and treatment globally.

References

1. Lacy BE, Mearin F, Chang L, Chey WD, Lembo AJ, Simren M, Spiller R. Bowel disorder. Gastroenterology. 2016;150:1393–407.

2. Drossman DA. Functional gastrointestinal disorders: history, pathophysiology, clinical features, and Rome IV. Gastroenterology. 2016;150:1262–79.
3. Drossman DA, Hasler WL. Rome IV –functional GI disorders: disorders of gut-brain interaction. Gastroenterology. 2016;150:1257–61.
4. Lovell RM, Ford AC. Global prevalence of and risk factors for irritable bowel syndrome: a meta-analysis. Clin Gastroenterol Hepatol. 2012;10:712–21.
5. Bockus HL, Bank J, Wilkinson SA. Neurogenic mucous colitis. Am J Med Sci. 1928;176:813–23.
6. Bockus HL. Gastroenterology, vol. II. Philadelphia: Saunders; 1944. p. 477–534.
7. Lacy BE, Lee RD. Irritable bowel syndrome. A syndrome in evolution. J Clin Gastroenterol. 2005;39(suppl 3):S230–42.
8. Manning AP, Thompson WG, Heaton KW, Morris AF. Towards positive diagnosis of the irritable bowel. Br Med J. 1978;2:653–4.
9. Ford AC, Talley NJ, Veldhuyzen Van Zanten SJ, Vakil NB, Simel DL, Moayyedi P. Will the history and physical examination help establish that irritable bowel syndrome is causing this patient's lower gastrointestinal tract symptoms? JAMA. 2008;300:1793–805.
10. Jellema P, van der Windt DA, Schellevis FG, van der Horst HE. Systematic review: accuracy of symptom-based criteria for diagnosis of irritable bowel syndrome in primary care. Aliment Pharmacol Ther. 2009;30:695–706.
11. Whitehead WE, Drossman DA. Validation of symptom-based diagnostic criteria for irritable bowel syndrome: a critical review. Am J Gastroenterol. 2010;105:814–20.
12. Lacy BE, Patel NK. Rome criteria and a diagnostic approach to irritable bowel syndrome. J Clin Med. 2017;6:99.
13. Kruis W, Thieme CH, Weinzierl M, Schüssler P, Holl J, Paulus W. A diagnostic score for the irritable bowel syndrome: its value in the exclusion of organic disease. Gastroenterology. 1984;87:1–7.
14. Thompson WG, Dotevall G, Drosman DA, Heaton KW, Kruis W. Irritable bowel syndrome: guidelines for the diagnosis. Gastroenterol Int. 1989;2:92–5.
15. Tibble JA, Sigthorsson G, Foster R, Forgacs I, Bjarnason I. Use of surrogate markers of inflammation and Rome criteria to distinguish organic from nonorganic intestinal disease. Gastroenterology. 2002;123:450–60.
16. Hammer J, Talley NJ. Value of different diagnostic criteria for the irritable bowel syndrome among men and women. J Clin Gastroenterol. 2008;42:160–6.
17. Thompson WG, Longstreth GF, Drossman DA, Heaton KW, Irvine EJ, Müller-Lissner SA. Functional bowel disorders and functional abdominal pain. Gut. 1999;45(Suppl 2):1143–7.
18. Drossman DA, Corazziari E, Talley NJ, Thompson WG, Whitehead WE, Rome II Multinational Working Teams. The functional gastrointestinal disorders. In: Diagnosis, pathophysiology and treatment: a multinational consensus. 2nd ed. McLean: Degnon; 2000.
19. Longstreth GF, Thompson WG, Chey WD, Houghton LA, Mearin F, Spiller RC. Functional bowel disorders. Gastroenterology. 2006;130:1480–91.
20. Levis SJ, Heaton KW. Stool form scale as a useful guide to intestinal transit time. Scand J Gastroenterol. 1997;32:920–4.
21. O'Donnell LJ, Virjee J, Heaton KW. Detection of pseudodiarrhoea by simple clinical assessment of intestinal transit rate. BMJ. 1990;300:439–40.
22. Sood R, Camilleri M, Gracie DJ, Gold MJ, To N, Law GR, Ford AC. Enhancing diagnostic performance of symptom-based criteria for irritable bowel syndrome by additional history and limited diagnostic evaluation. Am J Gastroenterol. 2016;111:1446–54.
23. Grad S, Dumitrascu DL. Irritable bowel syndrome subtypes: new names for old medical conditions. Dig Dis. 2020;38:122–7.
24. Palsson OS, Whitehead W, Tomblom H, Sperber AD, Simren M. Prevalence of Rome IV functional bowel disorders among adult in the United State, Canada, and the United Kingdom. Gastroenterology. 2020;100:1–11.

25. Aziz I, Tornblom H, Palsson OS, Whitehead WE, Simren M. How the change in IBS criteria from Rome III to Rome IV impacts on clinical characteristics and key pathophysiological factors. Am J Gastroenterol. 2018;113:1017–25.
26. Gwee KA, Bak YT, Ghoshal UC, Gonlachanvit S, Lee OY, Fock KM, Chua AS, Lu CL, Goh KL, Kositchaowat C, Makharia G, Park HJ, Chang FY, Fukudo S, Choi MG, Bhatia S, Ke M, Hou X, Hongo M, Asian Neurogastroenterology and Motility Association. Asian consensus on irritable bowel syndrome. J Gastroenterol Hepatol. 2010;25:1189–205.
27. Gwee KA, Gonlachanvit S, Ghoshal UC, Chua ASB, Miwa H, Wu J, Bak YT, Lee OY, Lu CL, Park HJ, Chen M, Syam AF, Abaham P, Sollano J, Chang CS, Suzuki H, Fang X, Fukudo S, Choi MG, Hou X, Hongo M. Second Asian consensus on irritable bowel syndrome. J Neurogastroenterol Motil. 2019;25:343–62.
28. Fukudo S, Kaneko H, Akiho H, Inamori M, Endo Y, Okumura T, Kanazawa M, Kamiya T, Sato K, Chiba T, Furuta K, Yamato S, Arakawa T, Fujiyama Y, Azuma T, Fujimoto K, Mine T, Miura S, Kinoshita Y, Sugano K, Shimosegawa T. Evidence-based clinical practice guidelines for irritable bowel syndrome. J Gastroenterol. 2015;50:11–50.
29. Fukudo S, Okumura T, Inamori M, Okuyama Y, Kanazawa M, Kamiya T, Sato K, Shiotani A, Naito Y, Fujikawa Y, Hokari R, Masaoka T, Fujimoto K, Kaneko H, Torii A, Matsueda K, Miwa H, Enomoto N, Shimosegawa T, Koike K. Evidence-based clinical practice guidelines for irritable bowel syndrome 2020. J Gastroenterol. 2021;56:193–217.

Chapter 2
The Epidemiology of Irritable Bowel Syndrome

Takeshi Kamiya, Akiko Shime, and Hidekatsu Fukuta

Abstract Irritable bowel syndrome (IBS) is a very common functional gastrointestinal disease, and it is likely various factors contribute to the causation of IBS symptoms. The prevalence of IBS are greatly affected by the IBS diagnostic criteria such as Manning, Rome III, and Rome IV. The worldwide prevalence of IBS ranges from 8% to 20% of the general population before the Rome IV criteria publication in 2016, whereas a recent study reported a 3.8% IBS prevalence with the Rome IV criteria. The Rome IV IBS criteria are thought to be more restrictive and severe than the Rome III and other criteria.

Numerous studies have reported that IBS is more prevalent in women than in men. Additionally, IBS is the most prevalent in patients with less than 50 years old, and this prevalence decrease with age. Several other factors including races, geographic location, eating habits, and body mass index influence the epidemiology of IBS.

Keywords Irritable bowel syndrome · Prevalence · Risk factors

2.1 Introduction

Irritable bowel syndrome (IBS) is one of the most prevalent functional bowel disorders. It is a symptom-based disease characterized by chronic and recurrent abdominal pain with altered bowel habits, and without any other organic disease or biochemical abnormality that could cause these symptoms [1–3]. Several factors such as disturbed gastrointestinal motility, colonic microbiome dysbiosis, sensory hypersensitivity, and psychosomatic factors may contribute to its pathogenesis;

T. Kamiya (✉) · A. Shime · H. Fukuta
Department of Medical Innovation, Nagoya City University Graduate School of Medical Sciences, Nagoya, Japan
e-mail: kamitake@med.nagoya-cu.ac.jp; crshime@med.nagoya-cu.ac.jp; fukuta-h@med.nagoya-cu.ac.jp

© The Editor(s) (if applicable) and The Author(s), under exclusive license to Springer Nature Singapore Pte Ltd. 2024

T. Kamiya, S. Fukudo (eds.), *Irritable Bowel Syndrome*,
https://doi.org/10.1007/978-981-97-8410-3_2

however, the etiology of IBS remains unclear. These constitutional or environmental factors could be directory or indirectly attributed to the prevalence of IBS.

This article summarizes the epidemiology, including the prevalence and risk factors, of IBS in Japan and globally.

2.2 Prevalence

Numerous studies have reported the prevalence of IBS, and prevalence rates are greatly affected by the diagnostic criteria. The Manning criteria [4] are the first symptom-based diagnostic criteria. In 1988, international experts gathered in Rome and created the Rome Foundation to classify and establish diagnostic criteria for all disorders of gut-brain interaction (DGBI), previously known as functional gastrointestinal disorders. These were followed by the Rome Foundation; subsequently, the Rome criteria, Rome I [5] in 1989, Rome II [6] in 1999, and Rome III [7] in 2006, were published following a consensus among these international experts. Most recently, the Rome IV [1] criteria were published in 2016. The worldwide prevalence of IBS is approximately 11.2% [8] based on a meta-analysis, with most estimates ranging from 8% to 20% [8–11] of the general population in major civilized countries before the Rome IV criteria publication. The systematic review by Lovell et al. [8] demonstrated pooled IBS prevalence values of 14.0%, 8.8%, 9.4%, and 11.3% by the Manning, Rome I, Rome II, and Rome III criteria, respectively. Conversely, IBS prevalence was substantially lower with the Rome IV criteria. A recent study on the worldwide prevalence of DGBI [12] reported a 3.8% IBS prevalence with the Rome IV criteria. This study was conducted in 33 countries, and data were collected by internet survey, personal intervention, and both methods in 24, 7, and 2 countries, respectively. This study included the Rome III IBS questions in 22 countries to compare IBS prevalence between the Rome III and Rome IV criteria. The overall IBS prevalence was 3.8% by the Rome IV criteria and 10.1% by the Rome III criteria in the 14 internet countries where the Rome III questions were included. Furthermore, the Rome III IBS prevalence rates in all countries range from 4.3% to 16.5%, which are substantially higher than the Rome IV IBS rates. Another meta-analysis of the global IBS prevalence [13] revealed a 9.2% pooled IBS prevalence among 53 studies with the Rome III criteria from 38 countries and comprising 395,385 participants and a 3.8% pooled IBS prevalence among 6 studies with the Rome IV criteria from 34 countries and comprising 82,476 individuals. A population-based survey [14] of adults in the United States, Canada, and the United Kingdom demonstrated a Rome IV IBS prevalence of 4.6% in the entire study sample, ranging from 4.5% in Canada to 4.7% in the United States. IBS was half as prevalent using the Rome IV criteria as it was using the Rome III criteria. The Rome III IBS rate was 9.0% in the total three country sample, ranging from 8.6% in the United States to 9.5% in Canada. Moreover, one online survey [15] on bowel symptoms reported that self-reported IBS is three times more prevalent than the Rome IV criteria. These results indicate that the Rome IV IBS criteria are more restrictive and

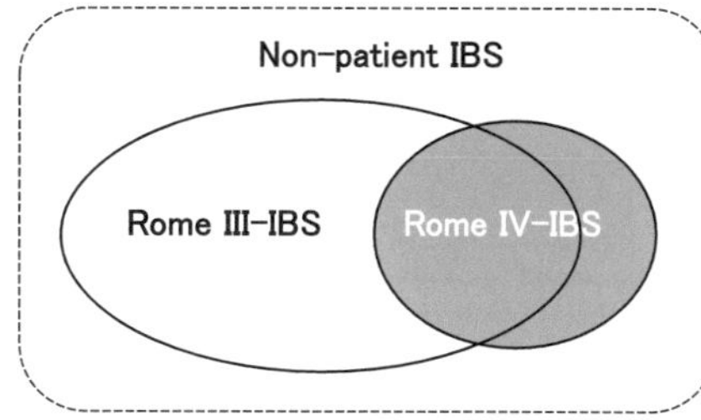

Fig. 2.1 The relationship between the Rome III IBS, Rome IV IBS, and non-patient IBS

severe than Rome III and that the Rome IV criteria are not better at identifying more masked IBS (non-patient IBS) cases (Fig. 2.1).

IBS prevalence in Japanese patients before using Rome IV criteria ranges from 13.1% to 14.2% in individuals who have health check-ups [16, 17] or internet surveys [18]. The worldwide prevalence study [12] revealed that the IBS prevalence in Japan was 2.2% by the Rome IV criteria and 9.3% by the Rome III criteria. The prevalence of IBS in Japan demonstrated a similar trend to other countries globally.

2.3 Subtype

IBS is classified into four subtypes [1] according to the predominant disorder in bowel habits. Predominant bowel habits are based on stool form [19]—the Bristol Stool Form Scale—used to record stool consistency on days with at least one abnormal bowel movement. The four subtypes in Rome III criteria are IBS with constipation (IBS-C), IBS with diarrhea (IBS-D), mixed IBS (IBS-M), and IBS unclassified (IBS-U). Pooling data from 23 studies of 102171 patients [13] revealed that 20.0%, 27.8%, 33.8%, and 14.1% of participants fulfilling the Rome III IBS criteria had IBS-C, IBS-D, IBS-M, and IBS-U, respectively. Furthermore, the term "predominant" was added to the IBS definition in the Rome IV criteria with the three main subtypes of IBS with predominant constipation (IBS-C), IBS with predominant diarrhea (IBS-D), and IBS with mixed bowel habits (IBS-M), with the additional subtype IBS-U.

A systematic review [13] reported IBS subtype prevalence based on the Rome IV criteria, with 29.3%, 31.5%, 26.4%, and 11.9% for IBS-C, IBS-D, IBS-M, and IBS-U, respectively, in patients with IBS. A global prevalence study [12] in an internet survey reported the overall Rome IV IBS subtype distribution as 1.3%, 1.2%, 1.3%, and 0.3% for IBS-C, IBS-D. IBS-M, and IBS-U, respectively (Fig. 2.2).

Miwa conducted a large-scale internet survey [18] of 10,000 subjects across Japan to determine IBS prevalence based on the Rome III criteria and revealed 13.1% IBS prevalence, with IBS-C, IBS-D, and IBS-M accounting for 24%, 29%, and 47% of cases, respectively. A sub-analysis of a worldwide study on Japanese patients [20] revealed that the IBS prevalence was IBS-C 3.0%, IBS-D 3.1%, IBS-M 2.7%, and IBS-U 0.6% with the Rome III criteria, whereas that of Rome IV was as

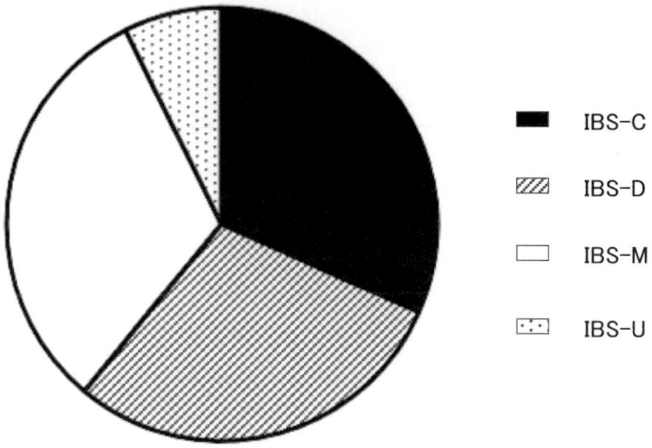

Fig. 2.2 Overall IBS subtype prevalence based on the Rome IV criteria (adapted from Sperber et al. [11])

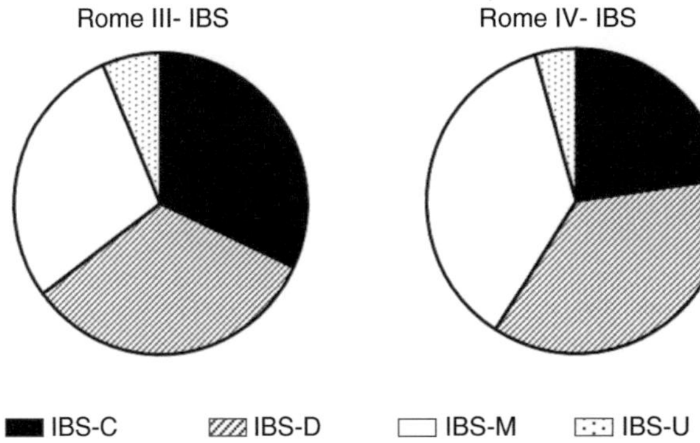

Fig. 2.3 IBS subtype prevalence in Japanese IBS patients based on the criteria of the Rome III and that of the Rome IV (adapted from Fukudo et al. [20])

follows: IBS-C 0.5%, IBS-D 0.8%, IBS-M 0.8%, and IBS-U 0.1% (Fig. 2.3). Slight differences in the prevalence of Japanese patients with IBS subtype were observed between the diagnostic criteria of Rome III and the Rome IV.

2.4 Epidemiological Factors

2.4.1 Sex and Age

Most of the studies indicate that IBS is more prevalent in women than in men. The pooled IBS prevalence based on the Rome III criteria [13] was higher in women compared with men, with an odds ratio (OR) of 1.46 for women. A worldwide study [12] revealed higher IBS prevalence rates with the Rome IV criteria among women with a women-to-men OR of 1.8 in an internet survey. Another report [8] demonstrated a 1.6 times higher prevalence of IBS among women than among men. IBS-C prevalence is especially characterized by female predominance, although all subtypes of IBS prevalence in women are higher than in men. A meta-analysis of 22 studies [21] measured gender differences in IBS symptoms and revealed that women with IBS were more likely to report abdominal pain (relative risk (RR) = 1.12) and constipation-related symptoms (RR = 1.12) than men with IBS. However, men were more likely to report diarrhea-related symptoms than women (RR = 0.84) in patients with IBS. Additionally, several studies in Asia [22–24], except Japan, revealed no significant sex difference in IBS prevalence.

Regarding age, IBS is the most prevalent in patients with less than 50 years old [8, 14, 15], and this prevalence decreases with age. IBS prevalence decreased with age in the internet survey [12], from 5.3% in 18–39 to 3.7% in 40–64 to 1.7% in the >65 age group. Other Japanese studies [18, 20] also revealed that younger age was predominant compared with older age in both the Rome III and Rome IV IBS. IBS is characterized by the predominance of young people over old people, and this characteristic is different from other lifestyle diseases, such as hypertension and diabetes.

Japanese studies reported female predominance similar to that in other countries. Okami et al. [25] reported IBS prevalence in 35.5% of nursing and medical school students as a whole, including 25.2% in men and 41.5% in women. The IBS prevalence rate using the Rome IV criteria was 5.2% in women and 2.9% in men, and the OR was 1.8 [20] in women versus men. Another study [18] reported 10.7% and 15.5% IBS prevalence among 5000 men and 5000 women, respectively. The subtypes in Japanese men and women were as follows [18]: IBS-C: 1.0% and 5.3%; IBS-D: 5.0% and 2.7%; and IBS-M: 4.7% and 7.5%, respectively.

Furthermore, ovarian hormones, such as estrogen and progesterone, may play a role either directly or indirectly in the mechanisms of these gender differences in IBS. One review article [26] by Heitkemper et al. demonstrated that the increase in gastrointestinal symptoms, including abdominal pain or discomfort, bloating, and bowel pattern alterations, during menstruation and early menopause occurs at times of declining or low ovarian hormones in women with IBS. Visceral pain sensitivity was significantly higher during menstruation [27] than at other phases of the menstrual cycle. Another meta-analysis [21] revealed that women with IBS were more likely to report abdominal pain and constipation-related symptoms than men, whereas men with IBS were more likely to report diarrhea-related symptoms than women with IBS. Further, both menstrual cycles and menopausal status affect IBS symptoms and female sex hormones influence the severity of IBS symptoms. Additionally, hormone supplements may affect IBS symptoms. Leuprolide, which is a gonadotropin-releasing hormone agonist, may be protective against IBS symptoms [28] by stimulating the release of the follicular-stimulating hormone and luteinizing hormone, which suppress ovarian hormone secretion. Further studies are needed to determine the effect of supplements on IBS symptoms.

2.4.2 Races and Geographic Location

Race may affect IBS development. Many studies [8, 11, 29] indicate that IBS prevalence differs by geographic area and country.

IBS prevalence may be different by race and geographic area, although these findings remain debated. An analysis in the United States [29] reported an IBS prevalence of 7.9% in African Americans and 13.1% in Whites. Another meta-analysis [8] indicated that the prevalence of IBS varied, ranging from 2.6% to 32% according to country. The literature review [11] revealed a pooled regional IBS prevalence rate ranging from 17.5% in Latin America; 9.6% in Asia; 8.1% in North America, Europe, Australia, and New Zealand; to 5.8% in the Middle East and Africa. A statistically significant degree of heterogeneity was found among the geographical regions. However, there were no statistical differences in IBS prevalence between the United State, United Kingdom, and Canada [14], and the recent global survey [12] of worldwide prevalence by the internet revealed 1.3–7.6% IBS prevalence diagnosed using the Rome IV criteria among countries. This survey revealed the highest IBS prevalence at 7.1% in Egypt and the lowest at 1.3% in Singapore, and the statistical differences among geographic areas, including West and East Europe, North and South America, Asia, Africa, and Australia, were not observed.

2.4.3 Food

Dietary habits are thought to be one of the factors associated with IBS development. A Japanese study [25] among nursing and medical students revealed that men with IBS ate less fish, fruit, milk, and green-yellow vegetables than those with no IBS. Furthermore, the rates of missed meals and irregular mealtimes were significantly higher in the IBS group. A recent randomized control trial [30, 31] revealed that a low fermentable oligo-di-monosaccharide and polyol (FODMAP) diet is beneficial for patients with IBS compared with a normal diet. In addition, several studies [32, 33] demonstrating the usefulness of a low-FODMAP diet have been reported. Each country has specific lifestyles and eating habits. Therefore, eating habits are closely related to the difference in the geographic area of IBS prevalence.

2.4.4 Other Factors

Several studies reported other factors investigating IBS development. Obesity is considered a risk factor for IBS. Talley et al. revealed [34] that IBS was not significantly associated with an increased body mass index (BMI), although an increased BMI was associated with diarrhea and abdominal pain. Another report [35] revealed that higher visceral adipose tissue and waist circumference are associated with an increased risk of IBS. However, there are a few reports that BMI is not associated with a higher risk of IBS. Conversely, people suffering from IBS were, on average, shorter, weighed less, and had a lower BMI than those with no signs of IBS [36]. Additionally, a negative statically significant linear association between BMI and IBS was observed for men [37] but not for women. The results of the relationships between IBS and obesity were controversial, and further studies were needed.

Regarding occupation, women veterans have a high IBS prevalence, which is highly associated with people with depression, anxiety, and combat-related post-traumatic stress disorder, according to a United States study [38]. Nojkov et al. [39] reported the association between rotating shift work for nurses and IBS development. Further, circadian rhythm disturbance may be a factor in its pathogenesis.

A Japanese internet survey [40] reported higher socioeconomic status among men with IBS compared with those without IBS. However, the effects of socioeconomic status have not been well described [8] in systematic reviews and meta-analyses. More studies are needed to demonstrate the relationship between IBS prevalence and socioeconomic status.

2.5 Conclusion

IBS represents one of the most prevalent DGBI disorders, and we often observe patients with IBS in clinical settings. This article has demonstrated a global IBS prevalence, but this varied considerably according to the diagnostic criteria used to define IBS. Furthermore, many factors including geographic region, age, gender, eating habits, lifestyle, and psychosocial background may influence the difference in IBS prevalence. These data are important to establish treatment strategies and future planning for the health care process. This article is expected to be of interest not only to gastroenterologist but also to general physicians, public health experts, and co-medical workers, such as nurses.

References

1. Lacy BE, Mearin F, Chang L, et al. Bowel disorder. Gastroenterology. 2016;150:1393–407.
2. Drossman DA. Functional gastrointestinal disorders: history, pathophysiology, clinical features, and Rome IV. Gastroenterology. 2016;150:1262–79.
3. Drossman DA, Hasler WL. Rome IV–functional GI disorders: disorders of gut-brain interaction. Gastroenterology. 2016;150:1257–61.
4. Manning AP, Thompson WG, Heaton KW, et al. Towards positive diagnosis of the irritable bowel. Br Med J. 1978;2:653–4.
5. Thompson WG, Dotevall G, Drosman DA, et al. Irritable bowel syndrome: guidelines for the diagnosis. Gastroenterol Int. 1989;2:92–5.
6. Thompson WG, Longstreth GF, Drossman DA, et al. Functional bowel disorders and abdominal pain. Gut. 1999;45(II):1143–7.

7. Longstreth GF, Thompson WG, Chey WD, et al. Functional bowel disorders. Gastroenterology. 2006;130:1480–91.
8. Lovell RM, Ford AC. Global prevalence of and risk factors for irritable bowel syndrome: a meta-analysis. Clin Gastroenterol Hepatol. 2012;10:712–21.
9. Saito YA, Schoenfeld P, Locke GR. The epidemiology of irritable bowel syndrome in North America: a systematic review. Am J Gastroenterol. 2002;97:1910–5.
10. Oshima T, Miwa H. Epidemiology of functional gastrointestinal disorders in Japan and in the world. J Neurogastroenterol Motil. 2015;21:320–9.
11. Sperber AD, Dumitrascu D, Fukudo S, et al. The global prevalence of IBS in adults remains elusive due to the heterogeneity of studies: a Rome foundation working team literature review. Gut. 2017;66:1075–82.
12. Sperber AD, Bangdiwala SI, Drossman DA, et al. Worldwide prevalence and burden of functional gastrointestinal disorders, results of Rome Foundation global study. Gastroenterology. 2021;160:99–114.
13. Oka P, Parr H, Barberio B, et al. Global prevalence if irritable bowel syndrome according to Rome III or IV criteria: a systematic review and meta-analysis. Lancet Gastroenterol Hepatol. 2020;5:908–17.
14. Paisson OS, Whitehead W, Sperber AD, et al. Prevalence of Rome IV functional bowel disorders among adults in the United State, Canada, and the United Kingdom. Gastroenterology. 2020;158:1262–73.
15. van den Houte K, Carbone F, Pannemans J, et al. Prevalence and impact of self-reported irritable bowel symptoms in the general population. United Eur Gastroentrol J. 2019;7:307–15.
16. Kanazawa M, Endo Y, Whitehead WE, et al. Patients and nonconsulters with irritable bowel syndrome reporting a parental history of bowel problems have more impaired psychological distress. Dig Dis Sci. 2004;49:1046–53.
17. Kubo M, Fujiwara Y, Shibata M, et al. Differences between risk factors among irritable bowel syndrome subtypes in Japanese adults. Neurogastroenterol Motil. 2011;23:249–54.
18. Miwa H. Prevalence of irritable bowel syndrome in Japan: Internet survey using Rome III criteria. Patient Prefer Adherence. 2008;2:143–7.
19. Lewis SJ, Heaton KW. Stool form scale as a useful guide to intestinal transit time. Scand J Gastroenterol. 1997;32:920–4.
20. Fukudo S, Nakaya K, Muratsubaki T, et al. Characteristics of disorders of gut-brain interaction in the Japanese population in the Rome foundation global epidemiological study. Neurogastroenterol Motil. 2023;35:e 014581.
21. Adeyemo MA, Spiegel BM, Chang L. Meta-analysis: to irritable bowel syndrome symptoms vary between men and women? Aliment Pharmacol Ther. 2010;32:738–55.
22. Siah KT, Wong RK, Chan YH, et al. Prevalence of irritable bowel syndrome in Singapore and its association with dietary, lifestyle, and environmental factors. J Neurogastroenterol Motil. 2016;22:670–6.
23. Gwee KA, Ghoshal UC, Chen M. Irritable bowel syndrome in Asia: pathogenesis, natural history, epidemiology, and management. J Gastroenterol Hepatol. 2018;33:99–110.
24. Gwee KA, Gonlachanvit S, Ghoshal UC, et al. Second Asian consensus on irritable bowel syndrome. J Neurogastroenterol Motil. 2019;25:343–62.
25. Okami Y, Kato T, Nin G, et al. Lifestyle and psychological factors related to irritable bowel syndrome in nursing and medical school students. J Gastroenterol. 2011;46:1403–10.
26. Heitkemper MM, Chang L. Do fluctuations in ovarian hormones affect gastrointestinal symptoms in women with irritable bowel syndrome? Genet Med. 2009;6(2):152–67.
27. Houghton LA, Lea R, Jackson N, et al. The menstrual cycle affects rectal sensitivity in patients with irritable bowel syndrome but not healthy volunteers. Gut. 2002;50:471–4.
28. Palomba S, Orio F, Manguso F, et al. Leuprolide acetate treatment with and without coadministration of tibolone in premenopausal women with menstrual cycle-related irritable bowel syndrome. Fertil Steril. 2005;83:1012–20.

29. Wigington WC, Johnson WD, Minocha A. Epidemiology of irritable bowel syndrome among African Americans as compared with whites: a population-based study. Clin Gastroenterol Hepatol. 2005;3:647–53.
30. Staudacher HM, Whelan K, Irving PM, et al. Comparison of symptom response following advice for low in fermentable carbohydrates (FODMAPs) versus standard dietary advice in patients with irritable bowel syndrome. J Hum Nutr Diet. 2011;24:487–95.
31. Halmons EP, Power VA, Shepherd SJ, et al. A diet low in FODMAPs reduce s symptoms of irritable bowel syndrome. Gastroenterology. 2014;146:67–75.
32. Altobelli E, Del Negro V, Angeletti PM, et al. Low-FODMAP diet improves irritable bowel syndrome symptoms: a meta-analysis. Nutrients. 2017;26:940.
33. Black CJ, Staudacher HM, Ford AC. Efficacy of a low FODMAP diet in irritable bowel s symptom: systematic review and network meta-analysis. Gut. 2022;71:1117–26.
34. Talley NJ, Howell S, Poulton R. Obesity and chronic gastrointestinal tract symptoms in young adults: a birth cohort study. Am J Gastroenterol. 2004;99:1807–14.
35. Lee CG, Lee JK, Kang YS, et al. Visceral abdominal obesity is associated with an increased risk of irritable bowel syndrome. Am J Gastroenterol. 2015;110:310–9.
36. Ebling B, Jurcic D, Gmajnic R, et al. Anthropological, demographic and socioeconomic characteristics of irritable bowel syndrome. Coll Antropol. 2011;35:513–21.
37. Le Pluart D, Sabate JM, Bouchoucha M, et al. Functional gastrointestinal disorders in 35447 adults and their association with body mass index. Aliment Pharmacol Ther. 2015;41:758–67.
38. Savas LS, White DL, Wieman M, et al. Irritable bowel syndrome and dyspepsia among women veterans: prevalence and association with psychological distress. Aliment Pharmacol Ther. 2009;29:115–25.
39. Nojkov B, Rubenstein JH, Chey WD, et al. The impact of rotating shift work on the prevalence of irritable bowel syndrome in nurses. Am J Gastroenterol. 2010;105:842–7.
40. Miwa H. J-ROAD II: Japanese research of abdominal symptoms for irritable bowel syndrome II. J New Rem Clin. 2010;59:32–6.

Part II
Pathophysiology

Chapter 3
Neurogastroenterology: Brain-Gut Axis, Stress, and Psychological Factors

Shin Fukudo, Yuhei Yamaguchi, Yasuhiro Sato, Yuka Endo, Tomotaka Shoji, Daisaku Tamura, Hiromichi Tsushima, Tomohiko Muratsubaki, Michiko Kano, and Motoyori Kanazawa

Abstract Irritable bowel syndrome (IBS) is now conceptualized with disorders of gut-brain interaction (DGBI). It should be noted that interactions between the brain and the gut are reciprocal. Microbiota and mucosal inflammation relate to pathophysiology of IBS. Visceral afferent neurons are mainly ascend via the sympathetic nervous system and parasympathetic nervous system (vagus nerve). Increase in intraluminal pressure of the colon causes a reflex action and gastrointestinal perception. This activity comprises (1) the peristaltic reflex, (2) the colo-colonic inhibitory reflex, and (3) colonic perception. The nociceptive signal ascends the primary afferent neurons whose cell bodies are in the dorsal root ganglia. They form synapse with the lamina I neurons of the dorsal horn of the spinal cord. Then the parabrachial nucleus,

---

S. Fukudo (✉)
Department of Behavioral Medicine, Tohoku University Graduate School of Medicine, Sendai, Japan

Department of Psychosomatic Medicine, Tohoku University Hospital, Sendai, Japan

Research Center for Accelerator and Radioisotope Science, Tohoku University, Sendai, Japan

Department of Psychosomatic Medicine, Japanese Red Cross Ishinomaki Hospital, Ishinomaki, Japan
e-mail: shin.fukudo.c6@tohoku.ac.jp

Y. Yamaguchi · Y. Sato · Y. Endo · T. Shoji · D. Tamura
Department of Psychosomatic Medicine, Tohoku University Hospital, Sendai, Japan
e-mail: yassat@hosp.tohoku.ac.jp; yendo@hosp.tohoku.ac.jp; tshoji@hosp.tohoku.ac.jp; d-tamura@hosp.tohoku.ac.jp

H. Tsushima · T. Muratsubaki · M. Kano
Department of Behavioral Medicine, Tohoku University Graduate School of Medicine, Sendai, Japan
e-mail: t-mura@med.tohoku.ac.jp

M. Kanazawa
Department of Behavioral Medicine, Tohoku University Graduate School of Medicine, Sendai, Japan

Department of Psychosomatic Medicine, Tohoku University Hospital, Sendai, Japan
e-mail: m-kanazawa@med.tohoku.ac.jp

© The Editor(s) (if applicable) and The Author(s), under exclusive license to Springer Nature Singapore Pte Ltd. 2024

T. Kamiya, S. Fukudo (eds.), *Irritable Bowel Syndrome*,
https://doi.org/10.1007/978-981-97-8410-3_3

the thalamus, the hypothalamus, and the amygdala are activated. A meta-analysis showed that colorectal distension in IBS patients activates the anterior cingulate cortex, amygdala, and midbrain but deactivates the medial and lateral prefrontal cortex, thereby revealing an association between IBS symptoms and functional changes in the neuronal network centering on the amygdala. Psychosocial stress activates paraventricular nucleus of the hypothalamus. Moreover, hormones, especially the main stress-related peptide corticotropin-releasing hormone (CRH), contribute to the pathological state of IBS patients. In IBS patiments, bowel movement, visceral perception, mucosal permeability, and low-grade inflammation are exaggerated when CRH is released. Possibly relating to the common neurotransmission and/or neuroendocrine changes, IBS patients have high comorbidity with anxiety disorder or depressive disorder. Further research of IBS based on the neurogastroenterology especially brain-gut axis, stress, and psychological factors is warranted in the future.

Keywords Irritable bowel syndrome · Brain-gut interaction · Gut-brain interaction · Stress · Psychological factor · Neurogastroenterology · Serotonin · Corticotropin-releasing hormone · Visceral perception · Amygdala · Anterior cingulate cortex

Abbreviations

ACTH	Adrenocorticotropic hormone
CRH	Corticotropin-releasing hormone
DGBI	Disorders of gut-brain interaction
FD	Functional dyspepsia
FGIDs	Functional gastrointestinal disorders
5-HT	5-hydroxytryptamine
IBS	Irritable bowel syndrome
IL	Interleukin
MDvc	Ventrocaudal part of medial dorsal nucleus
QOL	Quality of life
VMb	Basal ventral medial nucleus
VMpo	Posterior part of ventromedial nucleus

3.1 Introduction: Brain-Gut Axis in IBS

Irritable bowel syndrome (IBS) is one of the representative functional gastrointestinal disorders (FGIDs) [1]. IBS is now conceptualized with disorders of gut-brain interaction (DGBI) [2]. It should be noted that interactions between the brain and the gut are reciprocal [3]. Therefore, gut-brain interaction, brain-gut interactions, and brain-gut axis essentially mean the same phenomena.

3.2 Signal Originated from the Gut

How does the signal from the gut originate? Microbiota and mucosal inflammation relate to pathophysiology of IBS (Fig. 3.1) [4]. IBS develops after the insult of acute gastroenteritis (i.e., post-infectious IBS) [5]. Risk factors of postinfectious IBS are not only local inflammatory factors including lymphocytosis, hyperplasia of the enterochromaffin cells, bacteria with elongating toxin, and longer duration of initial

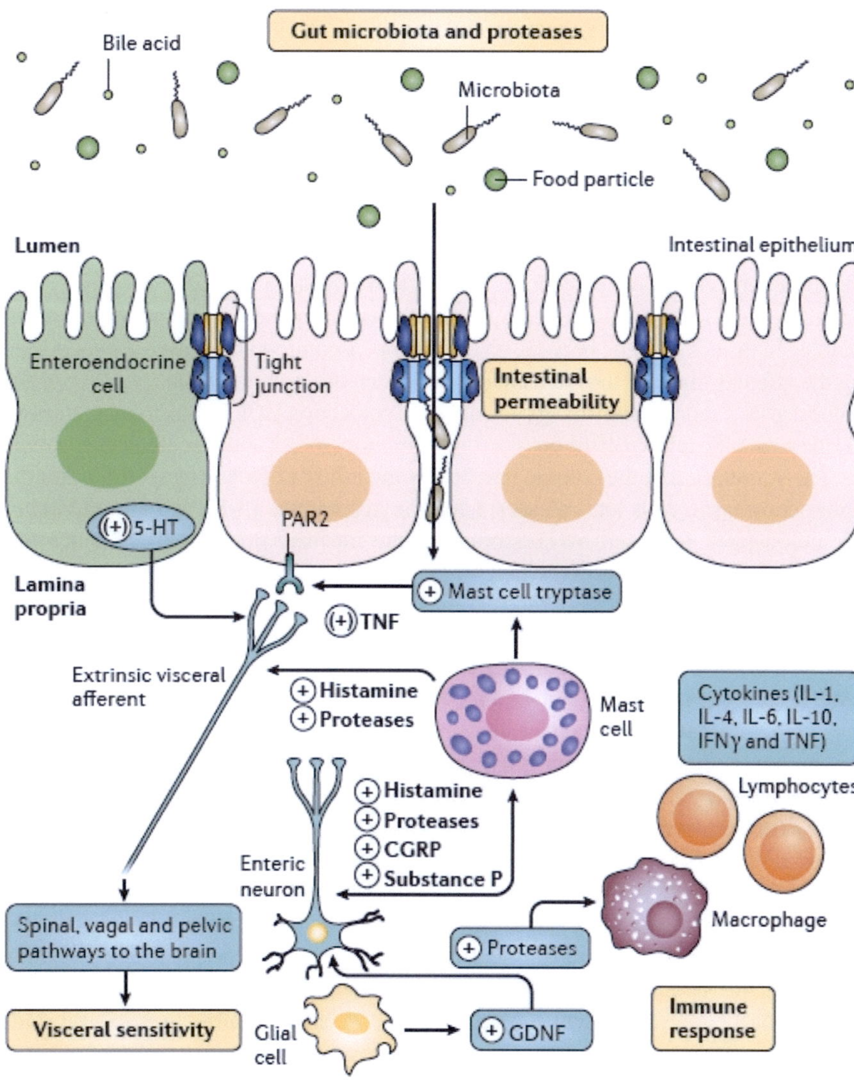

Fig. 3.1 How the signal is originated from the gut lumen in IBS. Altered gut microbiota, increased mucosal permeability, low-grade inflammation cause visceral hypersensitivity in IBS patients. Reproduced from the [4] with permission

illness but also systemic factors including adverse life events, depression, hypochondriasis, younger age below 60, female gender, and smoking [6]. Gut microbiota in IBS patients differ from those in healthy individuals [7]. Moreover, the composition of gut microbiota differs among IBS with diarrhea (IBS-D), IBS with constipation (IBS-C), and IBS with mixed bowel habits (IBS-M) [7]. In Japan, gut microbiota in IBS patients also differ from those observed in healthy individuals and short-chain fatty acid (SCFA) observed in the patients correlated with main symptoms [8]. The numbers of intraepithelial lymphocytes (1.8-fold), CD3+ cells (2.0-fold), and CD25+ cells (6.5-fold) are increased in the colon mucosa of IBS patients, indicating that the patients are in an immunostimulatory state [9].

3.3 Gut Signal Conducted to the Brain

How are the gut signals conducted to the brain? Mechanical and/or chemical stimulation to the gut activates visceral afferent neurons [10]. Visceral afferent neurons are mainly ascend via the sympathetic nervous system and parasympathetic nervous system (vagus nerve) [11]. Usually visceral pain is conducted by the visceral afferent neurons running in the sympathetic nervous system, while discomfort and nausea are conducted by the afferent fibers of the vagus nerve [10]. Increase in intraluminal pressure of the colon causes a reflex action and gastrointestinal perception [10]. This activity comprises (1) the peristaltic reflex, (2) the colo-colonic inhibitory reflex, and (3) colonic perception.

The stimulation of the colonic mucosa by the influx of feces or gas stimulates the enterochromaffin cells and releases 5-hydroxytryptamine (5-HT) in the mucosa of the colon [10]. Released 5-HT stimulates the intrinsic primary afferent neurons which have bipolar axons in the myenteric plexus with oral and aboral direction. In the oral site, the 5-HT interneuron is stimulated, and 5-HT is released to the synapse with the AH-type 2 neuron, which is the colonic motor neuron, and 5-HT3 and 5-HT4 receptors on the cell membrane play an important role in mediating acetylcholine release [10]. The neurotransmitter acetylcholine is finally released and causes ascending circular muscle contractions. On the other hand, at the aboral side, the inhibitory neuron like the nitric oxide neuron is stimulated, and descending circular muscle relaxations occur. This peristaltic reflex makes the bowel contents migrate in the rostral to caudal direction [10].

Next, the colo-colonic inhibitory reflex occurs when the bowel receives distension stimuli from the influx of feces and gas [10]. The parallel receptor of the sensory nerve endings, which have their cell bodies in the myenteric plexus, are stimulated, and a signal is transmitted via the nicotinic receptor due to acetylcholine release at the sympathetic ganglia in the celiac ganglion, the superior mesenteric ganglia, or the inferior mesenteric ganglia [10]. When the inhibitory neurotransmitter noradrenaline, which suppresses acetylcholinergic neurons, is released at these sympathetic postganglionic neurons, it causes colonic relaxation [10]. Somatostatin and neuropeptide Y are also known to be present in postganglionic neurons [11]. The parallel receptor in the intrinsic sensory neurons does not fire in response to active contraction of the circular muscle and is responsible for monitoring the state of bowel relaxation and contraction [10].

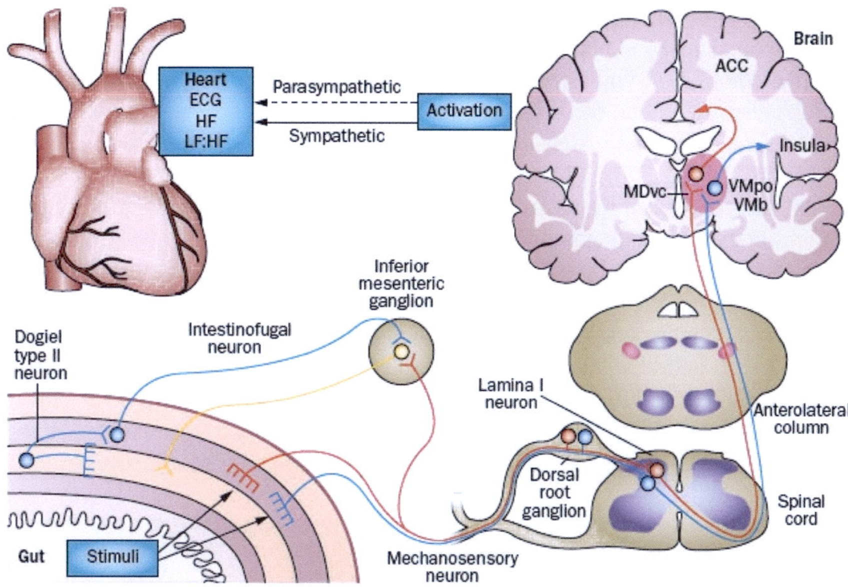

Fig. 3.2 How the pain signal from the gut is conducted to the brain in IBS. The nociceptive signals from the colorectum ascend the fine sympathetic afferent fibers which pass dorsal root ganglia. This primary afferent neurons have synapses with the second-order neurons in the lamina I of the dorsal horn of the spinal cord. The visceral afferent signals via lamina I pass the thalamus. Pathways bypassing thalamus via parabrachial nucleus, hypothalamus, and amygdala are also present. The signals are processed in the homeostatic afferent network and emotional afferent network including insula and anterior cingulate cortex. Then autonomic efferent pathways are activated and result in cardiac sympathetic arousal detected by increase in the ratio of low frequency (LF)/high frequency (HF) and/or cardiac vagal withdrawal detected decrease in HF component of heart rate variability. Reproduced from the [12] with permission

When distension stimuli increase, colonic perception is ultimately produced [12]. The spinal sensory neurons, which have receptors arranged serially in the longitudinal muscle, fire and transmit a signal via the viscerosomatic neurons that lie between the dorsal spinal nerve root and the dorsal horn of the spinal cord [12]. Their axons ascend via the contralateral spinothalamic tract and spinoreticular tract and cause central visceral sensations (Fig. 3.2) [12]. Therefore, luminal stimuli cause signals which enable monitoring of visceral events, in addition to reflex actions, to the brain. Either a high-intensity stimulus or a low sensory threshold will give rise to colonic perception [12].

3.4 Intracerebral Pathway in IBS

The nociceptive signal of the lamina I neurons mainly ascends the anterolateral column and stimulates the parabrachial nucleus and ventrocaudal part of medial dorsal (MDvc), posterior part of ventromedial (VMpo), and basal ventral medial (VMb) nuclei of the thalamus [12]. The signal is processed by the posterior insula and then sent to the anterior insula as well as the anterior cingulate cortex, amygdala, hypothalamus, and hippocampus [12]. Thus emotional circuit is activated and negative emotion is synthesized by the way of subjective feeling as well as bodily changes via the autonomic efferent nerves and neuroendocrines. A meta-analysis showed that colorectal distension in IBS patients activates the anterior cingulate cortex, amygdala, and midbrain but deactivates the medial and lateral prefrontal cortex, thereby revealing an association between IBS symptoms and functional changes in the neuronal network centering on the amygdala (Fig. 3.3) [13].

One of the intracerebral mechanisms of leading neurotransmitter responsible for the pathology of IBS is serotonin. Depletion of tryptophan, a serotonin precursor, causes visceral hypersensitivity [14] and elicits fear [15] in IBS patients. The administration of an antidepressant that inhibits the reuptake of serotonin in IBS patients suppresses hyperactivity of the anterior cingulate gyrus [16] and improves clinical IBS symptoms [17].

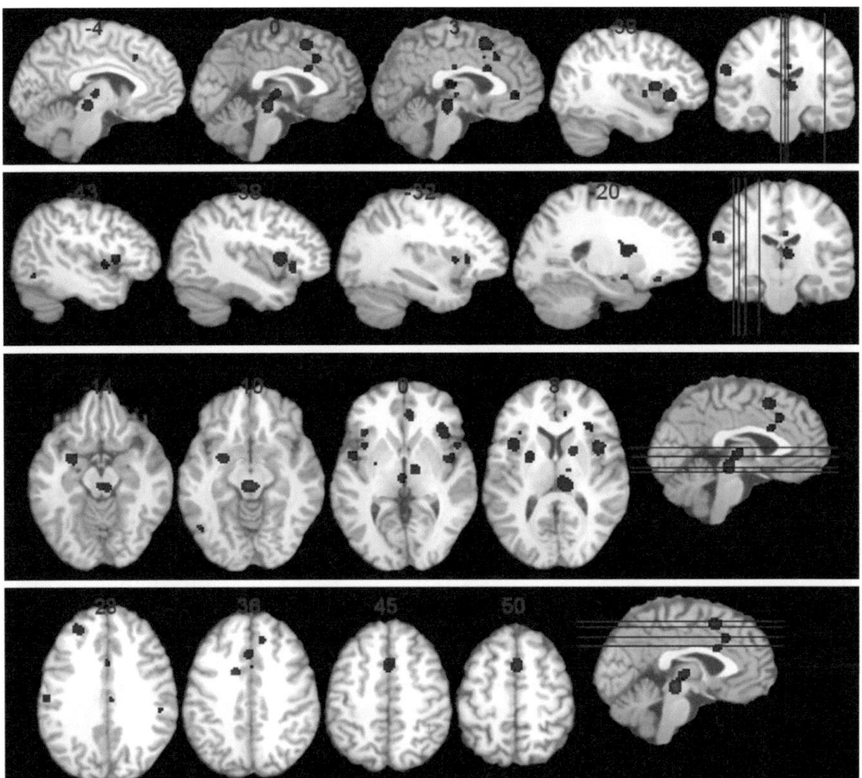

Fig. 3.3 Intracerebral processing of the pain signal in IBS. Meta-analysis showed differentially activated brain regions in response to colorectal distention in IBS patients from those in control subjects. Red color means more activated area in IBS patients than controls. Blue area implies more activated area in controls than IBS patients. Reproduced from the [13] with permission

Moreover, hormones, especially the main stress-related peptide corticotropin-releasing hormone (CRH), contribute to the pathological state of IBS patients. Bowel movement is activated when CRH is loaded on IBS patients [18], and CRH antagonists suppress stress-induced colonic motility [19]. In IBS patients, CRH-induced secretion of adrenocorticotropic hormone (ACTH) is proportional to the serum interleukin (IL)-6 as a marker of mucosal inflammation [20]. Serum cortisol secretion under the stress is exaggerated in IBS patients [21]. Exogenous administration of CRH induces greater activation of the amygdala in IBS patients than in controls [22]. IBS patients show exaggerated colonic barostat response to CRH administration [23]. The magnitude of ACTH response to CRH administration is negatively correlated with visceral stimulation-induced activation of the anterior cingulate cortex in healthy individuals but not in IBS patients [23]. These findings suggest the existence of the allostatic load relating CRH system in the specific brain regions in IBS patients.

There are some other candidates of intracerebral substances relating IBS. Oxytocin has an opposite action against CRH and increases thresholds of colonic visceral perception in IBS patients [24]. The administration of melatonin biosynthesized from serotonin improves abdominal pain in IBS patients [25]. In addition to the substances mentioned above, several neurotransmitters including histamine [26] and nitric oxide [27] play a role in the manifestations of IBS. In fact, pregabalin, an $\alpha_2\delta$ ligand that inhibits the release of a number of excitatory neurotransmitters, alleviates visceral pain in IBS patients [28].

3.5 Stress

Stress plays a role in the manifestation of IBS. Clinically, gastrointestinal symptoms in IBS patients worsen at the time of self-perceived stress, and this phenomenon has been confirmed psychometrically. Previous research showed that the correlation coefficient between stress loading and exacerbation of gastrointestinal symptoms is higher for IBS patients than that for healthy individuals [29]. Traumatic stress loaded to individuals in their earlier life increases risk for IBS [30]. Meta-analysis of 71 articles showed that odds ratio of functional somatic syndrome including IBS is 2.7 with 95% confidence interval 2.27–3.10 [31]. Meta-analysis from 8 articles which limited 648,375 IBS patients revealed that odds ratio of IBS is 2.8 with 95% confidence interval 2.06–3.54 [32]. Therefore, psychosocial stress plays important roles in causing and aggravating IBS.

When psychosocial stress is loaded on IBS patients in an examination room, bowel movement is activated, as determined by measurements of colonic manometry [33]. In IBS patients, the stimulation of the gastrointestinal system enhances the response of the brain, to varying degrees between the sexes, with the activation of brain areas that regulate the stress responses (i.e., the amygdala, anterior cingulate cortex, and insula) [34]. The inability of IBS patients to adapt quickly to circumstantial changes and the relatively low level of activation in their right dorsolateral prefrontal cortex are thought to play a role in the stress responses specific to IBS patients [35]. A report in which IBS patients interpret their life events worse than healthy individuals [36] supports this neurological findings.

3.6 Psychological Factors

The influence of psychological disorders in the pathology of IBS increases as the severity of IBS increases [37]. Representative psychological conditions in IBS are depression and anxiety, followed by somatization [37]. A cohort study revealed that depressive or anxiety disorder is a risk factor for the development of IBS (Table 3.1, upper) [38]. Although IBS alone was not a risk factor for depressive or anxiety disorder, functional gastrointestinal disorders as a whole including IBS increase the incidence of depressive or anxiety disorder (Table 3.1, lower) [38]. Here again, the brain-gut pathway in IBS is bidirectional.

The severity of IBS (especially abdominal pain or diarrhea) and psychological disturbance in IBS patients determine health care-seeking behaviors [39, 40]. Almost all IBS patients who visit clinic or hospital or 18% of IBS subjects in the general population have at least one or more psychological disturbance(s) [41]. There is no specific psychological disturbance(s) which is comorbid with IBS, but anxiety and depression are common comorbidity with IBS. Functional dyspepsia and gastroesophageal reflux disease as comorbid disorders with IBS impair the quality of life (QOL) [42]. Other extraintestinal disorders or psychological comorbidities with IBS may also impair QOL, but they need further research. Psychological comorbidities with IBS are possible risk factor of bad prognosis [43].

Table 3.1 Epidemiological evidence of reciprocal brain-gut axis in IBS

Upper: Brain-to-gut pathway. Baseline anxiety and depression significantly more odds ratio (OR) of IBS at 12 years later than baseline control

FGID diagnosis	Psychological distress variable	Baseline clinically elevated psychological distress		OR (95% CI)	*p* value[a]
		Yes, mean (SD)	No, mean (SD)		
Any FGID[b]	Anxiety	2.7 (2.6)	1.9 (2.4)	1.11 (1.03 to 1.19)	0.006
	Depression	1.3 (2.2)	1.1 (2.2)	1.04 (0.96 to 1.13)	0.293
IBS[c]	Anxiety	4.0 (3.7)	2.7 (3.0)	1.11 (1.03 to 1.18)	0.005
	Depression	2.6 (3.5)	1.5 (2.7)	1.10 (1.03 to 1.18)	0.007
FD[d]	Anxiety	3.9 (3.1)	2.8 (3.1)	1.09 (1.0 to 1.20)	0.057
	Depression	2.8 (3.7)	1.6 (2.9)	1.09 (1.0 to 1.20)	0.043

Lower: Gut-to-brain pathway. Baseline FGID significantly more mean difference coefficient in anxiety and depression at 12 years later than baseline control

FGID diagnosis	Psychological distress variable	Baseline FGID diagnosis		Mean difference coefficient[a] (95% CI)	*p* value
		Yes, mean (SD)	No, mean (SD)		
FGID	Anxiety	2.1 (2.2)	1.3 (2.0)	0.76 (0.37 to 1.14)	<0.001
	Depression	0.9 (1.9)	0.6 (1.7)	0.30 (–0.03 to 0.63)	0.010
IBS	Anxiety	1.6 (1.6)	1.5 (2.1)	0.02 (–0.86 to 0.90)	0.644
	Depression	0.7 (1.1)	0.7 (1.8)	0.01 (–0.73 to 0.75)	0.454
FD	Anxiety	1.7 (2.2)	1.5 (2.1)	0.31 (–0.58 to 1.19)	0.309
	Depression	0.8 (1.9)	0.7 (1.8)	0.11 (–0.63 to 0.85)	0.741

Data were analyzed from cohort samples with a total of 1002 subjects including 376 functional gastrointestinal disorders (FGID) and 626 controls for 12 years Reproduced from the [38] with permission

[a] Controlling for age and gender

[b] Controls defined as no FGID

[c] Controls defined as no IBS

[d] Controls defined as no FD

3.7 Conclusion

Brain-gut axis which means reciprocal communication between the brain and the gut plays an important role in pathogenesis and pathophysiology of IBS. Psychological factors especially psychosocial stress contribute to this process. Further research of IBS based on the neurogastroenterology especially brain-gut axis, stress, and psychological factors is warranted in the future.

Grant Support This research was supported by Grant-in-Aid for Scientific Research from the Ministry of Education, Science, Culture of Japan and Grant-in-Aid for Scientific Research from the Ministry of Health, Welfare, and Labor of Japan, SRF, and AMED-Moon Shot 20356688.

Employment No conflict of interests.

Personal Financial Interests No conflict of interest.

References

1. Lacy BE, Mearin F, Chang L, Chey WD, Lembo AJ, Simren M, Spiller R. Bowel disorders. Gastroenterology. 2016;150:1393–407.
2. Drossman DA, Hasler WL. Rome IV - functional GI disorders: disorders of gut-brain interaction. Gastroenterology. 2016;150:1257–61.
3. Fukudo S, Kanazawa M. Gene, environment, and brain-gut interactions in irritable bowel syndrome. J Gastroenterol Hepatol. 2011;26(Suppl 3):110–5.
4. Enck P, Aziz Q, Barbara G, Farmer A, Fukudo S, Mayer E, Niesler B, Quigley E, Rajilic-Stojanović M, Schemann M, Schwille-Kiuntke J, Simren M, Zipfel S, Spiller R. Irritable bowel syndrome (IBS). Nat Rev Dis Prim. 2016;2:16014.
5. Thabane M, Kottachchi DT, Marshall JK. Systematic review and meta-analysis: the incidence and prognosis of post-infectious irritable bowel syndrome. Aliment Pharmacol Ther. 2007;26:535–44.
6. Spiller R, Garsed K. Postinfectious irritable bowel syndrome. Gastroenterology. 2009;136:1979–88.
7. Kassinen A, Krogius-Kurikka L, Mäkivuokko H, et al. The fecal microbiota of irritable bowel syndrome patients differs significantly from that of healthy subjects. Gastroenterology. 2007;133:24–33.
8. Tana C, Umesaki Y, Imaoka A, et al. Altered profiles of intestinal microbiota and organic acids may be the origin of symptoms in irritable bowel syndrome. Neurogastroenterol Motil. 2010;22:512–9.
9. Ford AC, Talley NJ. Mucosal inflammation as a potential etiological factor in irritable bowel syndrome: a systematic review. J Gastroenterol. 2011;46:421–31.
10. Fukudo S, Machida T, Endo Y, Shoji T, Kano M, Kanazawa M. When and how should we study colonic motility? In: Quigley EM, Hongo M, Fukudo S, editors. Functional and GI motility disorders. Frontiers of gastrointestinal research, vol. 33. Basel: Karger; 2014. p. 65–81. https://doi.org/10.1159/000356745.
11. Kandel ER, Schwartz JH, Jessel TM. Principles of neural science. 5th ed. New York: McGraw-Hill; 2013.

12. Fukudo S. IBS: autonomic dysregulation in IBS. Nat Rev Gastroenterol Hepatol. 2013;10(10):569–71.
13. Tillisch K, Mayer EA, Labus JS. Quantitative meta-analysis identifies brain regions activated during rectal distension in irritable bowel syndrome. Gastroenterology. 2011;140:91–100.
14. Kilkens TO, Honig A, van Nieuwenhoven MA, et al. Acute tryptophan depletion affects brain-gut responses in irritable bowel syndrome patients and controls. Gut. 2004;53:1794–800.
15. Shufflebotham J, Hood S, Hendry J, et al. Acute tryptophan depletion alters gastrointestinal and anxiety symptoms in irritable bowel syndrome. Am J Gastroenterol. 2006;101:2582–7.
16. Morgan V, Pickens D, Gautam S, et al. Amitriptyline reduces rectal pain related activation of the anterior cingulate cortex in patients with irritable bowel syndrome. Gut. 2005;54:601–7.
17. Creed F, Fernandes L, Guthrie E, et al. The cost-effectiveness of psychotherapy and paroxetine for severe irritable bowel syndrome. Gastroenterology. 2003;124:303–17.
18. Fukudo S, Nomura T, Hongo M. Impact of corticotropin-releasing hormone on gastrointestinal motility and adrenocorticotropic hormone in normal controls and patients with irritable bowel syndrome. Gut. 1998;42:845–9.
19. Sagami Y, Shimada Y, Tayama J, et al. Effect of a corticotropin releasing hormone receptor antagonist on colonic sensory and motor function in patients with irritable bowel syndrome. Gut. 2004;53:958–64.
20. Dinan TG, Quigley EM, Ahmed SM, et al. Hypothalamic-pituitary-gut axis dysregulation in irritable bowel syndrome: plasma cytokines as a potential biomarker? Gastroenterology. 2006;130:304–11.
21. Chang L, Sundaresh S, Elliott J, et al. Dysregulation of the hypothalamic-pituitary-adrenal (HPA) axis in irritable bowel syndrome. Neurogastroenterol Motil. 2009;21:149–59.
22. Tanaka Y, Kanazawa M, Kano M, Morishita J, Hamaguchi T, Van Oudenhove L, Ly HG, Dupont P, Tack J, Yamaguchi T, Yanai K, Tashiro M, Fukudo S. Differential activation in amygdala and plasma noradrenaline during colorectal distention by administration of corticotropin-releasing hormone between healthy individuals and patients with irritable bowel syndrome. PLoS One. 2016;11:e0157347.
23. Kano M, Muratsubaki T, Van Oudenhove L, Morishita J, Yoshizawa M, Kono K, Yagihashi M, Tanaka Y, Mugikura S, Dupont P, Ly HG, Takase K, Kanazawa M, Fukudo S. Altered brain and gut responses to corticotropin-releasing hormone (CRH) in patients with irritable bowel syndrome. Sci Rep. 2017;7:12425.
24. Louvel D, Delvaux M, Felez A, et al. Oxytocin increases thresholds of colonic visceral perception in patients with irritable bowel syndrome. Gut. 1996;39:741–7.
25. Song GH, Leng PH, Gwee KA, et al. Melatonin improves abdominal pain in irritable bowel syndrome patients who have sleep disturbances: a randomised, double blind, placebo controlled study. Gut. 2005;54:1402–7.
26. Hattori T, Watanabe S, Kano M, et al. Differential responding of autonomic function to histamine H antagonism in irritable bowel syndrome. Neurogastroenterol Motil. 2010;22:1284–91.
27. Kuiken SD, Klooker TK, Tytgat GN, et al. Possible role of nitric oxide in visceral hypersensitivity in patients with irritable bowel syndrome. Neurogastroenterol Motil. 2006;18:115–22.
28. Houghton LA, Fell C, Whorwell PJ, et al. Effect of a second-generation alpha2delta ligand (pregabalin) on visceral sensation in hypersensitive patients with irritable bowel syndrome. Gut. 2007;56:1218–25.
29. Whitehead WE, Crowell MD, Robinson JC, et al. Effects of stressful life events on bowel symptoms: subjects with irritable bowel syndrome compared with subjects without bowel dysfunction. Gut. 1992;33:825–30.
30. Chitkara DK, van Tilburg MA, Blois-Martin N, et al. Early life risk factors that contribute to irritable bowel syndrome in adults: a systematic review. Am J Gastroenterol. 2008;103:765–74.
31. Afari N, Ahumada SM, Wright LJ, Mostoufi S, Golnari G, Reis V, Cuneo JG. Psychological trauma and functional somatic syndromes: a systematic review and meta-analysis. Psychosom Med. 2014;76:2–11.

32. Ng QX, Soh AYS, Loke W, Venkatanarayanan N, Lim DY, Yeo WS. Systematic review with meta-analysis: the association between post-traumatic stress disorder and irritable bowel syndrome. J Gastroenterol Hepatol. 2019;34:68–73.
33. Fukudo S, Suzuki J. Colonic motility, autonomic function, and gastrointestinal hormones under psychological stress on irritable bowel syndrome. Tohoku J Exp Med. 1987;151:373–85.
34. Naliboff BD, Berman S, Chang L, et al. Sex-related differences in IBS patients: central processing of visceral stimuli. Gastroenterology. 2003;124:1738–47.
35. Aizawa E, Sato Y, Kochiyama T, et al. Altered cognitive function of prefrontal cortex during error feedback in patients with irritable bowel syndrome, based on FMRI and dynamic causal modeling. Gastroenterology. 2012;143:1188–98.
36. Parker CH, Naliboff BD, Shih W, Presson AP, Videlock EJ, Mayer EA, Chang L. Negative events during adulthood are associated with symptom severity and altered stress response in patients with irritable bowel syndrome. Clin Gastroenterol Hepatol. 2019;17:2245–52.
37. Spiller R, Aziz Q, Creed F, et al. Guidelines on the irritable bowel syndrome: mechanisms and practical management. Gut. 2007;56:1770–98.
38. Koloski NA, Jones M, Kalantar J, et al. The brain-gut pathway in functional gastrointestinal disorders is bidirectional: a 12-year prospective population-based study. Gut. 2012;61:1284–90.
39. Drossman DA, McKee DC, Sandler RS, et al. Psychosocial factors in the irritable bowel syndrome: a multivariate study of patients and nonpatients with irritable bowel syndrome. Gastroenterology. 1988;95:701–8.
40. Talley NJ, Boyce PM, Jones M. Predictors of health care seeking for irritable bowel syndrome: a population based study. Gut. 1997;41:394–8.
41. Whitehead WE, Palsson O, Jones KR. Systematic review of the comorbidity of irritable bowel syndrome with other disorders: what are the causes and implications? Gastroenterology. 2002;122:1140–56.
42. Kaji M, Fujiwara Y, Shiba M, et al. Prevalence of overlaps between GERD, FD and IBS and impact on health-related quality of life. J Gastroenterol Hepatol. 2010;25:1151–6.
43. Creed F, Ratcliffe J, Fernandez L, et al. Health-related quality of life and health care costs in severe, refractory irritable bowel syndrome. Ann Intern Med. 2001;134(9 Pt 2):860–8.

Chapter 4
The Role of Brain Orexin in the Regulation of Gastrointestinal Functions such as Intestinal Motility, Visceral Sensation, and Intestinal Barrier Function

T. Okumura

Abstract Neuropeptide orexin acts in the brain to stimulate gastrointestinal secretion and motility and improve visceral sensation. These results suggest that orexin plays a role in the pathophysiology of functional gastrointestinal disorders.

Keywords Orexin · Brain · Gastrointestinal secretion · Gastrointestinal motility · Visceral sensation

4.1 Introduction

Altered intestinal motility, visceral hypersensitivity, and leaky gut are the major pathophysiology in functional gastrointestinal disorders such as irritable bowel syndrome (IBS) [1]. Accumulating evidence has indicated that a number of peripheral and central factors are involved in the regulation of intestinal motility, visceral sensation, and intestinal barrier function [1]. We could get a novel approach for IBS treatment if the mechanisms of the altered intestinal functions would be clarified. In this review, we have focused on neuropeptide, orexin that plays a role in the regulation of gut motility, visceral sensation, and intestinal permeability.

T. Okumura (✉)
Division of Gastroenterology and Hematology/Oncology, Department of Medicine, Asahikawa Medical University, Asahikawa, Japan
e-mail: okumurat@asahikawa-med.ac.jp

© The Editor(s) (if applicable) and The Author(s), under exclusive license to Springer Nature Singapore Pte Ltd. 2024

T. Kamiya, S. Fukudo (eds.), *Irritable Bowel Syndrome*,
https://doi.org/10.1007/978-981-97-8410-3_4

4.2 Orexin and Gut Motility

Orexins are novel neuropeptides that are localized in neurons in the lateral hypothalamus [2, 3]. Despite their highly restricted origin, orexin nerve fibers are identified widely throughout the central nervous system (CNS) [4, 5]. It has been reported that orexins are implicated in a wide variety of physiological functions such as feeding [2, 6], sleep/awake [7], and anxiety/depression [8–11]. In addition, orexin acts centrally to regulate gastrointestinal functions such as gastric secretion [12, 13]. Bülbül et al. demonstrated intracerebroventricular orexin-A-stimulated gastric contractions in non-fasted conscious rats [14]. Kobashi et al. [15] showed that intracisternal administration of orexin-A enhanced phasic contractions of the distal stomach, and this action was blocked by vagotomy in anesthetized rats. We have demonstrated that intravenous injection of 2-deoxy-D-glucose (2-DG), a central vagal stimulant, significantly increased gastric motility. Intracisternal injection of SB-334687, a selective orexin 1 receptor (OX1R) antagonist [16], did not modify basal motility, but the antagonist significantly suppressed this stimulated action of 2-DG, suggesting that endogenous orexin-A in the brain is involved in the vagal-dependent stimulation of gastric contractions [17]. We have also shown that orexin acts centrally to increase colonic motility [18]. Thus, orexin acts in the brain to stimulate gastrointestinal motility.

4.3 Orexin and Visceral Sensation

We have also examined the effect of central orexin on visceral sensation in rats [19]. Intracisternal but not intraperitoneal injection of orexin-A increased the threshold volume of abdominal withdrawal reflex (AWR), suggesting that orexin-A acts centrally to induce visceral antinociception. Intracisternal SB334867, an OX1R antagonist injected centrally, completely blocked the morphine-induced antinociceptive action, supporting the involvement of OX1R in central orexin-induced visceral hyposensitivity, and that endogenous orexin indeed mediates the antinociceptive effect of morphine on visceral sensation through the OX1R. The brain orexin signaling to induce visceral antinociception against colonic distension mediates visceral hyposensitivity by not only morphine but levodopa [20] or central ghrelin [21] because OX1R antagonist administered into the cisterna magna significantly blocked visceral antinociception induced by levodopa or ghrelin. We would therefore speculate that brain orexin signaling plays a vital role in providing a visceral antinociceptive action.

The Wistar-Kyoto (WKY) rat is an animal model with a genetic predisposition toward an exaggerated stress response and is used to study disorders such as IBS, where stress plays a substantial role [22–26]. WKY rats displayed visceral hypersensitivity compared to control rats [27]. Taheri et al. have demonstrated that compared to control rats, WKY rats had significantly lower orexin A-immunoreactivity and prepro-orexin mRNA levels in the brain [28]. Allard et al. have revealed fewer orexin-A positive neurons in the hypothalamus of WKY rats compared to control [29]. These findings together with the evidence that orexin acts centrally in the brain to induce visceral hyposensitivity as described above suggest that decreased orexin signaling in the brain in WKY rats may explain the reason why WKY rats, an animal model for IBS, displayed visceral hypersensitivity.

Dopamine system in the CNS is capable of inducing an antinociceptive action for visceral pain [30]. Intracisternal but not subcutaneous injection of D1 (SKF38398) or D2 (quinpirole) dopamine receptor agonist dose-dependently increased the threshold volume of colonic distension-induced AWR, respectively. Pretreatment with D1 (SCH23390) or D2 (sulpiride) dopamine receptor antagonist injected subcutaneously potently blocked the centrally injected orexin-A-induced antinociceptive action against colonic distension, suggesting that dopaminergic signaling via D1 and D2 dopamine receptors in the brain may induce visceral antinociception and the dopaminergic signaling may be involved in the central orexin-induced antinociceptive action against colonic distension [31].

Biological effects of cannabinoids (CB) are mediated primarily through specific cannabinoid receptors (CB_1 and CB_2). CB system may be implicated in the visceral antinociception through CB_1 and CB_2 receptors [32]. In addition, we have demonstrated that intraperitoneal injection of either $CB_{1/2}$ agonist, WIN 55212 or O-arachidonoyl ethanolamine, increased the threshold volume of colonic distension-induced abdominal withdrawal reflex in rats, suggesting CB could induce visceral antinociception. Pretreatment with either the CB_1 or CB_2 antagonist potently blocked the centrally injected orexin-A-induced antinociceptive action [33], suggesting that the CB signaling may be involved in the central orexin-induced antinociceptive action vis CB_1 and CB_2 receptors.

Adenosine is an ubiquitous endogenous neuromodulator or neurotransmitter, which plays an important role in pain modulation [34]. Central or systemic administration of adenosine and its analogs leads to antinociception in various animal models. We examined the effect of central adenosine on visceral sensation [35]. Intracisternal injection of N(6)-cyclopentyladenosine (CPA), an adenosine A1 receptor agonist, dose-dependently increased the threshold volume of colonic distension-induced AWR, respectively, suggesting that CPA acts centrally to induce antinociceptive action. Pretreatment with DPCPX, an adenosine A1 receptor antagonist, injected subcutaneously potently blocked the centrally injected orexin-A-induced antinociceptive action, suggesting that adenosinergic signaling via adenosine A1 receptors in the CNS may induce visceral antinociception and the adenosinergic signaling may be involved in the central orexin-induced antinociceptive action.

Thus, orexin in the brain is capable of inducing visceral antinociception at least in three different pathways. Dopamine, cannabinoid, adenosine, or oxytocin plays a vital role in the visceral hyposensitivity by orexinergic signaling.

4.4 Orexin and Intestinal Barrier Function

We have very recently examined the role of brain orexin in the regulation of intestinal barrier function [36]. Intracisternally administered orexin-A but not orexin-B dose-dependently blocked the increased intestinal permeability by lipopolysaccharide (LPS), while intraperitoneally injected orexin-A failed to block it. Atropine or vagotomy abolished the action by central orexin-A. Intravenous injection of 2-DG, a central vagal stimulant, significantly blocked the LPS-induced increased in intestinal permeability and atropine prevented the action of 2-DG. Intracisternal injection of SB-334687, a selective orexin 1 receptor antagonist, significantly blocked the action of 2-DG-induced improvement of intestinal hyperpermeability. These results suggest that exogenously administered or endogenously released orexin acts centrally to improve the intestinal hyperpermeability by LPS via the vagal cholinergic pathway. The findings also suggest for the first time that the brain could control intestinal permeability.

4.5 Orexin and IBS

IBS is a functional disorder of the gastrointestinal (GI) tract [1]. Brain-gut interaction plays an important role in the pathophysiology of IBS. Since brain orexin plays a regulatory role in gastrointestinal motility, visceral sensation, and intestinal barrier function as described above, we would suggest that orexin in the central nervous system might be involved in the development of IBS. The speculation may be further supported by the following reasons. Orexin neurons project their axon terminals to a wide variety of neuronal systems. Through these neuronal connections, orexin acts in the brain to control sleep/awake cycle, have antidepressive effect, stimulate gastrointestinal motility, and induce antinociceptive action against colonic distension. Additionally, we have very recently demonstrated that orexin acts in the brain to improve intestinal barrier function in rats [36]. Considering these findings, if the orexinergic signaling were inhibited, decreased orexin signaling may induce sleep disturbance, depressive state, and also disturbance of GI functions such as colonic motility, visceral sensation, and intestinal barrier function. In addition to gastrointestinal motility disturbance, visceral hypersensitivity and intestinal hyperpermeability the so-called leaky gut, sleep disturbance, and depression are closely associated with the clinical characteristics of IBS [1], suggesting that pathophysiology in a part of IBS patients could be explained by decreased orexin signaling in the brain. Based upon these speculation, we would suggest that orexinergic signaling in the brain may be a novel therapeutic target for patients with IBS.

4.6 Conclusion

The neuronal rapid regulation in intestinal motility, visceral sensation, and intestinal barrier function by central orexin may help us understand the brain-gut interaction in stress-sensitive gastrointestinal disorders like IBS deeply associated with the gastrointestinal function. Decreased orexin signaling in the brain may be involved in the development of IBS. In addition, increased orexin signaling may be considered to be a therapeutic option for IBS.

References

1. Drossman DA. Functional gastrointestinal disorders: history, pathophysiology, clinical features and Rome IV. Gastroenterology. 2016;2016:16.
2. Sakurai T, Amemiya A, Ishii M, et al. Orexins and orexin receptors: a family of hypothalamic neuropeptides and G protein-coupled receptors that regulate feeding behavior. Cell. 1998;92:573–85.
3. de Lecea L, Kilduff TS, Peyron C, et al. The hypocretins: hypothalamus-specific peptides with neuroexcitatory activity. Proc Natl Acad Sci USA. 1998;95:322–7.
4. Peyron C, Tighe DK, van den Pol AN, et al. Neurons containing hypocretin (orexin) project to multiple neuronal systems. J Neurosci. 1998;18:9996–10015.
5. Date Y, Ueta Y, Yamashita H, et al. Orexins, orexigenic hypothalamic peptides, interact with autonomic, neuroendocrine and neuroregulatory systems. Proc Natl Acad Sci USA. 1999;96:748–53.
6. Yamada H, Okumura T, Motomura W, et al. Inhibition of food intake by central injection of anti-orexin antibody in fasted rats. Biochem Biophys Res Commun. 2000;267:527–31.
7. Chemelli RM, Willie JT, Sinton CM, et al. Narcolepsy in orexin knockout mice: molecular genetics of sleep regulation. Cell. 1999;98:437–51.
8. Suzuki M, Beuckmann CT, Shikata K, et al. Orexin-A (hypocretin-1) is possibly involved in generation of anxiety-like behavior. Brain Res. 2005;1044:116–21.
9. Brundin L, Björkqvist M, Petersén A, et al. Reduced orexin levels in the cerebrospinal fluid of suicidal patients with major depressive disorder. Eur Neuropsychopharmacol. 2007;17:573–9.
10. Lutter M, Krishnan V, Russo SJ, et al. Orexin signaling mediates the antidepressant-like effect of calorie restriction. J Neurosci. 2008;28:3071–5.
11. Ito N, Yabe T, Gamo Y, et al. I.c.v. administration of orexin-A induces an antidepressive-like effect through hippocampal cell proliferation. Neuroscience. 2008;157:720–32.
12. Takahashi N, Okumura T, Yamada H, et al. Stimulation of gastric acid secretion by centrally administered orexin-A in conscious rats. Biochem Biophys Res Commun. 1999;254:623–7.
13. Yamada H, Takahashi N, Tanno S, et al. A selective orexin-1 receptor antagonist, SB334867, blocks 2-DG-induced gastric acid secretion in rats. Neurosci Lett. 2005;376:137–42.
14. Bülbül M, Babygirija R, Ludwig K, et al. Central orexin-A increases gastric motility in rats. Peptides. 2010;31:2118–22.
15. Kobashi M, Furudono Y, Matsuo R, et al. Central orexin facilitates gastric relaxation and contractility in rats. Neurosci Lett. 2002;332:171–4.
16. Smart D, Sabido-David C, Brough SJ, et al. SB-334867-A: the first selective orexin-1 receptor antagonist. Br J Pharmacol. 2001;132:1179–82.
17. Nozu T, Tuchiya Y, Kumei S, et al. Endogenous orexin-A in the brain mediates 2-deoxy-D-glucose-induced stimulation of gastric motility in freely moving conscious rats. J Gastroenterol. 2012;47:404–11.

18. Nozu T, Kumei S, Takakusaki K, et al. Central orexin-A increases colonic motility in conscious rats. Neurosci Lett. 2011;498:143–6.
19. Okumura T, Nozu T, Kumei S, et al. Antinociceptive action against colonic distension by brain orexin in conscious rats. Brain Res. 2015;1598:12–7.
20. Okumura T, Nozu T, Kumei S, et al. Levodopa acts centrally to induce an antinociceptive action against colonic distension through activation of D2 dopamine receptors and the orexinergic system in the brain in conscious rats. J Pharmacol Sci. 2016;130:123–7.
21. Okumura T, Nozu T, Kumei S, Takakusaki K, Ohhira M. Ghrelin acts centrally to induce an antinociceptive action during colonic distension through the orexinergic, dopaminergic and opioid systems in conscious rats. Brain Res. 2018;1686:48–54.
22. Courvoisier H, Moisan MP, Sarrieau A, et al. Behavioral and neuroendocrine reactivity to stress in the WKHA/WKY inbred rat strains: a multifactorial and genetic analysis. Brain Res. 1996;743:77–85.
23. Gunter WD, Shepard JD, Foreman RD, et al. Evidence for visceral hypersensitivity in high-anxiety rats. Physiol Behav. 2000;69:379–82.
24. Johnson AC, Tran L, Schulkin J, et al. Importance of stress receptor-mediated mechanisms in the amygdala on visceral pain perception in an intrinsically anxious rat. Neurogastroenterol Motil. 2012;24:479–86.
25. O'Malley D, Dinan TG, Cryan JF. Interleukin-6 modulates colonic transepithelial ion transport in the stress-sensitive wistar kyoto rat. Front Pharmacol. 2012;3:190.
26. Rittenhouse PA, López-Rubalcava C, Stanwood GD, et al. Amplified behavioral and endocrine responses to forced swim stress in the Wistar-Kyoto rat. Psychoneuroendocrinology. 2002;27:303–18.
27. O'Mahony SM, Clarke G, McKernan DP, et al. Differential visceral nociceptive, behavioural and neurochemical responses to an immune challenge in the stress-sensitive Wistar Kyoto rat strain. Behav Brain Res. 2013;253:310–7.
28. Taheri S, Gardiner J, Hafizi S, et al. Orexin A immunoreactivity and preproorexin mRNA in the brain of Zucker and WKY rats. Neuroreport. 2001;12:459–64.
29. Allard JS, Tizabi Y, Shaffery JP, Trouth CO, Manaye K. Stereological analysis of the hypothalamic hypocretin/orexin neurons in an animal model of depression. Neuropeptides. 2004;38:311–5.
30. Wood PB. Role of central dopamine in pain and analgesia. Expert Rev Neurother. 2008;8:781–97.
31. Okumura T, Nozu T, Kumei S, et al. Involvement of the dopaminergic system in the central orexin-induced antinociceptive action against colonic distension in conscious rats. Neurosci Lett. 2015;605:34–8.
32. Malik Z, Baik D, Schey R. The role of cannabinoids in regulation of nausea and vomiting, and visceral pain. Curr Gastroenterol Rep. 2015;17:429.
33. Okumura T, Nozu T, Kumei S, st al. Role of the cannabinoid signaling in the brain orexin- and ghrelin-induced visceral antinociception in conscious rats. J Pharmacol Sci. 2018;137:230–2.
34. Sawynok J. Adenosine receptor activation and nociception. Eur J Pharmacol. 1998;347:1–11.
35. Okumura T, Nozu T, Kumei S, Takakusaki K, Miyagishi S, Ohhira M. Adenosine A1 receptors mediate the intracisternal injection of orexin-induced antinociceptive action against colonic distension in conscious rats. J Neurol Sci. 2016;362:106–10.
36. Okumura T, Nozu T, Ishioh M, Igarashi S, Kumei S, Ohhira M. Brain orexin improves intestinal barrier function via the vagal cholinergic pathway. Neurosci Lett. 2020;714:134592.

Chapter 5
The Role of Microbiota in the Pathophysiology of Irritable Bowel Syndrome

Akifumi Fukui, Yuji Naito, Kazuhiro Kamada, and Tomohisa Takagi

Abstract Irritable bowel syndrome (IBS) is a functional gastrointestinal disorder, the physiology of which is not well understood. There are multiple factors and pathways involved in the pathophysiology of IBS. Among all, increased epithelial hyperpermeability, inflammation, and altered brain-gut interactions play a major role. These findings could be mediated by gut microbiota. Recent studies have shown that the changes in the composition and function of the gut dysbiosis may be associated with several symptoms in patients with IBS. It has been established that host immune system and its interaction with metabolic products of gut microbiota play an important role in the gastrointestinal tract. Therefore, probiotics, prebiotics, and antibiotics have shown some promising results in managing IBS symptoms via modulating the interaction between the above. This paper especially discusses the role of microbiota in the pathophysiology of IBS.

Keywords Irritable bowel syndrome · Gut dysbiosis · Mucosa-associated microbiota · Postinfectious irritable bowel syndrome · Inflammation · Metabolites

5.1 Introduction

New technology known as microbial DNA sequencing has allowed us to better characterize the human gut microbiota. Although interactions between a host and its commensal microbiota and their metabolites are symbiotic, changes in the composition and function of the gut microbiota, called "gut dysbiosis," are thought to be associated with various kinds of diseases [1, 2].

A. Fukui · Y. Naito (✉) · K. Kamada · T. Takagi
Department of Molecular Gastroenterology and Hepatology, Kyoto Prefectural University of Medicine, Kyoto, Japan
e-mail: afukui@koto.kpu-m.ac.jp; ynaito@koto.kpu-m.ac.jp; k-kamada@koto.kpu-m.ac.jp; takatomo@koto.kpu-m.ac.jp

© The Editor(s) (if applicable) and The Author(s), under exclusive license to Springer Nature Singapore Pte Ltd. 2024

T. Kamiya, S. Fukudo (eds.), *Irritable Bowel Syndrome*,
https://doi.org/10.1007/978-981-97-8410-3_5

Several lines of recent evidence indicate that gut microbiota may be involved in the pathogenesis and pathophysiology of functional gastrointestinal disorders, including irritable bowel syndrome (IBS), through the metabolic capacity of the luminal microbiota to influence the host via inflammatory, immune, and metabolic pathways [3–5]. For example, chronic functional intestinal dysfunction can develop following bacterial and viral infections, such as acute infectious gastroenteritis, and some microscopic and biochemical changes in the epithelial cells and immunocompetent cells have been shown, which are known as "postinfectious IBS (PI-IBS)" [6, 7].

Of the factors that may modify the gastrointestinal barrier and affect its immune activation, the gut microbiota is presently the main suspect [3, 8]. Gut dysbiosis has previously been linked with predisposition to immune system activation that can trigger aberrant immune responses, resulting in inflammation in the gastrointestinal tract. These factors likely sensitize the neurons, which conduct signals from the gut to the central nervous system, called "gut-brain-microbiota" [3].

Recently, several studies have pointed out substantial alterations in the composition of the microbiota in subjects with IBS [9]. However, truly little is known about the effect of this dysbiosis on the gastrointestinal tract and how it may link to its function. In this chapter, recent evidence in the role of microbiota in the pathophysiology of IBS are reviewed (Fig. 5.1).

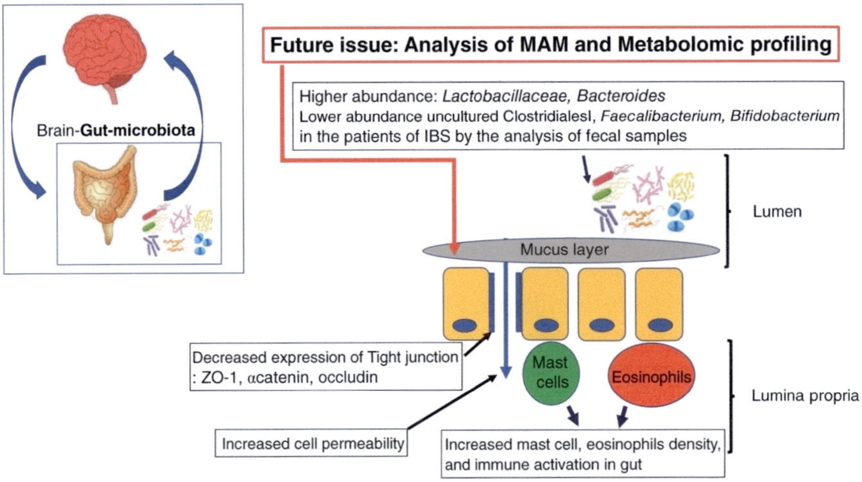

Fig. 5.1 The role of microbiota in the pathophysiology of IBS: Among the factors that may modify the gastrointestinal barrier and affect its immune activation, the gut dysbiosis is presently the main suspect. These factors likely sensitize the neurons, which conduct signals from the gut to the central nervous system, called "gut-brain-microbiota"

5.2 The Role of Microbiota in the Pathophysiology of Postinfectious IBS

Previously, Thabane et al. [10] analyzed databases to identify the studies of PI-IBS epidemiology. They reported that gastroenteritis was associated with increased odds of developing IBS (POR = 5.86; 95% CI: 3.60–9.54). In subgroup analysis, the odds of developing IBS were increased at 3 months (POR = 7.58; 95% CI: 4.27–13.45), 6 months (POR = 5.18; 95%CI: 3.24–8.26), 12 months (POR = 6.37; 95% CI: 2.63–15.40), and 24–36 months (POR = 3.85; 95% CI: 2.95–5.02). Kanazawa et al. [11] also reported that IBS patients and IBS non-consulters were more likely to report an infective history compared with controls (44.6 vs 16.1%, $P < 0.001$, for patients and 32.6 vs 16.1%, $P < 0.01$, for non-consulters), supporting the notion that a history of acute gastroenteritis is a significant risk factor for the development of IBS in Japan, as reported in other countries. Recently, the Rome Foundation produced a working team report to summarize the available evidence on the pathophysiology of PI-IBS and provide guidance for diagnosis and treatment, based on findings reported in the literature and clinical experience [12]. In this paper, it was reported that PI-IBS develops in about 10% of patients after infectious gastroenteritis. Risk factors included female sex, younger age, psychological distress during or before acute gastroenteritis, and severity of the acute episode.

As evidenced by the analysis of patients who developed PI-IBS, infective gastroenteritis could cause systemic inflammation and altered microbiome diversity, which in turn perpetuates a cycle of chronic and low-grade inflammation [12]. The pathogenesis of PI-IBS was thought to involve changes in the gastrointestinal microbiome, as well as epithelial permeability and immune system factors. Until now, IL-1β is a proinflammatory cytokine that drives cellular inflammation. Upregulated expression of IL-1β mRNA has been reported in rectal biopsies of patients who developed PI-IBS. This phenomenon was not observed in patients who did not develop PI-IBS [13]. Patients who developed PI-IBS also had significantly higher CD3+, CD4+, and CD8+ T-cell counts in the gastrointestinal mucosa [14]. Taken together, these findings support an inflammation-immunological etiopathogenesis of PI-IBS.

Furthermore, using 16S rRNA sequencing, studies have found reduced microbial diversity in patients who developed PI-IBS. The relative abundance of the genera *Bacteroides* and genera *Prevotella* has been found to be increased in PI-IBS patients compared to healthy controls [15]. However, these mechanisms are incompletely understood.

5.3 The Role of Microbiota in the Pathophysiology of Gastrointestinal Inflammation in IBS

The gastrointestinal mucosa is part of a complicated immune system and contributes a large variety of immune cells. Exposure to food, bacteria, and viruses may cause sensitization of the enteric immune system and activation of the inflammatory cascade. According to an in vivo study, experiments with animal models have shown that colonization of germ-free animals with microbiota from IBS patients can induce visceral hypersensitivity, impair intestinal permeability, and alter gastrointestinal transit time [8].

Increased gastrointestinal permeability is considered an early event in the pathogenesis of IBS that leads to low-grade immune cell infiltration of the gut mucosa [16, 17]. Indeed, increased epithelial permeability has been primarily described in PI-IBS and IBS. Vivinus-Nebot et al. [18] reported that IBS patients have increased mucosal permeability regardless of subtype with decreased expression of tight junctions (TJs), such as zonula occludens-1(ZO-1), α-catenin, and occludin as adhesion molecules of the gut epithelium, as well as low-grade inflammation in the gut. TJs changes are probably the results of bacterial-mediated and proteasome-mediated degeneration triggered by low-grade enteric inflammation. Cell populations in low-grade inflammatory infiltrates in the colonic mucosa of IBS patients consist of mast cells, eosinophils, macrophages, CD3+ cells, CD25+ cells, and intraepithelial lymphocytes (Fig. 5.1) [3, 19].

Recently, the evidence for involvement of altered gut microbiota composition in IBS pathophysiology has been accumulating. Kassinen et al. [20] compared the microbiota structure in the fecal samples of IBS patients and healthy controls by PCR amplification of the 16S rRNA gene. They reported that the coverage of the clone libraries of IBS subtypes and control subjects was significantly different ($P < 0.0253$). The samples were also distinguishable by Bayesian analysis of bacterial population structure, and significant ($P < 0.05$) differences between the clone libraries were found in several bacterial genera, which could be verified by quantitative PCR assays of phylotypes belonging to the genera *Coprococcus*, *Collinsella*, and *Coprobacillus*. Tana et al. [21] also performed microbiota analysis of fecal samples using quantitative real-time PCR and culture methods in Japanese persons and the determination of organic acid levels using high-performance liquid chromatography in IBS patients. In this report, they showed that gut dysbiosis and some short-chain fatty acids were correlated with gastrointestinal symptoms in IBS. They demonstrated that IBS patients had significantly higher abundance of genera *Veillonella* ($P = 0.046$) and *Lactobacillus* ($P = 0.031$) than controls. They also expressed significantly higher levels of acetic acid ($P = 0.049$), propionic acid ($P = 0.025$), and total organic acids ($P = 0.014$) than controls. Furthermore, IBS patients with higher levels of acetic acid or propionic acid showed significantly worse IBS symptoms, quality of life (QOL), and negative emotions than those with lower levels of acetic acid or propionic acid or healthy controls. Genera *Veillonella* and *Lactobacillus* are known to produce acetic and propionic acids. Therefore, higher levels of acetic and propionic acids may be associated with abdominal symptoms, impaired QOL, and negative emotions in IBS.

Recently, another systematic review of gut microbiota composition of IBS patients, based on 22 articles selected from among 2631 studies, was published by the Rome Foundation [4]. In this working team report, most studies assessed adults with a combination of IBS subtypes and collected microbiota from fecal samples. However, two articles collected mucosal-associated microbiota (MAM) using biopsy samples from the rectal membrane. Interestingly, although the microbial diversity and composition in luminal-microbiota and MAM were different [22], fecal samples were nearly the same in all studies. Rangel et al. [23] also reported that the composition of the MAM and the fecal-associated microbiota in unprepared sigmoid colon differs significantly ($P = 0.002$). However, clinical characteristics of IBS did not correlate with this difference. Phylum *Bacteroidetes* dominate MAM, and *Firmicutes*, *Actinobacteria*, and *Proteobacteria* dominate the fecal-associated microbiota. On the other hand, healthy subjects had a significantly higher abundance of the bacterial group uncultured *Clostridiales* I in the MAM than IBS patients ($P < 0.005$). Both types of collection are relevant, since both fecal microbiota and MAM can affect the host via immune-microbial interactions and subsequently influence IBS symptoms. The diversity of the microbiota was either decreased or not different in IBS patients compared with healthy controls.

Now, recent studies have shown that the microbial compositions of the luminal microbiota and the MAM differ, suggesting that these two distinct microbial populations play different roles within the intestinal microbiota ecosystem [4, 24]. MAM, in close contact with the host, is considered to affect epithelial and mucosal function to a greater degree than luminal bacteria. The analysis of MAM may be more deeply involved in the pathophysiology of gastrointestinal diseases, as well as systemic diseases [2, 25]. In the future, further accumulation of MAM samples is necessary to elucidate the physiology of dysbiosis in IBS [4, 24, 26].

To clarify the role of gut dysbiosis in the patients with IBS, the working team performed a detailed analysis at the phylum and genus levels using fecal samples and discussed in this report. In the phylogenetic analysis, genus *Enterobacteriaceae* (phylum *Proteobacteria*), *Lactobacillaceae* (phylum *Bacteroidetes*), and *Bacteroides* (phylum *Bacteroidetes*) were increased and demonstrated potentially harmful microbiota in IBS patients compared with healthy controls, whereas uncultured *Clostridiales* I, genus *Faecalibacterium*, and genus *Bifidobacterium* were decreased and the potentially protective microbiota in IBS patients (Fig. 5.1).

The family of *Enterobacteriaceae* contains several pathogenic bacteria, for example, *Escherichia*, *Campylobacter*, *Shigella*, and *Salmonella*. The higher abundance of genera *Enterobacteriaceae* may reflect previous gastroenteritis in these patients, such as PI-IBS [3]. Another possible hypothesis to explain these findings is the change in the gastrointestinal environment affected by potential inflammation, cell hyperpermeability, and increased gastrointestinal motility could allow for the expanding of facultative, non-fastidious bacteria, such as the family of *Enterobacteriaceae*. The family of *Lactobacillaceae* can produce organic acids, including lactic acid and/or acetic acid, from glucose or fructose, depending on patterns of fermentation and be associated with abdominal pain and bloating in IBS patients [21, 27]. The family of *Bacteroides* was increased in IBS patients, especially in the IBS-diarrhea type. Previously, Le Chatelier et al. [28] reported that some species, including enterotoxigenic strains of *Bacteroides fragilis*, can produce toxins and this may be due to low-grade inflammation. Because *Bacteroides fragilis* toxin can dissolve mucosal glycoproteins, thus affecting the microenvironment, colonic mucosal inflammation, and increased gastrointestinal motility, which can cause abdominal pain and diarrhea.

On the other hand, a potentially "protective" bacterial group in IBS patients was found in the group uncultured *Clostridiales* I. Indeed, there is a protective effect for IBS symptoms. However, the mechanism of the protective effect is unclear. The genera *Faecalibacterium*, which belong to a similar order as uncultured *Clostridial* I, have been associated with maintenance of normal gut microbiota. Lopez-Siles et al. [29] reported genera *Faecalibacterium* were considered the main butyrate-producing and anti-inflammatory organisms and reduced IBS symptoms via mediation of interleukin-17 expression in a rat model, as well as maintained gut-barrier integrity [29, 30]. Genus *Bifidobacterium* was decreased significantly in IBS patients, regardless of IBS subtype. In fact, IBS patients who received *Bifidobacterium longum* had reduced depression scores and improved QOL affected by decreasing 4-cresolsulfate levels. This substance is produced by host-bacterial interactions and influences the dopamine/noradrenaline pathway in depression [31]. Interestingly, a systematic review of probiotics in IBS highlighted that *Bifidobacterium*-containing interventions reduce IBS symptoms, which is not seen in products that contain *Lactobacillus* alone [32].

5.4 Conclusion

Gut dysbiosis is thought to modulate mucosal inflammation and act either directly or indirectly through microbial metabolites. Recently, new technology known as microbial DNA sequencing provide a kind of big data for fecal samples; this allows a detailed description of the luminal environment, but we cannot still define a causative process that leads to the development of IBS. Further investigates are needed to determine whether this inflammation is a cause or a consequence of immune-inflammatory processes and how it is related to alterations of microbiota or gut permeability. The analysis of MAM and metabolomic profiling might help answer these questions.

References

1. Andoh A. Physiological role of gut microbiota for maintaining human health. Digestion. 2016;93(3):176–81. https://doi.org/10.1159/000444066.

2. Fukui A, Takagi T, Naito Y, et al. Higher levels of streptococcus in upper gastrointestinal mucosa associated with symptoms in patients with functional dyspepsia. Digestion. 2020;101(1):38–45. https://doi.org/10.1159/000504090.
3. Enck P, Aziz Q, Barbara G, et al. Irritable bowel syndrome. Nat Rev Dis Primers. 2016;2:16014. https://doi.org/10.1038/nrdp.2016.14.
4. Pittayanon R, Lau JT, Yuan Y, et al. Gut microbiota in patients with irritable bowel syndrome-a systematic review. Gastroenterology. 2019;157(1):97–108. https://doi.org/10.1053/j.gastro.2019.03.049.
5. Gu Y, Zhou G, Qin X, et al. The potential role of gut mycobiome in irritable bowel syndrome. Front Microbiol. 2019;10:1894. https://doi.org/10.3389/fmicb.2019.01894.
6. Marshall JK, Thabane M, Borgaonkar MR, et al. Postinfectious irritable bowel syndrome after a food-borne outbreak of acute gastroenteritis attributed to a viral pathogen. Clin Gastroenterol Hepatol. 2007;5(4):457–60. https://doi.org/10.1016/j.cgh.2006.11.025.
7. Quigley EM. Gut microbiome as a clinical tool in gastrointestinal disease management: are we there yet? Nat Rev Gastroenterol Hepatol. 2017;14(5):315–20. https://doi.org/10.1038/nrgastro.2017.29.
8. Chong PP, Chin VK, Looi CY, et al. The microbiome and irritable bowel syndrome - a review on the pathophysiology, current research and future therapy. Front Microbiol. 2019;10:1136. https://doi.org/10.3389/fmicb.2019.01136.
9. Simren M, Barbara G, Flint HJ, et al. Intestinal microbiota in functional bowel disorders: a Rome foundation report. Gut. 2013;62(1):159–76. https://doi.org/10.1136/gutjnl-2012-302167.
10. Thabane M, Kottachchi DT, Marshall JK. Systematic review and meta-analysis: the incidence and prognosis of post-infectious irritable bowel syndrome. Aliment Pharmacol Ther. 2007;26(4):535–44. https://doi.org/10.1111/j.1365-2036.2007.03399.
11. Kanazawa M, Endo Y, Whitehead WE, et al. Patients and nonconsulters with irritable bowel syndrome reporting a parental history of bowel problems have more impaired psychological distress. Dig Dis Sci. 2004;49(6):1046–53. https://doi.org/10.1023/b:ddas.0000034570.52305.10.
12. Barbara G, Grover M, Bercik P, et al. Rome Foundation Working Team report on post-infection irritable bowel syndrome. Gastroenterology. 2019;156(1):46–58. https://doi.org/10.1053/j.gastro.2018.07.011.
13. Gwee KA, Collins SM, Read NW, et al. Increased rectal mucosal expression of interleukin 1beta in recently acquired post-infectious irritable bowel syndrome. Gut. 2003;52(4):523–6. https://doi.org/10.1136/gut.52.4.523.
14. Spiller RC, Jenkins D, Thornley JP, et al. Increased rectal mucosal enteroendocrine cells, T lymphocytes, and increased gut permeability following acute Campylobacter enteritis and in post-dysenteric irritable bowel syndrome. Gut. 2000;47(6):804–11. https://doi.org/10.1136/gut.47.6.804.
15. Jalanka-Tuovinen J, Salojarvi J, Salonen A, et al. Faecal microbiota composition and host-microbe cross-talk following gastroenteritis and in postinfectious irritable bowel syndrome. Gut. 2014;63(11):1737–45. https://doi.org/10.1136/gutjnl-2013-305994.
16. Qin HY, Xavier Wong HL, Zang KH, et al. Enterochromaffin cell hyperplasia in the gut: factors, mechanism and therapeutic clues. Life Sci. 2019;239:116886. https://doi.org/10.1016/j.lfs.2019.116886.
17. Ng QX, Soh AYS, Loke W, et al. The role of inflammation in irritable bowel syndrome (IBS). J Inflamm Res. 2018;11:345–9. https://doi.org/10.2147/JIR.S174982.
18. Vivinus-Nebot M, Frin-Mathy G, Bzioueche H, et al. Functional bowel symptoms in quiescent inflammatory bowel diseases: role of epithelial barrier disruption and low-grade inflammation. Gut. 2014;63(5):744–52. https://doi.org/10.1136/gutjnl-2012-304066.
19. Fritscher-Ravens A, Pflaum T, Mosinger M, et al. Many patients with irritable bowel syndrome have atypical food allergies not associated with immunoglobulin E. Gastroenterology. 2019;157(1):109–18. https://doi.org/10.1053/j.gastro.2019.03.046.

20. Kassinen A, Krogius-Kurikka L, Makivuokko H, et al. The fecal microbiota of irritable bowel syndrome patients differs significantly from that of healthy subjects. Gastroenterology. 2007;133(1):24–33. https://doi.org/10.1053/j.gastro.2007.04.005.
21. Tana C, Umesaki Y, Imaoka A, et al. Altered profiles of intestinal microbiota and organic acids may be the origin of symptoms in irritable bowel syndrome. Neurogastroenterol Motil. 2010;22(5):512–9. https://doi.org/10.1111/j.1365-2982.2009.01427.
22. Li G, Yang M, Jin Y, et al. Involvement of shared mucosal-associated microbiota in the duodenum and rectum in diarrhea-predominant irritable bowel syndrome. J Gastroenterol Hepatol. 2018;33(6):1220–6. https://doi.org/10.1111/jgh.14059.
23. Rangel I, Sundin J, Fuentes S, et al. The relationship between faecal-associated and mucosal-associated microbiota in irritable bowel syndrome patients and healthy subjects. Aliment Pharmacol Ther. 2015;42:1211–21.
24. Sundin J, Aziz I, Nordlander S, et al. Evidence of altered mucosa-associated and fecal microbiota composition in patients with irritable Bowel Syndrome. Sci Rep. 2020;10(1):593. https://doi.org/10.1038/s41598-020-57468-y.
25. Ringel Y, Maharshak N, Ringel-Kulka T, et al. High throughput sequencing reveals distinct microbial populations within the mucosal and luminal niches in healthy individuals. Gut Microbes. 2015;6(3):173–81. https://doi.org/10.1080/19490976.2015.1044711.
26. Zhong W, Lu X, Shi H, et al. Distinct microbial populations exist in the mucosa-associated microbiota of diarrhea predominant irritable bowel syndrome and ulcerative colitis. J Clin Gastroenterol. 2019;53(9):660–72. https://doi.org/10.1097/MCG.0000000000000961.
27. Hegazi FZ, Abo-Elnaga IG. Degradation of organic acids by dairy lactic acid bacteria. Zentralbl Bakteriol Naturwiss. 1980;135(3):212–22. https://doi.org/10.1016/s0323-6056(80)80025-5.
28. Le Chatelier E, Nielsen T, Qin J, et al. Richness of human gut microbiome correlates with metabolic markers. Nature. 2013;500(7464):541–6. https://doi.org/10.1038/nature12506.
29. Lopez-Siles M, Duncan SH, Garcia-Gil LJ, et al. Faecalibacterium prausnitzii: from microbiology to diagnostics and prognostics. ISME J. 2017;11(4):841–52. https://doi.org/10.1038/ismej.2016.176.
30. Zhang M, Qiu X, Zhang H, et al. Faecalibacterium prausnitzii inhibits interleukin-17 to ameliorate colorectal colitis in rats. PLoS One. 2014;9(10):e109146. https://doi.org/10.1371/journal.pone.0109146.
31. Pinto-Sanchez MI, Hall GB, Ghajar K, et al. Probiotic Bifidobacterium longum NCC3001 reduces depression scores and alters brain activity: a pilot study in patients with irritable bowel syndrome. Gastroenterology. 2017;153(2):448–59. https://doi.org/10.1053/j.gastro.2017.05.003.
32. Ford AC, Harris LA, Lacy BE, et al. Systematic review with meta-analysis: the efficacy of prebiotics, probiotics, synbiotics and antibiotics in irritable bowel syndrome. Aliment Pharmacol Ther. 2018;48(10):1044–60. https://doi.org/10.1111/apt.15001.

Chapter 6
Mucosal Inflammation and Visceral Hypersensitivity in Irritable Bowel Syndrome

Keishi Komori, Eikichi Ihara, and Hirotada Akiho

Abstract Mucosal inflammation and visceral hypersensitivity are considered to be closely related factors that contribute to the pathogenesis of irritable bowel syndrome. Mucosal inflammation can be induced by factors such as diet, food allergies, psychological stress, changes in intestinal permeability, and alterations of the intestinal flora. Visceral hypersensitivity results from aberrant activation of peripheral nerves. These events, which may also be associated with an increase in the abundance and/or activation of mast cells, are considered to be the major causes of irritable bowel syndrome.

Keywords Irritable bowel syndrome · Mucosal inflammation · Visceral hypersensitivity

---

K. Komori
Department of Medicine and Bioregulatory Science, Graduate School of Medical Sciences, Kyushu University, Fukuoka, Japan
e-mail: kkomori@med.kyushu-u.ac.jp

E. Ihara
Department of Medicine and Bioregulatory Science, Graduate School of Medical Sciences, Kyushu University, Fukuoka, Japan

Department of Gastroenterology and Metabolism, Graduate School of Medical Sciences, Kyushu University, Fukuoka, Japan
e-mail: eikichi@intmed3.med.kyushu-u.ac.jp

H. Akiho (✉)
Department of Gastroenterology, Kitakyushu Municipal Medical Center, Kitakyushu, Japan
e-mail: akiho@med.kyushu-u.ac.jp

© The Editor(s) (if applicable) and The Author(s), under exclusive license to Springer Nature Singapore Pte Ltd. 2024

T. Kamiya, S. Fukudo (eds.), *Irritable Bowel Syndrome*,
https://doi.org/10.1007/978-981-97-8410-3_6

6.1 Introduction

Irritable bowel syndrome (IBS) is characterized by abdominal pain and discomfort accompanied by diarrhea and constipation. Changes in gut motility, the so-called irritability, are perceived by the brain of patients with IBS as pain and/or discomfort. Although the precise pathogenesis of IBS is still unclear, many factors are known to contribute to changes in gut motility, including mucosal inflammation and visceral hypersensitivity associated with gut infections, gut immune responses, alterations in the gut commensal microbiota, diet, food allergies, and psychosocial factors [1]. Indeed, mucosal inflammation, visceral hypersensitivity, and possible links between them have drawn much attention in efforts to understand the pathogenesis of IBS [2].

Visceral hypersensitivity results from allodynia and hyperalgesia. Allodynia is defined as pain sensation caused by stimuli that would not normally provoke pain, while hyperalgesia is defined as increased sensitivity to stimuli that normally do cause pain. For example, using a colonic barostat to induce varying degrees of intestinal pressure, Ritchie showed that patients with IBS not only felt abdominal pain upon balloon dilation to a degree that did not induce pain in healthy subjects but also exhibited elevated abdominal pain upon balloon dilation that did cause abdominal pain in healthy subjects [3].

In this section, we describe how mucosal inflammation and visceral hypersensitivity are involved in the pathogenesis of IBS, with a particular focus on the contribution of immune cells, especially mast cells, which are present at higher abundance in the gut mucosa of patients with IBS compared with healthy subjects (Fig. 6.1).

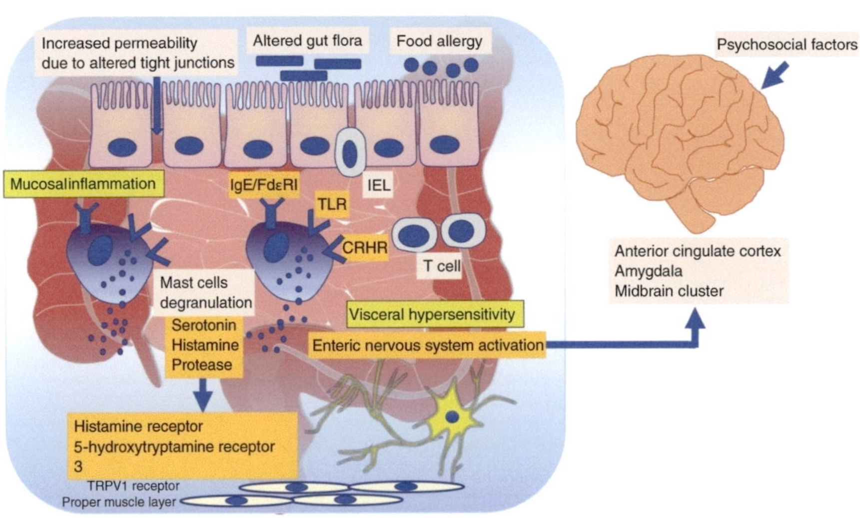

Fig. 6.1 Schematic illustration of putative factors related to mucosal inflammation and visceral hypersensitivity involved in the pathogenesis of bowel syndrome. Mast cell degranulation is considered to be a major cause of IBS symptoms. *TLR* toll-like receptor, *CRHR* corticotropin-releasing hormone receptor, *IEL* intraepithelial lymphocyte, *FcεRI* high-affinity IgE receptor

6.2 Mucosal Inflammation in IBS

6.2.1 Significance of Low-Grade Inflammation in IBS

Serum high-sensitivity C-reactive protein levels are abnormally high in patients with IBS, particularly those whose main symptoms include diarrhea, and the levels correlate with the severity of abdominal symptoms [4], suggesting that inflammatory changes might be involved in the pathogenesis of IBS. Several studies have analyzed gut mucosal tissue biopsies from patients with IBS to identify changes in subsets of immune cells (Tables 6.1 and 6.2) [2, 5–44]. These studies demonstrated that the abundance of mast cells is increased in the mucosa of all regions of the

Table 6.1 Studies examining the abundance of immune cells in the intestine of patients with IBS

	Large intestine				
	Recto/sigmoid	Descending	Transverse	Ascending	Cecum
Mast cell					
↑	[5, 6, 8, 17, 23, 29, 34, 36]	[2, 7, 10, 11, 14–17]		[17, 34]	[17, 23, 32, 35, 39]
→	[11–13, 18–20, 26, 32, 41]	[12, 32]	[12, 17]	[12, 32]	[26]
↓	[27]	[9, 27]		[9]	
IEL					
↑	[12, 37]	[12]	[12]	[12]	
→	[18, 19]				[35, 39]
T cell					
↑	[6, 12, 18, 19, 29, 37]	[12, 16]	[12]	[12]	[35]
→	[13]	[9]		[9]	
B cell					
→	[22]	[16]			
↓				[22]	
NK					
→	[12]	[12]	[12]	[9, 12]	
Macrophage					
→	[32]	[32]		[32]	[32]
↓	[37]	[9]			
Neutrophil					
→	[12, 17, 32–34, 44]	[12, 17, 32]	[12, 17]	[12, 17, 32–34]	[17, 32, 35]
Eosinophil					
↑					[17]
→	[17, 26, 32–34]	[17, 32]	[17]	[17, 32–34]	[26, 32, 35, 39]
Plasma cell					
→	[32–34]	[32]		[32–34]	[32, 35]

Table summarizes information from [25, 28, 47]. Reference numbers refer to citations in the present article

Table 6.2 Studies examining the abundance of immune cells in the intestine of patients with IBS

	Small intestine		
	Ileum	Jejunum	Duodenum
Mast cell			
↑	[17, 34, 41–43]	[24, 30, 31]	[21, 40]
→	[26]	[38, 42]	[42]
IEL			
↑		[24]	[21]
→		[31]	
Neutrophil			
→	[33, 34]		
Eosinophil			
→	[17, 26, 33, 34]		[40]
Plasma cell			
→	[33, 34]		

Table summarizes information from [25, 28, 47]. Reference numbers refer to citations in the present article

gastrointestinal (GI) tract, including the rectum, colon, jejunum, ileum, and duodenum (Tables 6.1 and 6.2). Intraepithelial lymphocytes (IELs) and various T-cell subsets are also increased in the gut mucosa of IBS patients [45]; specifically, the numbers of $CD3^+$, $CD4^+$, $CD25^+$, and $CD8^+$ T lymphocytes are higher in the large intestine of IBS patients compared with healthy subjects [12, 16]. Similarly, the GI tracts of patients with postinfection IBS (PI-IBS), in which IBS is elicited by an acute episode of gastroenteritis, have been reported to contain increased numbers of $CD45RO^+$ $CD4^+$ activated/memory T lymphocyte and $CD4^+CD8^+$ double-positive T lymphocyte and decreased numbers of B lymphocytes compared with healthy subjects [46]. However, a systematic review found no evidence of a significant difference in the number of regulatory T cells in the GI tracts of IBS patients and healthy subjects [28, 47]. The aberrant numbers of activated lymphocytes in the gut are thought to contribute to the symptoms of diarrhea [18] via the release of interleukin (IL) 1β [48], nitric oxide [49], and prostaglandin (PG) D2 [50]. In contrast to lymphocytes and mast cells, eosinophils are not increased in the gut mucosa of IBS patients [47]. This contrasts with patients with functional dyspepsia, a disorder of the upper abdominal region, in whom duodenal eosinophilia has been shown to be pathogenic [51]. The guts of IBS patients also show no significant difference from healthy subjects with respect to the abundance of other immune cells, including neutrophils, plasma cells, B cells, and natural killer cells (Tables 6.1 and 6.2), although it is not yet clear whether antigen-presenting cells such as macrophages and dendritic cells are involved in IBS [28]. Among all of the immune cells elevated in the gut mucosa of IBS patients, mast cells have most clearly been shown to be associated with IBS pathogenesis [28, 47].

6.2.2 Involvement of Mast Cells in IBS

Mast cells play a key role in the host defense against pathogens via recruitment of other immune cells, secretion of agents that promote vascular permeability, and induction of allergic inflammatory responses [52]. Most mast cells in the GI tract are found in the mucosal lamina propria and the submucosa [53] and have been suggested to be physically associated with peripheral nerves of the colonic mucosa. Electron microscopy of the mucosa of patients with IBS showed that the proximity of mast cells to peripheral nerves correlated positively with mast cell degranulation, and the severity of IBS abdominal symptoms correlated with the number of mast cells located within 5 μm of peripheral nerves [2]. Consistent with this, the levels of histamine, proteases, and PGE2, presumably released from mast cells, were elevated in the colonic mucosa of IBS patients compared with healthy subjects [7]. Supernatants from gut biopsy samples from IBS patients, but not from healthy subjects, caused an increase in the discharge of mesenteric afferent nerves. In addition, the discharge correlated significantly with the number of mast cells in the lamina propria and the release of histamine and proteases, which are known to contribute significantly to sensory neuron excitation. Other components of supernatants from colonic biopsy samples from IBS patients, including serotonin, histamine, and tryptase, have been shown to increase the rate of spike discharge in human submucosal neurons [10]. Given that mast cells are the major source of histamine [54], it is conceivable that the increased number and/or activity of mast cells in the intestinal mucosa play an important role in the pathogenesis of IBS.

6.2.3 Development, Migration, and Activation of GI-Associated Mast Cells in IBS

Mast cells are derived from bone marrow hematopoietic stem cells; these cells develop into multipotent progenitors, which, in turn, differentiate into common myeloid progenitors [55], and then mast cells. Mast cells are long-lived, surviving for months and even years, and can replenish their granules following inflammation-induced degranulation [56]. These cells release numerous biologically active products, including tryptase, chymase, histamine, serotonin, IL-1, IL-3, IL-4, IL-6, IL-18, tumor necrosis factor-α, transforming growth factor-β, chemokines, and lipid metabolites [53]. Mast cells also contribute to the recruitment of other immune cells, such as neutrophils, eosinophils, and basophils, via the release of inflammatory mediators such as monocyte chemotactic protein 1 and macrophage inflammatory protein $1\alpha_{(CCL3)}$ and $1_{\beta(CCL4)}$. Small numbers of mast cell progenitors circulate in the blood and, if necessary, are recruited to target tissues where they mature into mast cells. Integrin α4β7, its ligand vascular cell adhesion molecule 1, and the α-chemokine receptor CXCR2 play important roles in homing of mast cell progenitors to the gut [52, 57]. The differentiation and proliferation of mast cells depends on stem cell factor produced by fibroblasts and endothelial cells, which is increased by exposure to Th2 cytokines, including IL-5 and IL-9, but suppressed by exposure to the Th1 cytokine interferon-γ [58]. Th2 cytokines are thought to be upregulated in IBS patients who have increased numbers and/or activation of mast cells; however, this remains to be formally established. A few reports have shown that mucosal tissues from IBS patients contain elevated levels of IL-1β and IL-8 and decreased levels of IL-10 compared with mucosal tissues from healthy subjects, but as yet there is no consensus [28].

Mast cells can be activated via several mechanisms. These cells play a role in IgE-mediated allergic inflammation and act as regulatory and effector cells in innate and adaptive immunity [53]. Mast cells can be activated to degranulate via IgE binding to the high-affinity IgE receptor $Fc_{\varepsilon}RI$ [59], and increasing evidence suggest that mast cells can also be activated via IgG, IgA, free Ig light chains, complement C3a and C5a [60], substance P, calcitonin gene-related peptide, corticotropin-releasing hormone (CRH), and Toll-like receptors (TLRs) [54, 61–63]. Among these stimuli, the most important for IBS are IgE and CRH, which are produced in a stress-related manner, and TLRs, which are activated by microbial molecules and are thus relevant to changes in intestinal flora. A population-based study found that diet and food allergies play an important role in the pathogenesis of IBS [64]. Although food allergies have also been linked to psychological distress [65], their relationship with IBS was found to be independent of psychological factors [64]. This finding implicates food allergen-specific IgE in the pathogenesis of IBS. Malabsorption of certain foods, such as fructose and sorbitol, carbohydrate-rich foods, fatty foods, coffee, alcohol, and spices, have been associated with abdominal symptoms in patients with disorders of bowel function, especially IBS [66, 67]. Intravenous administration of CRH caused a greater effect on contractions of the descending colon in patients with IBS than in healthy controls [68]. Moreover, a nonselective CRH receptor antagonist has been found to improve distension-induced changes in gut motility and visceral perception in IBS patients [69]. CRH is a crucial molecule secreted by the hypothalamus in response to stress. In the GI, the stress-mast cell axis is thought to be involved in the regulation of motor and visceral responses [61]. Activation of CRH receptors on mast cells leads to the selective release of cytokines and other proinflammatory mediators [61]. CRH interaction with its receptors CRH-R1 and CRH-R2 on subepithelial mast cells [70] induces the release of mucin, ions, and water, leading to an increase in intestinal epithelial permeability [71–73]. TLRs are expressed on a wide variety of immune cells, including mast cells, and their recognition of bacterial molecules plays an important role in innate immunity [74]. Colonic biopsy samples from patients with IBS contain higher levels of TLR4 and TLR5 mRNA and decreased levels of TLR7 and TLR8 mRNA compared with tissues from healthy subjects [75]. Murine mast cells have been shown to express TLR4 protein and TLR7 and TLR8 mRNA [76]. Lipopolysaccharides produced by Gram-negative bacteria are ligands for TLR4; flagellin, the major structural subunit of flagella, is a ligand for TLR5; and TLR7 and TLR8 both recognize viral or bacterial single-stranded RNA [77, 78]. Thus, stimulation of intestinal mast cells by allergens, psychological stress, viruses, and bacteria can contribute to IBS symptoms. Further study will be required to clarify the precise roles of these stimuli in IBS.

6.2.4 *Altered Microbiota in IBS and PI-IBS*

The gut microbiota of IBS patients differs from that of healthy subjects. For example, *Veillonella* and *Lactobacillus* are present at significantly higher proportions in fecal samples from IBS patients compared with healthy subjects [79]. Similarly, the fecal and gut mucosal microbial composition of patients with PI-IBS differ from that of both healthy subjects and patients with IBS [80]. A large Canadian cohort study examined the nature and epidemiology of PI-IBS. The Rome I criteria were met by 10.1% of healthy subjects, 27.5% of patients with self-reported gastroenteritis, and 36.2% of subjects with clinically suspected gastroenteritis [81]. That study also implicated *Escherichia coli* and *Campylobacter jejuni* in the development of PI-IBS. In addition to bacteria (*Salmonella*, *Shigella* spp., *C. jejuni*), infection by several parasites (*Trichinella britovi*, *Giardia duodenalis*) and viruses (*Norovirus*, Epstein-Barr virus) may be associated with PI-IBS [81]. Notably, the number of mast cells in the terminal ileum mucosa of PI-IBS patients infected with *Shigella* spp. was significantly higher than the numbers in healthy subjects [37].

The gut mucosa of IBS patients and PI-IBS patients have higher numbers of mast cells associated with nerves than the gut mucosa of healthy subjects, as illustrated by co-staining of neuron-specific enolase, substance P, and 5-hydroxytryptamine [41]. In addition, enteroendocrine cells (including 5-hydroxytryptamine-containing cells) and T lymphocytes are more abundant in the rectal mucosa of PI-IBS patients suffering from *Campylobacter* enteritis [37]. Thus, mast cells appear to be involved in eliciting the symptoms of PI-IBS in addition to IBS. Changes in the gut microbiota alter the intestinal composition of secondary bile acids, which in turn, may be associated with diarrhea and/or constipation in patients with IBS. Bile acids are known to affect gut peristalsis via activation of the TGR5 receptor [82]. Thus, changes in the gut microbiota, whether dependent on or independent of acute infection, may affect the development of IBS symptoms via mast or lymphoid cell hyperplasia.

6.3 Visceral Hypersensitivity in IBS

6.3.1 *Visceral Hypersensitivity in Patients with IBS*

Abdominal pain resulting from visceral hypersensitivity is an essential symptom of IBS [83]. Patients with IBS experience abdominal pain in response to colonic barostat dilation that does not cause pain in healthy subjects [3]. Intraduodenal infusion of lipids also causes visceral hypersensitivity in IBS patients, as evaluated by stimulation of rectal distension [84]. Barostat stimulation-induced rectal extension results in activation of sympathetic nerves and increased heart rate, indicating that the distention is perceived by the insula in the right brain [85]. Accumulated evidence has demonstrated a role for visceral hypersensitivity in IBS.

6.3.2 Activity of the Transient Receptor Potential Vanilloid 1 (TRPV1) in IBS-Associated Visceral Hypersensitivity

Sensory neurons of the thoracic and abdominal regions of the gut are controlled by two pathways; the sympathetic large splanchnic nerve, which connects to the spinal cord, and the parasympathetic vagus nerve, which connects directly to the brainstem, where vagal afferents terminate close to the mucosal epithelium [86]. In contrast, in the lower abdominal regions of the gut, the sensory neurons are controlled by spinal nerves, such as the pelvic and lumbar splanchnic nerves. Spinal afferents terminate in the serosa and muscle layers of the intestine. Both vagal and spinal sensory afferents are exposed to agents absorbed from the lumen and/or mediators released from enteroendocrine cells and immune cells [79, 86].

TRPV1 is a pain-sensing nociceptive receptor expressed by sensory nerves and plays a crucial role in pain sensing in patients with IBS. TRPV1 was first cloned as a capsaicin receptor in 1997 [87], and it was later recognized to be a temperature-activated ion channel in the pain pathway that is sensitive not only to capsaicin but also to heat, acids, and lipids. In the lower gut, TRPV1 is expressed in peripheral nerves such as gut ganglia and interganglionic nerves of the mucous membrane, submucosal layer, and muscular layer. The response of TRPV1 in colonic nerve fibers is elevated in IBS patients compared with healthy subjects [88]. In IBS patients, inflammatory mediators, including PGs, trypsin, and tryptase, decrease the temperature activation threshold of TRPV1 to a degree where they can be activated even at body temperature. Sensitization of TRPV1 by serotonin may also reduce the temperature threshold for TRPV1 activation [89]. Thus, it is reasonable to assume that visceral hypersensitivity can be caused by a decrease in the activation threshold of TRPV1 associated with inflammatory cell infiltration and elevated release of mediators. Indeed, mast cell degranulation has been shown to increase the excitability of vagal, splanchnic, and mesenteric afferents, thereby contributing to nociceptive processes associated with visceral pain [90]. MicroRNAs, which play crucial roles in regulating gene expression, have also been implicated in visceral hypersensitivity; for example, decreased expression of miR-199 in the colon contributes to chronic visceral pain and nociception via upregulation of TRPV1 expression [88]. Collectively, these studies support a role for TRPV1 in visceral hypersensitivity.

6.3.3 Increased Gut Mucosal Permeability in IBS-Associated Visceral Hypersensitivity

IBS patients with increased gut mucosal permeability experience more severe symptoms and hypersensitivity to both visceral and thermal nociceptive pain stimuli compared with IBS patients with normal gut permeability or healthy subjects [91]. Increased gut mucosal permeability facilitates the penetration of bacterial products, such as serine and cysteine proteases and bile salts, into the mucosa, and may be associated with mild immune activation and IBS symptoms [92]. Mucosal inflammation has been reported to be closely associated with mucosal barrier function. Expression of zonula occludens 1 (ZO-1), a key component of the intercellular tight junctions that maintain mucosal barrier function, is reduced at both the mRNA and protein level in patients with IBS. Another study showed that the IBS severity score correlated significantly with the degree of paracellular permeability in IBS patients [39]. Interestingly, mast cell activation was shown to affect the expression of ZO-1 and to increase gut mucosal permeability, which was associated with abdominal symptoms in IBS patients [31]. Thus, it seems reasonable to assume that alterations in mucosal barrier function may play a role in the visceral hypersensitivity of IBS.

6.3.4 Psychological Factors in IBS-Associated Visceral Hypersensitivity

As noted above, the gut receives dual sensory innervation. Sensory fibers contained in the vagus and pelvic nerves terminate in the brain stem and lumbosacral spinal cord, respectively, whereas the majority of visceral sensory fibers terminate in the spinal cord [93]. The emotional component of with abdominal pain is transmitted to the anterior cingulate cortex and the island, and recognition of the location and quality of the pain is transmitted to the cortical sensory areas [94]. A case report of a woman with IBS who had a history of sexual abuse described psychosocial impairment, high life stress, visceral hypersensitivity, and activation of the corresponding brain areas associated with pain intensity. Both the visceral hypersensitivity and activation of the brain area were diminished when the patient's psychological condition had clinically improved [95]. This finding indicated that activation of certain brain areas responding to rectal distension is not affected by factors related to the disease state itself, but instead depends on the patient's emotional state [95]. Some studies have used functional magnetic resonance imaging (fMRI) and positron emission tomography (PET) to observe changes in brain activity during rectal extension stimulation. A meta-analysis of brain imaging studies performed during rectal distension stimulation (13 studies using fMRI and 5 studies using PET) revealed that activation of the brain regions associated with visceral afferent processing, such as the thalamus, insula, and anterior midcingulate, was similar in patients with IBS and healthy subjects. However, the two cohorts exhibited significant differences in activation of regions associated with emotional arousal, such as the pregenual anterior cingulate cortex and amygdala. Moreover, the midbrain cluster, which is involved in endogenous pain modulation, was also activated in IBS patients, whereas activation of the medial and lateral prefrontal cortex was observed in healthy subjects [96]. These results suggest that emotional changes or an innate predisposition may cause changes in brain pain sensitivity in IBS patients that lead to visceral hypersensitivity.

6.4 Conclusion

In this section, we focused on how mucosal inflammation and visceral hypersensitivity are associated with the pathogenesis of IBS. Although the etiology of IBS has yet to be precisely delineated, mucosal inflammation and visceral hypersensitivity are linked and are associated with an increased abundance and/or activation of mast cells, altered gut microbiota, diet, food allergies, sensory neuron receptor expression, impaired gut mucosal permeability, and psychological stress. Additional studies will be necessary to clarify the link between mucosal inflammation and visceral hypersensitivity in the pathogenesis of IBS.

References

1. Barbara G, De Giorgio R, Stanghellini V, Cremon C, Salvioli B, Corinaldesi R. New pathophysiological mechanisms in irritable bowel syndrome. Aliment Pharmacol Ther. 2004;20(2):1–9. https://doi.org/10.1111/j.1365-2036.2004.02036.x. PubMed PMID: 15335408.
2. Barbara G, Stanghellini V, De Giorgio R, Cremon C, Cottrell GS, Santini D, et al. Activated mast cells in proximity to colonic nerves correlate with abdominal pain in irritable bowel syndrome. Gastroenterology. 2004;126(3):693–702. https://doi.org/10.1053/j.gastro.2003.11.055. PubMed PMID: 14988823.
3. Ritchie J. Pain from distension of the pelvic colon by inflating a balloon in the irritable colon syndrome. Gut. 1973;14(2):125–32. https://doi.org/10.1136/gut.14.2.125. PubMed PMID: 4696535; PubMed Central PMCID: PMCPMC1412559.
4. Hod K, Ringel-Kulka T, Martin CF, Maharshak N, Ringel Y. High-sensitive C-reactive protein as a marker for inflammation in irritable bowel syndrome. J Clin Gastroenterol. 2016;50(3):227–32. https://doi.org/10.1097/MCG.0000000000000327. PubMed PMID: 25930973; PubMed Central PMCID: PMCPMC4950940.
5. Ahn JY, Lee KH, Choi CH, Kim JW, Lee HW, Kim JW, et al. Colonic mucosal immune activity in irritable bowel syndrome: comparison with healthy controls and patients with ulcerative colitis. Dig Dis Sci. 2014;59(5):1001–11. https://doi.org/10.1007/s10620-013-2930-4. PubMed PMID: 24282051.
6. Akbar A, Yiangou Y, Facer P, Walters JR, Anand P, Ghosh S. Increased capsaicin receptor TRPV1-expressing sensory fibres in irritable bowel syndrome and their correlation with abdominal pain. Gut. 2008;57(7):923–9. https://doi.org/10.1136/gut.2007.138982. PubMed PMID: 18252749; PubMed Central PMCID: PMCPMC2564830.

7. Barbara G, Wang B, Stanghellini V, de Giorgio R, Cremon C, Di Nardo G, et al. Mast cell-dependent excitation of visceral-nociceptive sensory neurons in irritable bowel syndrome. Gastroenterology. 2007;132(1):26–37. https://doi.org/10.1053/j.gastro.2006.11.039. PubMed PMID: 17241857.
8. Bhuiyan MR, Majumder TK, Raihan AA, Roy PK, Farha N, Kamal M. Histopathological alterations in post-infectious irritable bowel syndrome in Bangladeshi population. Mymensingh Med J. 2010;19(2):275–81. PubMed PMID: 20395926.
9. Braak B, Klooker TK, Wouters MM, Welting O, van der Loos CM, Stanisor OI, et al. Mucosal immune cell numbers and visceral sensitivity in patients with irritable bowel syndrome: is there any relationship? Am J Gastroenterol. 2012;107(5):715–26. https://doi.org/10.1038/ajg.2012.54. PubMed PMID: 22488080.
10. Buhner S, Li Q, Vignali S, Barbara G, De Giorgio R, Stanghellini V, et al. Activation of human enteric neurons by supernatants of colonic biopsy specimens from patients with irritable bowel syndrome. Gastroenterology. 2009;137(4):1425–34. https://doi.org/10.1053/j.gastro.2009.07.005. PubMed PMID: 19596012.
11. Cenac N, Andrews CN, Holzhausen M, Chapman K, Cottrell G, Andrade-Gordon P, et al. Role for protease activity in visceral pain in irritable bowel syndrome. J Clin Invest. 2007;117(3):636–47. https://doi.org/10.1172/JCI29255. PubMed PMID: 17304351; PubMed Central PMCID: PMCPMC1794118.
12. Chadwick VS, Chen W, Shu D, Paulus B, Bethwaite P, Tie A, et al. Activation of the mucosal immune system in irritable bowel syndrome. Gastroenterology. 2002;122(7):1778–83. https://doi.org/10.1053/gast.2002.33579. PubMed PMID: 12055584.
13. Chang L, Adeyemo M, Karagiannides I, Videlock EJ, Bowe C, Shih W, et al. Serum and colonic mucosal immune markers in irritable bowel syndrome. Am J Gastroenterol. 2012;107(2):262–72. https://doi.org/10.1038/ajg.2011.423. PubMed PMID: 22158028; PubMed Central PMCID: PMCPMC3297737.
14. Coeffier M, Gloro R, Boukhettala N, Aziz M, Lecleire S, Vandaele N, et al. Increased proteasome-mediated degradation of occludin in irritable bowel syndrome. Am J Gastroenterol. 2010;105(5):1181–8. https://doi.org/10.1038/ajg.2009.700. PubMed PMID: 19997094.
15. Cremon C, Carini G, Wang B, Vasina V, Cogliandro RF, De Giorgio R, et al. Intestinal serotonin release, sensory neuron activation, and abdominal pain in irritable bowel syndrome. Am J Gastroenterol. 2011;106(7):1290–8. https://doi.org/10.1038/ajg.2011.86. PubMed PMID: 21427712.
16. Cremon C, Gargano L, Morselli-Labate AM, Santini D, Cogliandro RF, De Giorgio R, et al. Mucosal immune activation in irritable bowel syndrome: gender-dependence and association with digestive symptoms. Am J Gastroenterol. 2009;104(2):392–400. https://doi.org/10.1038/ajg.2008.94. PubMed PMID: 19174797.
17. De Silva AP, Nandasiri SD, Hewavisenthi J, Manamperi A, Ariyasinghe MP, Dassanayake AS, et al. Subclinical mucosal inflammation in diarrhea-predominant irritable bowel syndrome (IBS) in a tropical setting. Scand J Gastroenterol. 2012;47(6):619–24. https://doi.org/10.3109/00365521.2012.666672. PubMed PMID: 22486731.
18. Dunlop SP, Jenkins D, Neal KR, Spiller RC. Relative importance of enterochromaffin cell hyperplasia, anxiety, and depression in postinfectious IBS. Gastroenterology. 2003;125(6):1651–9. https://doi.org/10.1053/j.gastro.2003.09.028. PubMed PMID: 14724817.
19. Dunlop SP, Jenkins D, Spiller RC. Distinctive clinical, psychological, and histological features of postinfective irritable bowel syndrome. Am J Gastroenterol. 2003;98(7):1578–83. https://doi.org/10.1111/j.1572-0241.2003.07542.x. PubMed PMID: 12873581.
20. El-Salhy M, Gundersen D, Hatlebakk JG, Hausken T. Low-grade inflammation in the rectum of patients with sporadic irritable bowel syndrome. Mol Med Rep. 2013;7(4):1081–5. https://doi.org/10.3892/mmr.2013.1320. PubMed PMID: 23417076.
21. Foley S, Garsed K, Singh G, Duroudier NP, Swan C, Hall IP, et al. Impaired uptake of serotonin by platelets from patients with irritable bowel syndrome correlates with duodenal immune activation. Gastroenterology. 2011;140(5):1434–43. https://doi.org/10.1053/j.gastro.2011.01.052. PubMed PMID: 21315720.

22. Forshammar J, Isaksson S, Strid H, Stotzer PO, Sjovall H, Simren M, et al. A pilot study of colonic B cell pattern in irritable bowel syndrome. Scand J Gastroenterol. 2008;43(12):1461–6. https://doi.org/10.1080/00365520802272126. PubMed PMID: 18663666.
23. Goral V, Kucukoner M, Buyukbayram H. Mast cells count and serum cytokine levels in patients with irritable bowel syndrome. Hepato-Gastroenterology. 2010;57(101):751–4. PubMed PMID: 21033222.
24. Guilarte M, Santos J, de Torres I, Alonso C, Vicario M, Ramos L, et al. Diarrhoea-predominant IBS patients show mast cell activation and hyperplasia in the jejunum. Gut. 2007;56(2):203–9. https://doi.org/10.1136/gut.2006.100594. PubMed PMID: 17005763; PubMed Central PMCID: PMCPMC1856785.
25. Hughes PA, Zola H, Penttila IA, Blackshaw LA, Andrews JM, Krumbiegel D. Immune activation in irritable bowel syndrome: can neuroimmune interactions explain symptoms? Am J Gastroenterol. 2013;108(7):1066–74. https://doi.org/10.1038/ajg.2013.120. PubMed PMID: 23649183.
26. Ishimoto H, Oshima T, Sei H, Yamasaki T, Kondo T, Tozawa K, et al. Claudin-2 expression is upregulated in the ileum of diarrhea predominant irritable bowel syndrome patients. J Clin Biochem Nutr. 2017;60(2):146–50. https://doi.org/10.3164/jcbn.16-92. PubMed PMID: 28366996; PubMed Central PMCID: PMCPMC5370533.
27. Klooker TK, Braak B, Koopman KE, Welting O, Wouters MM, van der Heide S, et al. The mast cell stabiliser ketotifen decreases visceral hypersensitivity and improves intestinal symptoms in patients with irritable bowel syndrome. Gut. 2010;59(9):1213–21. https://doi.org/10.1136/gut.2010.213108. PubMed PMID: 20650926.
28. Lazaridis N, Germanidis G. Current insights into the innate immune system dysfunction in irritable bowel syndrome. Ann Gastroenterol. 2018;31(2):171–87. https://doi.org/10.20524/aog.2018.0229. PubMed PMID: 29507464; PubMed Central PMCID: PMCPMC5825947.
29. Lee KJ, Kim YB, Kim JH, Kwon HC, Kim DK, Cho SW. The alteration of enterochromaffin cell, mast cell, and lamina propria T lymphocyte numbers in irritable bowel syndrome and its relationship with psychological factors. J Gastroenterol Hepatol. 2008;23(11):1689–94. https://doi.org/10.1111/j.1440-1746.2008.05574.x. PubMed PMID: 19120860.
30. Martinez C, Lobo B, Pigrau M, Ramos L, Gonzalez-Castro AM, Alonso C, et al. Diarrhoea-predominant irritable bowel syndrome: an organic disorder with structural abnormalities in the jejunal epithelial barrier. Gut. 2013;62(8):1160–8. https://doi.org/10.1136/gutjnl-2012-302093. PubMed PMID: 22637702.
31. Martinez C, Vicario M, Ramos L, Lobo B, Mosquera JL, Alonso C, et al. The jejunum of diarrhea-predominant irritable bowel syndrome shows molecular alterations in the tight junction signaling pathway that are associated with mucosal pathobiology and clinical manifestations. Am J Gastroenterol. 2012;107(5):736–46. https://doi.org/10.1038/ajg.2011.472. PubMed PMID: 22415197.
32. O'Sullivan M, Clayton N, Breslin NP, Harman I, Bountra C, McLaren A, et al. Increased mast cells in the irritable bowel syndrome. Neurogastroenterol Motil. 2000;12(5):449–57. https://doi.org/10.1046/j.1365-2982.2000.00221.x. PubMed PMID: 11012945.
33. Park JH, Rhee PL, Kim G, Lee JH, Kim YH, Kim JJ, et al. Enteroendocrine cell counts correlate with visceral hypersensitivity in patients with diarrhoea-predominant irritable bowel syndrome. Neurogastroenterol Motil. 2006;18(7):539–46. https://doi.org/10.1111/j.1365-2982.2006.00771.x. PubMed PMID: 16771769.
34. Park JH, Rhee PL, Kim HS, Lee JH, Kim YH, Kim JJ, et al. Mucosal mast cell counts correlate with visceral hypersensitivity in patients with diarrhea predominant irritable bowel syndrome. J Gastroenterol Hepatol. 2006;21(1):71–8. https://doi.org/10.1111/j.1440-1746.2005.04143.x. PubMed PMID: 16706815.
35. Piche T, Saint-Paul MC, Dainese R, Marine-Barjoan E, Iannelli A, Montoya ML, et al. Mast cells and cellularity of the colonic mucosa correlated with fatigue and depression in irritable bowel syndrome. Gut. 2008;57(4):468–73. https://doi.org/10.1136/gut.2007.127068. PubMed PMID: 18194987.

36. Sohn W, Lee OY, Lee SP, Lee KN, Jun DW, Lee HL, et al. Mast cell number, substance P and vasoactive intestinal peptide in irritable bowel syndrome with diarrhea. Scand J Gastroenterol. 2014;49(1):43–51. https://doi.org/10.3109/00365521.2013.857712. PubMed PMID: 24256141.
37. Spiller RC, Jenkins D, Thornley JP, Hebden JM, Wright T, Skinner M, et al. Increased rectal mucosal enteroendocrine cells, T lymphocytes, and increased gut permeability following acute Campylobacter enteritis and in post-dysenteric irritable bowel syndrome. Gut. 2000;47(6):804–11. https://doi.org/10.1136/gut.47.6.804. PubMed PMID: 11076879; PubMed Central PMCID: PMCPMC1728147.
38. Vicario M, Gonzalez-Castro AM, Martinez C, Lobo B, Pigrau M, Guilarte M, et al. Increased humoral immunity in the jejunum of diarrhoea-predominant irritable bowel syndrome associated with clinical manifestations. Gut. 2015;64(9):1379–88. https://doi.org/10.1136/gutjnl-2013-306236. PubMed PMID: 25209656.
39. Vivinus-Nebot M, Dainese R, Anty R, Saint-Paul MC, Nano JL, Gonthier N, et al. Combination of allergic factors can worsen diarrheic irritable bowel syndrome: role of barrier defects and mast cells. Am J Gastroenterol. 2012;107(1):75–81. https://doi.org/10.1038/ajg.2011.315.
40. Walker MM, Talley NJ, Prabhakar M, Pennaneac'h CJ, Aro P, Ronkainen J, et al. Duodenal mastocytosis, eosinophilia and intraepithelial lymphocytosis as possible disease markers in the irritable bowel syndrome and functional dyspepsia. Aliment Pharmacol Ther. 2009;29(7):765–73. https://doi.org/10.1111/j.1365-2036.2009.03937.x. PubMed PMID: 19183150; PubMed Central PMCID: PMCPMC4070654.
41. Wang LH, Fang XC, Pan GZ. Bacillary dysentery as a causative factor of irritable bowel syndrome and its pathogenesis. Gut. 2004;53(8):1096–101. https://doi.org/10.1136/gut.2003.021154. PubMed PMID: 15247174; PubMed Central PMCID: PMCPMC1774156.
42. Wang SH, Dong L, Luo JY, Gong J, Li L, Lu XL, et al. Decreased expression of serotonin in the jejunum and increased numbers of mast cells in the terminal ileum in patients with irritable bowel syndrome. World J Gastroenterol. 2007;13(45):6041–7. https://doi.org/10.3748/wjg.v13.45.6041. PubMed PMID: 18023097; PubMed Central PMCID: PMCPMC4250888.
43. Weston AP, Biddle WL, Bhatia PS, Miner PB Jr. Terminal ileal mucosal mast cells in irritable bowel syndrome. Dig Dis Sci. 1993;38(9):1590–5. https://doi.org/10.1007/bf01303164.
44. Willot S, Gauthier C, Patey N, Faure C. Nerve growth factor content is increased in the rectal mucosa of children with diarrhea-predominant irritable bowel syndrome. Neurogastroenterol Motil. 2012;24(8):734–9. https://doi.org/10.1111/j.1365-2982.2012.01933.x.
45. Tornblom H, Lindberg G, Nyberg B, Veress B. Full-thickness biopsy of the jejunum reveals inflammation and enteric neuropathy in irritable bowel syndrome. Gastroenterology. 2002;123(6):1972–9. https://doi.org/10.1053/gast.2002.37059.
46. Sundin J, Rangel I, Kumawat AK, Hultgren-Hornquist E, Brummer RJ. Aberrant mucosal lymphocyte number and subsets in the colon of post-infectious irritable bowel syndrome patients. Scand J Gastroenterol. 2014;49(9):1068–75. https://doi.org/10.3109/00365521.2014.926982.
47. Burns G, Carroll G, Mathe A, Horvat J, Foster P, Walker MM, et al. Evidence for local and systemic immune activation in functional dyspepsia and the irritable bowel syndrome: a systematic review. Am J Gastroenterol. 2019;114(3):429–36. https://doi.org/10.1038/s41395-018-0377-0.
48. Plaisancie P, Barcelo A, Moro F, Claustre J, Chayvialle JA, Cuber JC. Effects of neurotransmitters, gut hormones, and inflammatory mediators on mucus discharge in rat colon. Am J Phys. 1998;275(5):1073–84. https://doi.org/10.1152/ajpgi.1998.275.5.G1073.
49. Kuwahara A, Kuramoto H, Kadowaki M. 5-HT activates nitric oxide-generating neurons to stimulate chloride secretion in guinea pig distal colon. Am J Phys. 1998;275(4):829–34. https://doi.org/10.1152/ajpgi.1998.275.4.G829.
50. Frieling T, Rupprecht C, Kroese AB, Schemann M. Effects of the inflammatory mediator prostaglandin D2 on submucosal neurons and secretion in guinea pig colon. Am J Phys. 1994;266(1):132–9. https://doi.org/10.1152/ajpgi.1994.266.1.G132.

51. Ronkainen J, Aro P, Walker MM, Agreus L, Johansson SE, Jones M, et al. Duodenal eosinophilia is associated with functional dyspepsia and new onset gastro-oesophageal reflux disease. Aliment Pharmacol Ther. 2019;50(1):24–32. https://doi.org/10.1111/apt.15308.
52. Dahlin JS, Hallgren J. Mast cell progenitors: origin, development and migration to tissues. Mol Immunol. 2015;63(1):9–17. https://doi.org/10.1016/j.molimm.2014.01.018.
53. Albert-Bayo M, Paracuellos I, Gonzalez-Castro AM, Rodriguez-Urrutia A, Rodriguez-Lagunas MJ, Alonso-Cotoner C, et al. Intestinal mucosal mast cells: key modulators of barrier function and homeostasis. Cells. 2019;8(2):135. https://doi.org/10.3390/cells8020135. PubMed PMID: 30744042; PubMed Central PMCID: PMCPMC6407111.
54. Buhner S, Schemann M. Mast cell-nerve axis with a focus on the human gut. Biochim Biophys Acta. 2012;1822(1):85–92. https://doi.org/10.1016/j.bbadis.2011.06.004.
55. Akashi K, Traver D, Miyamoto T, Weissman IL. A clonogenic common myeloid progenitor that gives rise to all myeloid lineages. Nature. 2000;404(6774):193–7. https://doi.org/10.1038/35004599.
56. Abraham SN, St John AL. Mast cell-orchestrated immunity to pathogens. Nat Rev Immunol. 2010;10(6):440–52. https://doi.org/10.1038/nri2782. PubMed PMID: 20498670; PubMed Central PMCID: PMCPMC4469150.
57. Abonia JP, Austen KF, Rollins BJ, Joshi SK, Flavell RA, Kuziel WA, et al. Constitutive homing of mast cell progenitors to the intestine depends on autologous expression of the chemokine receptor CXCR2. Blood. 2005;105(11):4308–13. https://doi.org/10.1182/blood-2004-09-3578. PubMed PMID: 15705791; PubMed Central PMCID: PMCPMC1895025.
58. Elieh Ali Komi D, Grauwet K. Role of mast cells in regulation of T cell responses in experimental and clinical settings. Clin Rev Allergy Immunol. 2018;54(3):432–45. https://doi.org/10.1007/s12016-017-8646-z.
59. Zhang L, Song J, Hou X. Mast cells and irritable bowel syndrome: from the bench to the bedside. J Neurogastroenterol Motil. 2016;22(2):181–92. https://doi.org/10.5056/jnm15137. PubMed PMID: 26755686; PubMed Central PMCID: PMCPMC4819856.
60. Bischoff SC, Kramer S. Human mast cells, bacteria, and intestinal immunity. Immunol Rev. 2007;217:329–37. https://doi.org/10.1111/j.1600-065X.2007.00523.x.
61. Santos J, Alonso C, Guilarte M, Vicario M, Malagelada JR. Targeting mast cells in the treatment of functional gastrointestinal disorders. Curr Opin Pharmacol. 2006;6(6):541–6. https://doi.org/10.1016/j.coph.2006.08.001.
62. Santos J, Guilarte M, Alonso C, Malagelada JR. Pathogenesis of irritable bowel syndrome: the mast cell connection. Scand J Gastroenterol. 2005;40(2):129–40. https://doi.org/10.1080/00365520410009410.
63. Barbara G, Cremon C, Carini G, Bellacosa L, Zecchi L, De Giorgio R, et al. The immune system in irritable bowel syndrome. J Neurogastroenterol Motil. 2011;17(4):349–59. https://doi.org/10.5056/jnm.2011.17.4.349. PubMed PMID: 22148103; PubMed Central PMCID: PMCPMC3228974.
64. Koloski N, Jones M, Walker MM, Veysey M, Zala A, Keely S, et al. Population based study: atopy and autoimmune diseases are associated with functional dyspepsia and irritable bowel syndrome, independent of psychological distress. Aliment Pharmacol Ther. 2019;49(5):546–55. https://doi.org/10.1111/apt.15120.
65. Addolorato G, Marsigli L, Capristo E, Caputo F, Dall'Aglio C, Baudanza P. Anxiety and depression: a common feature of health care seeking patients with irritable bowel syndrome and food allergy. Hepato-Gastroenterology. 1998;45(23):1559–64.
66. Rumessen JJ, Gudmand-Hoyer E. Functional bowel disease: malabsorption and abdominal distress after ingestion of fructose, sorbitol, and fructose-sorbitol mixtures. Gastroenterology. 1988;95(3):694–700. https://doi.org/10.1016/s0016-5085(88)80016-7.
67. Simren M, Mansson A, Langkilde AM, Svedlund J, Abrahamsson H, Bengtsson U, et al. Food-related gastrointestinal symptoms in the irritable bowel syndrome. Digestion. 2001;63(2):108–15. https://doi.org/10.1159/000051878.

68. Fukudo S, Nomura T, Hongo M. Impact of corticotropin-releasing hormone on gastrointestinal motility and adrenocorticotropic hormone in normal controls and patients with irritable bowel syndrome. Gut. 1998;42(6):845–9. https://doi.org/10.1136/gut.42.6.845. PubMed PMID: 9691924; PubMed Central PMCID: PMCPMC1727153.
69. Sagami Y, Shimada Y, Tayama J, Nomura T, Satake M, Endo Y, et al. Effect of a corticotropin releasing hormone receptor antagonist on colonic sensory and motor function in patients with irritable bowel syndrome. Gut. 2004;53(7):958–64. https://doi.org/10.1136/gut.2003.018911. PubMed PMID: 15194643; PubMed Central PMCID: PMCPMC1774093.
70. Wallon C, Yang PC, Keita AV, Ericson AC, McKay DM, Sherman PM, et al. Corticotropin-releasing hormone (CRH) regulates macromolecular permeability via mast cells in normal human colonic biopsies in vitro. Gut. 2008;57(1):50–8. https://doi.org/10.1136/gut.2006.117549.
71. Vanuytsel T, van Wanrooy S, Vanheel H, Vanormelingen C, Verschueren S, Houben E, et al. Psychological stress and corticotropin-releasing hormone increase intestinal permeability in humans by a mast cell-dependent mechanism. Gut. 2014;63(8):1293–9. https://doi.org/10.1136/gutjnl-2013-305690.
72. Castagliuolo I, Wershil BK, Karalis K, Pasha A, Nikulasson ST, Pothoulakis C. Colonic mucin release in response to immobilization stress is mast cell dependent. Am J Phys. 1998;274(6):1094–100. https://doi.org/10.1152/ajpgi.1998.274.6.G1094.
73. Saunders PR, Maillot C, Million M, Tache Y. Peripheral corticotropin-releasing factor induces diarrhea in rats: role of CRF1 receptor in fecal watery excretion. Eur J Pharmacol. 2002;435(2-3):231–5. https://doi.org/10.1016/s0014-2999(01)01574-6.
74. Kaisho T, Akira S. Critical roles of toll-like receptors in host defense. Crit Rev Immunol. 2000;20(5):393–405.
75. Brint EK, MacSharry J, Fanning A, Shanahan F, Quigley EM. Differential expression of toll-like receptors in patients with irritable bowel syndrome. Am J Gastroenterol. 2011;106(2):329–36. https://doi.org/10.1038/ajg.2010.438.
76. Sandig H, Bulfone-Paus S. TLR signaling in mast cells: common and unique features. Front Immunol. 2012;3:185. https://doi.org/10.3389/fimmu.2012.00185. PubMed PMID: 22783258; PubMed Central PMCID: PMCPMC3389341.
77. Tanji H, Ohto U, Shibata T, Taoka M, Yamauchi Y, Isobe T, et al. Toll-like receptor 8 senses degradation products of single-stranded RNA. Nat Struct Mol Biol. 2015;22(2):109–15. https://doi.org/10.1038/nsmb.2943.
78. Zhang Z, Ohto U, Shibata T, Krayukhina E, Taoka M, Yamauchi Y, et al. Structural analysis reveals that toll-like receptor 7 Is a dual receptor for guanosine and single-stranded RNA. Immunity. 2016;45(4):737–48. https://doi.org/10.1016/j.immuni.2016.09.011.
79. Tana C, Umesaki Y, Imaoka A, Handa T, Kanazawa M, Fukudo S. Altered profiles of intestinal microbiota and organic acids may be the origin of symptoms in irritable bowel syndrome. Neurogastroenterol Motil. 2010;22(5):512–9. https://doi.org/10.1111/j.1365-2982.2009.01427.x.
80. Sundin J, Rangel I, Fuentes S, Heikamp-de Jong I, Hultgren-Hornquist E, de Vos WM, et al. Altered faecal and mucosal microbial composition in post-infectious irritable bowel syndrome patients correlates with mucosal lymphocyte phenotypes and psychological distress. Aliment Pharmacol Ther. 2015;41(4):342–51. https://doi.org/10.1111/apt.13055.
81. Spiller R, Garsed K. Postinfectious irritable bowel syndrome. Gastroenterology. 2009;136(6):1979–88. https://doi.org/10.1053/j.gastro.2009.02.074.
82. Kawamata Y, Fujii R, Hosoya M, Harada M, Yoshida H, Miwa M, et al. A G protein-coupled receptor responsive to bile acids. J Biol Chem. 2003;278(11):9435–40. https://doi.org/10.1074/jbc.M209706200.
83. Bueno L, Fioramonti J. Visceral perception: inflammatory and non-inflammatory mediators. Gut. 2002;51(1):19–23. https://doi.org/10.1136/gut.51.suppl_1.i19. PubMed PMID: 12077058; PubMed Central PMCID: PMCPMC1867723.

84. Caldarella MP, Milano A, Laterza F, Sacco F, Balatsinou C, Lapenna D, et al. Visceral sensitivity and symptoms in patients with constipation- or diarrhea-predominant irritable bowel syndrome (IBS): effect of a low-fat intraduodenal infusion. Am J Gastroenterol. 2005;100(2):383–9. https://doi.org/10.1111/j.1572-0241.2005.40100.x.
85. Suzuki H, Watanabe S, Hamaguchi T, Mine H, Terui T, Kanazawa M, et al. Brain activation associated with changes in heart rate, heart rate variability, and plasma catecholamines during rectal distention. Psychosom Med. 2009;71(6):619–26. https://doi.org/10.1097/PSY.0b013e31819b69ca.
86. Aerssens J, Hillsley K, Peeters PJ, de Hoogt R, Stanisz A, Lin JH, et al. Alterations in the brain-gut axis underlying visceral chemosensitivity in Nippostrongylus brasiliensis-infected mice. Gastroenterology. 2007;132(4):1375–87. https://doi.org/10.1053/j.gastro.2007.02.019.
87. Caterina MJ, Schumacher MA, Tominaga M, Rosen TA, Levine JD, Julius D. The capsaicin receptor: a heat-activated ion channel in the pain pathway. Nature. 1997;389(6653):816–24. https://doi.org/10.1038/39807.
88. Zhou Q, Yang L, Larson S, Basra S, Merwat S, Tan A, et al. Decreased miR-199 augments visceral pain in patients with IBS through translational upregulation of TRPV1. Gut. 2016;65(5):797–805. https://doi.org/10.1136/gutjnl-2013-306464. PubMed PMID: 25681400; PubMed Central PMCID: PMCPMC4853572.
89. Sugiuar T, Bielefeldt K, Gebhart GF. TRPV1 function in mouse colon sensory neurons is enhanced by metabotropic 5-hydroxytryptamine receptor activation. J Neurosci. 2004;24(43):9521–30. https://doi.org/10.1523/JNEUROSCI.2639-04.2004. PubMed PMID: 15509739; PubMed Central PMCID: PMCPMC6730150.
90. Rijnierse A, Nijkamp FP, Kraneveld AD. Mast cells and nerves tickle in the tummy: implications for inflammatory bowel disease and irritable bowel syndrome. Pharmacol Ther. 2007;116(2):207–35. https://doi.org/10.1016/j.pharmthera.2007.06.008.
91. Zhou Q, Zhang B, Verne GN. Intestinal membrane permeability and hypersensitivity in the irritable bowel syndrome. Pain. 2009;146(1-2):41–6. https://doi.org/10.1016/j.pain.2009.06.017. PubMed PMID: 19595511; PubMed Central PMCID: PMCPMC2763174.
92. Piche T. Tight junctions and IBS--the link between epithelial permeability, low-grade inflammation, and symptom generation? Neurogastroenterol Motil 2014; 26(3): 296-302. doi: https://doi.org/10.1111/nmo.12315.
93. Gebhart GF. Visceral pain-peripheral sensitisation. Gut. 2000;47(4):54–5. https://doi.org/10.1136/gut.47.suppl_4.iv54. PubMed PMID: 11076915; PubMed Central PMCID: PMCPMC1766818.
94. Mayer EA, Raybould HE. Role of visceral afferent mechanisms in functional bowel disorders. Gastroenterology. 1990;99(6):1688–704. https://doi.org/10.1016/0016-5085(90)90475-g.
95. Drossman DA, Ringel Y, Vogt BA, Leserman J, Lin W, Smith JK, et al. Alterations of brain activity associated with resolution of emotional distress and pain in a case of severe irritable bowel syndrome. Gastroenterology. 2003;124(3):754–61. https://doi.org/10.1053/gast.2003.50103.
96. Tillisch K, Mayer EA, Labus JS. Quantitative meta-analysis identifies brain regions activated during rectal distension in irritable bowel syndrome. Gastroenterology. 2011;140(1):91–100. https://doi.org/10.1053/j.gastro.2010.07.053. PubMed PMID: 20696168; PubMed Central PMCID: PMCPMC3253553.

Chapter 7
Genetic Factors

Ryo Katsumata and Akiko Shiotani

Abstract Irritable bowel syndrome (IBS) contains heterogeneous pathophysiology, and each factor of various pathophysiological factors might be partly connected with genetic status. A large number of studies investigating genetic factors have ranged from analysis of family history to molecular-based genetic analysis. The genetic factors are mainly described as single nucleotide polymorphisms (SNPs) and recently evaluated by new technic like genome-wide association studies (GWAS) and epigenetic analysis. In this captor, we summarized the candidate genes affecting IBS and the influence of genetic factors on therapeutic efficacy.

Keywords Serotonin · Tryptophan hydroxylase · Corticotropin-releasing hormone · Genome-wide association studies (GWAS)

The role of host genetics in irritable bowel syndrome (IBS) has been highlighted by epidemiological studies. The prevalence of patients with IBS is reported to be regionally different; the rate reaches 5.8% in African population, 9.6% in Asian, 8.1% in European, and 17.5% in South American [1]. In addition to food customs and social factors, genetic factors may play an important role in this difference, and there is genetic heterogeneity among races detected on a molecular basis. Moreover, familial aggregation and high prevalence of IBS in monozygotic twins compared with dizygotic twins strongly support genetic contribution to IBS onset [2–4]. In a large nationwide Swedish cohort study, a higher odds ratio of IBS was found in first-, second-, and third-degree relatives of IBS patients. It suggested that genes or shared environmental exposures contribute to the development of IBS [5]. The relationships between genetic factors and onset risks of IBS have been ascertained by accumulating molecular analysis.

R. Katsumata · A. Shiotani (✉)
Department of Gastroenterology and Hepatology, Kawasaki Medical School, Kurashiki City, Okayama Prefecture, Japan
e-mail: katsumata@med.kawasaki-m.ac.jp; shiotani@med.kawasaki-m.ac.jp

© The Editor(s) (if applicable) and The Author(s), under exclusive license to Springer Nature Singapore Pte Ltd. 2024

T. Kamiya, S. Fukudo (eds.), *Irritable Bowel Syndrome*,
https://doi.org/10.1007/978-981-97-8410-3_7

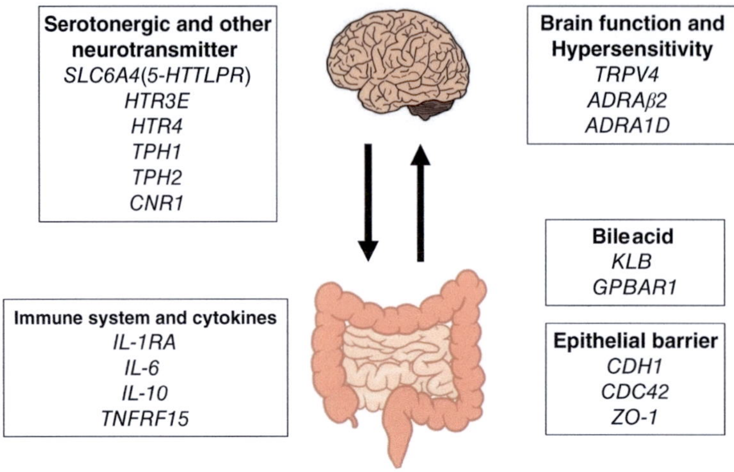

Fig. 7.1 Overview of IBS-related genes

7.1 Candidate Genes Affecting IBS

The polymorphism alterations of genes such as serotonergic, other neurotransmitter pathway, and cytokine-related proteins were confirmed to be associated with IBS onset. The other gene alterations were also considered in other various fields containing brain function, hypersensitivity, epithelial barrier functions, bile acid signaling genes, etc. [6, 7]. The overview of IBS-related genes is summarized in Fig. 7.1 [8]. However, the susceptible genetic factors are unlikely to be certain definite risk, and many other environmental factors also strongly contribute to pathophysiology of IBS.

7.1.1 Serotonin and Other Mediators

Polymorphism of serotonin (5-HT) transporter (5-HTT) gene: solute carrier family 6 member 4 (*SLC6A4*) also known as *5-HTTLPR* (serotonin-transporter-linked polymorphic region) with a short (S) variation of 14 repeats and a long (L) variation of 16 repeats has been proven to influence the activity of SERT. *5-HTTLPR* polymorphism was reported to be associated with IBS subtypes, which are classified based on stool habit [9]. *5-HTTLPR S/S* genotype as compared to other genotypes *L/L* and *S/L* has less 5-HT uptake resulting in higher blood levels of 5-HT and was expected to be associated with diarrhea dominant IBS (IBS-D). In contrast, *LL* genotype is expected to be a risk factor for constipation-predominant IBS (IBS-C) [10]. In a systematic review and meta-analysis, there was a positive association between *5-HTTLPR* polymorphism and IBS onset risk only in the East Asian population and not in the Caucasian [10]. Additionally, the impact of genetic factors can differ between genders. For example, men with IBS-D have been observed to have a reduced frequency of the *5-HTTLPR S/S* genotype compared to healthy men [11].

Tryptophan hydroxylase (TPH) is the rate-limiting enzyme in the synthesis of serotonin. The *TPH* promoter variant (11:g.18047335T>C, rs4537731), intron 3 variant (11:g.18033757T>G, rs211105), and intron 7 (11:g.18026269G>T, rs1800532) have been extensively studied with respect to psychiatric disorders such as borderline personality disorder [12, 13]. With respect to IBS, Jun S et al. [14] previously reported possible associations between two *TPH1* gene single-nucleotide polymorphisms (SNPs), rs4537731 and rs211105, and daily reporting of gastrointestinal (GI) symptoms including diarrhea, bloating, and loose stools. Similarly, IBS-D patients with *TPH* rs211105 T/T genotype showed severe diarrhea and lower score of QOL simultaneously [15].

A hypothalamic hormone, corticotropin-releasing hormone (CRH), mediates its effects through two receptors—CRH-R1 and CRH-R2—and CRH plays a crucial role in many stress-related disorders including IBS. The two SNPs of *CRH-R1* rs7209436 and rs242924 were reported to be significantly associated with IBS symptoms [16]. Furthermore, alpha adrenergic-1D (*ADRA1D*) plays an important role in sensory-afferent processing, and *ADRA1D* SNP rs1556832 was connected with severe GI symptom including abdominal pain and bloating and IBS symptom severity score [17, 18].

7.1.2 Immune System and Cytokines

Enhanced immune activation in intestinal mucosa and systemic micro-inflammation are considerable role in some patients with IBS [19, 20]. In a systematic review from 28 studies, TNF receptor superfamily member 15 (*TNFRF15*) rs4263839 and rs6478108 increased the risk of IBS onset. The prevalence of *IL23R* rs11465804 G allele was significantly higher in patients with IBS-C [21]. IL10 is known to be an anti-inflammatory cytokine, and a recent review indicated that *IL10* rs1800896 was associated with decreased IBS onset risk [22]. Interestingly, high-producer *IL10* SNPs decreased the risk of IBS in Caucasians (1082 G/A, rs1800870) and in Asians (819C/T rs1800872) [23].

Several factors such as female sex, psychical status, and specific bacterial type turned out to be risk factors of postinfectious IBS (PI-IBS). *TNF-α* (−308 G/A, rs1800629) genotypes associated with IBS in Asian [20], was confirmed to be associated with PI-IBS. In addition, *IL6* rs1800795 G allele significantly increased IBS risk in Caucasian subgroups and PI-IBS risk [23]. The alteration of immune status modulated by cytokines plays a key role in the pathophysiology of IBS.

7.1.3 Intestinal Barrier Function

Increased intestinal permeability is related with a visceral hypersensitivity that causes GI symptoms including abdominal pain and bloating, which are typical symptoms of IBS [24]. Gene polymorphisms involved in epithelial barrier function including cadherin 1 (*CDH1*) and cell division cycle 42 (*CDC42*) have been found to be associated with IBS onset [7]. In addition, *CDH1* (rs16260, -C160A) and Toll-like receptor 9 (*TLR9*) (rs352139, P545P) were also reported to be genetic risk factors of PI-IBS [25, 26].

Zonula occluden 1 (ZO-1) protein is one of the important tight junction proteins and the mRNA expression decrease in patients with IBS [27]. The ZO-1 protein expression in the colonic mucosa was reduced in HLA-DQ2/8-positive IBS patients compared with the negative patients [28].

7.1.4 Bile Acid Signaling Genes

Bile acids stimulate water and electrolyte secretion on intestinal mucosa and influence bowel habit by accelerating colonic transit [29]. The malabsorption of bile acid through an intestinal mucosa and following an increased level of total fecal bile acid were reported in a subset of patients with IBS [30]. Interestingly, several genes involved in bile acid metabolism and bile acid receptor gene have been reported to associate with clinical symptoms of IBS-D. Klotho-beta (KLB) is involved in a regulation of bile acid synthesis, and the membrane-bound bile acid receptor (TGR5), also known as the G protein-coupled bile acid receptor 1 (GpBAR1), is activated by primary and secondary bile acid associated with several metabolic functions including the control of lipids titers and obesity. Both KLB and TGR5 variants are connected with shorter colonic transit time among patients with IBS-D [31].

7.2 Genome-Wide Association Studies

A locus at 7p22. 1 and 9p31.2, which includes the genes *KDELR2* (KDEL endoplasmic reticulum protein retention receptor 2) and *GRID2IP* (glutamate receptor, ionotropic, delta 2 (Grid2) interacting protein), was newly reported to be associated with IBS risk in genome-wide association studies (GWAS) evaluation [32]. Over expression of *KDELR2* in IBS mucosa supported the speculation that *KDELR2* is affecting IBS predisposition through mediating the effects of bacterial toxins in the gut. In a GWAS meta-analysis of IBS, SNPs related with the regulation of ion channel activity such as SCN5A and sucrase-isomaltase (SI) were considered as one of the most plausible candidate of gene variation affecting IBS [33]. However, it is difficult to explain the function of these risk genes in the IBS pathogenesis.

7.3 Epigenetics and Micro-RNAs

Stress and other environmental factors such as food, microbiota, and following immune reaction including inflammation can trigger epigenetic changes such as DNA methylation and histone modification [34]. Mahurkar et al. [35] revealed that patients with IBS presented differential methylation status compared to healthy controls, and epigenetic modifications in novel targets such as subcommissural organ-spondin (*SSPO*) and glutathione-S-transferases mu 5 (*GSTM5*) were associated with IBS.

The level of circulating miR-150 and miR-342-3p in the blood of patients with IBS was reported to be elevated [36], and the level of miR-29a expression in the small bowel and colon tissues is correlated with the mucosal permeability in IBS [37]. A variation c.*76G>A(rs62625044) in the 3′ untranslated region (UTR) of *HTR3E* is dominantly found in patients with IBS than controls, and the variation is located in the miRNA-510 target site [38]. A variant c.*61T>C(rs201253747) within *HTR4* is predominantly present in patients with IBS-D, and the polymorphism is connected with a binding site of the miR-16 and miR-103/107 [39].

7.4 Treatment Efficacy

In the first study investigating specific SNPs for predicting the effect of 5-HT3R antagonists, *5-HTTLPR* was associated with colonic transit response to alosetron in IBS-D patients, and the *L/L* genotype demonstrates greater response. In contrast, with regard to 5-HT 3 agonist, tegaserod, IBS-C patients carrying *5-HTTLPR L/L* genotype, showed less efficiency compared to subjects with *S/S* and *L/S* genotype [40]. Among Japanese patients with IBS-D, the prevalence of *TPH1* rs4537731 and *TPH1* rs211105 genotype were significantly different between responders and non-responders of ramosetron [41]. In a recent study investigating responsiveness to ondansetron, rs6766410 of the *HTR3C* gene is associated with stool consistency responders [42]. Cannabinoid receptor type 1 (*CNR1*) AAT triplet genotype with more than ten repeats was associated with IBS risk in Korean, but the results were not consistent. However, *CNR1* rs806378 (CC vs CT/TT) and fatty acid amide hydrolase (*FAAH*) rs324420 are correlated with treatment effectiveness of nonselective cannabinoid receptor agonist, dronabinol, in IBS patients [43].

Food manipulation is also one of the therapy options of IBS, and several studies showed relationship between therapeutic efficacy and genetic factors. In IBS-D patients, clinical responses of gluten-free diet were reported to differ according to HLA-DQ2 genotype [44]. Recently, low fermentable oligosaccharides, disaccharides, monosaccharides, and polyols (FODMAP) diet as a treatment for patients with IBS is of current interest. The responses of low-FODMAP diet were different depending on gene variants of intestinal sucrase-isomaltase (*SI*) [45].

7.5 Conclusions

Besides several genetic markers seem to be related to modest increase in IBS onset risk, genetic status is widely connected to pathophysiologic factors of IBS. Accumulative data regarding genetic factors in IBS have provided a better understanding of IBS. Prevention or treatment based on individual genetic data might lead to optimal choices in a foreseeable future.

References

1. Enck P, Aziz Q, Barbara G, Farmer AD, Fukudo S, Mayer EA, et al. Irritable bowel syndrome. Nat Rev Dis Primers. 2016;24(2):16014.
2. Saito YA, Petersen GM, Larson JJ, Atkinson EJ, Fridley BL, de Andrade M, et al. Familial aggregation of irritable bowel syndrome: a family case-control study. Am J Gastroenterol. 2010;105(4):833–41.
3. Bengtson MB, Ronning T, Vatn MH, Harris JR. Irritable bowel syndrome in twins: genes and environment. Gut. 2006;55(12):1754–9.
4. Levy RL, Jones KR, Whitehead WE, Feld SI, Talley NJ, Corey LA. Irritable bowel syndrome in twins: heredity and social learning both contribute to etiology. Gastroenterology. 2001;121(4):799–804.
5. Waehrens R, Ohlsson H, Sundquist J, Sundquist K, Zoller B. Risk of irritable bowel syndrome in first-degree, second-degree and third-degree relatives of affected individuals: a nationwide family study in Sweden. Gut. 2015;64(2):215–21.
6. Gazouli M, Wouters MM, Kapur-Pojskic L, Bengtson MB, Friedman E, Nikcevic G, et al. Lessons learned-resolving the enigma of genetic factors in IBS. Nat Rev Gastroenterol Hepatol. 2016;13(2):77–87.
7. Enck P, Aziz Q, Barbara G, Farmer AD, Fukudo S, Mayer EA, et al. Irritable bowel syndrome. Nat Rev Dis Primers. 2016;2:16014.
8. Sperber AD, Dumitrascu D, Fukudo S, Gerson C, Ghoshal UC, Gwee KA, et al. The global prevalence of IBS in adults remains elusive due to the heterogeneity of studies: a Rome Foundation working team literature review. Gut. 2017;66(6):1075–82.
9. Drossman DA. Functional gastrointestinal disorders: history, pathophysiology, clinical features and Rome IV. Gastroenterology. 2016;150:1262–79.
10. Zhang ZF, Duan ZJ, Wang LX, Yang D, Zhao G, Zhang L. The serotonin transporter gene polymorphism (5-HTTLPR) and irritable bowel syndrome: a meta-analysis of 25 studies. BMC Gastroenterol. 2014;14:23.
11. Niesler B, Kapeller J, Fell C, Atkinson W, Moller D, Fischer C, et al. 5-HTTLPR and STin2 polymorphisms in the serotonin transporter gene and irritable bowel syndrome: effect of bowel habit and sex. Eur J Gastroenterol Hepatol. 2010;22(7):856–61.
12. Andreou D, Saetre P, Werge T, Andreassen OA, Agartz I, Sedvall GC, et al. Tryptophan hydroxylase gene 1 (TPH1) variants associated with cerebrospinal fluid 5-hydroxyindole

acetic acid and homovanillic acid concentrations in healthy volunteers. Psychiatry Res. 2010;180(2-3):63–7.
13. Wilson ST, Stanley B, Brent DA, Oquendo MA, Huang YY, Haghighi F, et al. Interaction between tryptophan hydroxylase I polymorphisms and childhood abuse is associated with increased risk for borderline personality disorder in adulthood. Psychiatr Genet. 2012;22(1):15–24.
14. Jun S, Kohen R, Cain KC, Jarrett ME, Heitkemper MM. Associations of tryptophan hydroxylase gene polymorphisms with irritable bowel syndrome. Neurogastroenterol Motil. 2011;23(3):233–9. e116
15. Katsumata R, Shiotani A, Murao T, Ishii M, Fujita M, Matsumoto H, et al. The TPH1 rs211105 gene polymorphism affects abdominal symptoms and quality of life of diarrhea-predominant irritable bowel syndrome. J Clin Biochem Nutr. 2018;62(3):270–6.
16. Sato N, Suzuki N, Sasaki A, Aizawa E, Obayashi T, Kanazawa M, et al. Corticotropin-releasing hormone receptor 1 gene variants in irritable bowel syndrome. PLoS One. 2012;7(9):e42450.
17. Orand A, Naliboff B, Gadd M, Shih W, Ju T, Presson AP, et al. Corticotropin-releasing hormone receptor 1 (CRH-R1) polymorphisms are associated with irritable bowel syndrome and acoustic startle response. Psychoneuroendocrinology. 2016;73:133–41.
18. Orand A, Gupta A, Shih W, Presson AP, Hammer C, Niesler B, et al. Catecholaminergic gene polymorphisms are associated with GI symptoms and morphological brain changes in irritable bowel syndrome. PLoS One. 2015;10(8):e0135910.
19. Ohman L, Simren M. Pathogenesis of IBS: role of inflammation, immunity and neuroimmune interactions. Nat Rev Gastroenterol Hepatol. 2010;7(3):163–73.
20. Ford AC, Talley NJ. Mucosal inflammation as a potential etiological factor in irritable bowel syndrome: a systematic review. J Gastroenterol. 2011;46(4):421–31.
21. Zhu S, Wang B, Jia Q, Duan L. Candidate single nucleotide polymorphisms of irritable bowel syndrome: a systemic review and meta-analysis. BMC Gastroenterol. 2019;19(1):165.
22. Qin SY, Jiang HX, Lu DH, Zhou Y. Association of interleukin-10 polymorphisms with risk of irritable bowel syndrome: a meta-analysis. World J Gastroenterol. 2013;19(48):9472–80.
23. Bashashati M, Rezaei N, Bashashati H, Shafieyoun A, Daryani NE, Sharkey KA, et al. Cytokine gene polymorphisms are associated with irritable bowel syndrome: a systematic review and meta-analysis. Neurogastroenterol Motil. 2012;24(12):1102–e566.
24. Zhou Q, Zhang B, Verne GN. Intestinal membrane permeability and hypersensitivity in the irritable bowel syndrome. Pain. 2009;146(1-2):41–6.
25. Villani AC, Lemire M, Thabane M, Belisle A, Geneau G, Garg AX, et al. Genetic risk factors for post-infectious irritable bowel syndrome following a waterborne outbreak of gastroenteritis. Gastroenterology. 2010;138(4):1502–13.
26. Spiller R, Lam C. An update on post-infectious irritable bowel syndrome: role of genetics, immune activation, serotonin and altered microbiome. J Neurogastroenterol Motil. 2012;18(3):258–68.
27. Piche T, Barbara G, Aubert P, Bruley des Varannes S, Dainese R, Nano JL, et al. Impaired intestinal barrier integrity in the colon of patients with irritable bowel syndrome: involvement of soluble mediators. Gut. 2009;58(2):196–201.
28. Vazquez-Roque MI, Camilleri M, Smyrk T, Murray JA, O'Neill J, Carlson P, et al. Association of HLA-DQ gene with bowel transit, barrier function, and inflammation in irritable bowel syndrome with diarrhea. Am J Physiol Gastrointest Liver Physiol. 2012;303(11):G1262-9.
29. Shin A, Camilleri M, Vijayvargiya P, Busciglio I, Burton D, Ryks M, et al. Bowel functions, fecal unconjugated primary and secondary bile acids, and colonic transit in patients with irritable bowel syndrome. Clin Gastroenterol Hepatol. 2013;11(10):1270–5.e1
30. Wedlake L, A'Hern R, Russell D, Thomas K, Walters JR, Andreyev HJ. Systematic review: the prevalence of idiopathic bile acid malabsorption as diagnosed by SeHCAT scanning in patients with diarrhoea-predominant irritable bowel syndrome. Aliment Pharmacol Ther. 2009;30(7):707–17.

31. Wong BS, Camilleri M, Carlson PJ, Guicciardi ME, Burton D, McKinzie S, et al. A Klothobeta variant mediates protein stability and associates with colon transit in irritable bowel syndrome with diarrhea. Gastroenterology. 2011;140(7):1934–42.
32. Ek WE, Reznichenko A, Ripke S, Niesler B, Zucchelli M, Rivera NV, et al. Exploring the genetics of irritable bowel syndrome: a GWA study in the general population and replication in multinational case-control cohorts. Gut. 2015;64(11):1774–82.
33. Bonfiglio F, Henstrom M, Nag A, Hadizadeh F, Zheng T, Cenit MC, et al. A GWAS meta-analysis from 5 population-based cohorts implicates ion channel genes in the pathogenesis of irritable bowel syndrome. Neurogastroenterol Motil. 2018;30(9):e13358.
34. Radley JJ, Kabbaj M, Jacobson L, Heydendael W, Yehuda R, Herman JP. Stress risk factors and stress-related pathology: neuroplasticity, epigenetics and endophenotypes. Stress. 2011;14(5):481–97.
35. Mahurkar S, Polytarchou C, Iliopoulos D, Pothoulakis C, Mayer EA, Chang L. Genome-wide DNA methylation profiling of peripheral blood mononuclear cells in irritable bowel syndrome. Neurogastroenterol Motil. 2016;28(3):410–22.
36. Fourie NH, Peace RM, Abey SK, Sherwin LB, Rahim-Williams B, Smyser PA, et al. Elevated circulating miR-150 and miR-342-3p in patients with irritable bowel syndrome. Exp Mol Pathol. 2014;96(3):422–5.
37. Zhou Q, Souba WW, Croce CM, Verne GN. MicroRNA-29a regulates intestinal membrane permeability in patients with irritable bowel syndrome. Gut. 2010;59(6):775–84.
38. Kapeller J, Houghton LA, Monnikes H, Walstab J, Moller D, Bonisch H, et al. First evidence for an association of a functional variant in the microRNA-510 target site of the serotonin receptor-type 3E gene with diarrhea predominant irritable bowel syndrome. Hum Mol Genet. 2008;17(19):2967–77.
39. Wohlfarth C, Schmitteckert S, Hartle JD, Houghton LA, Dweep H, Fortea M, et al. miR-16 and miR-103 impact 5-HT4 receptor signalling and correlate with symptom profile in irritable bowel syndrome. Sci Rep. 2017;7(1):14680.
40. Li Y, Nie Y, Xie J, Tang W, Liang P, Sha W, et al. The association of serotonin transporter genetic polymorphisms and irritable bowel syndrome and its influence on tegaserod treatment in Chinese patients. Dig Dis Sci. 2007;52(11):2942–9.
41. Shiotani A, Kusunoki H, Ishii M, Imamura H, Manabe N, Kamada T, et al. Pilot study of biomarkers for predicting effectiveness of ramosetron in diarrhea-predominant irritable bowel syndrome: expression of S100A10 and polymorphisms of TPH1. Neurogastroenterol Motil. 2015;27(1):82–91.
42. Gunn D, Garsed K, Lam C, Singh G, Lingaya M, Wahl V, et al. Abnormalities of mucosal serotonin metabolism and 5-HT3 receptor subunit 3C polymorphism in irritable bowel syndrome with diarrhoea predict responsiveness to ondansetron. Aliment Pharmacol Ther. 2019;50(5):538–46.
43. Wong BS, Camilleri M, Busciglio I, Carlson P, Szarka LA, Burton D, et al. Pharmacogenetic trial of a cannabinoid agonist shows reduced fasting colonic motility in patients with nonconstipated irritable bowel syndrome. Gastroenterology. 2011;141(5):1638–47.e1-7
44. Wahnschaffe U, Schulzke JD, Zeitz M, Ullrich R. Predictors of clinical response to gluten-free diet in patients diagnosed with diarrhea-predominant irritable bowel syndrome. Clin Gastroenterol Hepatol. 2007;5(7):844–50. quiz 769
45. Zheng T, Eswaran S, Photenhauer AL, Merchant JL, Chey WD, D'Amato M. Reduced efficacy of low FODMAPs diet in patients with IBS-D carrying sucrase-isomaltase (SI) hypomorphic variants. Gut. 2019;69(2):397–8.

Part III
Diagnosis

Chapter 8
Diagnostic Algorithm for IBS

Ryota Hokari and Nao Sugihara

Abstract Irritable bowel syndrome (IBS) have major economic effects on healthcare systems and adversely affect quality of life. However, usefulness of routine tests to identify IBS is very low. Thus, algorithms are useful to diagnose IBS patients efficiently. Diagnostic algorithms are used for patients with chronic abdominal pain or discomfort and/or abnormal bowel movement. Colonoscopy may be considered in patients with alarm symptoms. If all of them or colonoscopy is negative, Rome IV criteria is applied. Several noninvasive diagnostic markers are dissatisfied so far. Functional MRI will evolve promising diagnostic tools, although it is not suitable for daily practice. Psychological markers in combination with other biomarkers may help avoid unnecessary diagnostic testing in differentiating IBS from health.

Keywords Colonoscopy · Functional MRI · Psychological markers · Calprotectin · Fecal occult blood test · Tissue transglutaminase antibodies · Carbohydrate breath test · Serologic markers

8.1 Introduction

Irritable bowel syndrome (IBS) is a functional gastrointestinal (GI) disorder characterized by abdominal pain or discomfort and altered bowel habits [1]. Thus, IBS occurs in the absence of identifiable physical, radiologic, or laboratory indications of organic disease [2] A recent systematic review of IBS epidemiologic studies noted an IBS prevalence of 10–12% [3] IBS accounts for significant healthcare resource utilization and economic burden. The Rome Foundation has published diagnostic criteria for IBS [4]. However, diagnostic algorism for clinical practice is needed to support physicians and to reduce socioeconomic burden of IBS. Several clinical guidelines for IBS have been proposed, and the Japanese Society of

R. Hokari (✉) · N. Sugihara
National Defense Medical College, Tokorozawa, Saitama, Japan
e-mail: ryota@ndmc.ac.jp

© The Editor(s) (if applicable) and The Author(s), under exclusive license to Springer Nature Singapore Pte Ltd. 2024

T. Kamiya, S. Fukudo (eds.), *Irritable Bowel Syndrome*,
https://doi.org/10.1007/978-981-97-8410-3_8

Gastroenterology (JSGE) subsequently developed evidence-based clinical practice guidelines for IBS [5].

8.2 Clinical Presentation

Clinical feature of IBS is abdominal pain associated with changes in bowel habits [1]. Typically, no alarm features of organic disease, such as unintentional weight loss or rectal bleeding, are present. The clinical course of IBS is chronic although symptoms are extremely variable and fluctuate over time. The symptoms of IBS are heterogeneous, wax, and wane over time.

8.3 Alarm Symptoms of Organic Disease

The diagnosis of IBS relies on symptom-based criteria with normal results of complementary tests to rule out organic diseases. Only a limited number of laboratory tests are recommended without any need to perform invasive investigations, unless patient does not have alarm features. Alarm features that have traditionally increased suspicion for organic disease include a bloody stool, weight loss, iron-deficiency anemia, nocturnal symptoms, and a family history of such organic diseases as colorectal cancer, inflammatory bowel disease (IBD), and celiac disease [6–8]. However, most alarm features have poor overall accuracy for organic pathology, including colorectal cancer with the exception of anemia and weight loss, which have good specificity for organic disease. Certain percentage of IBS patients lacking alarm features have organic colonic diseases. Thus, physicians may not refuse patient's requirement to have colonic examination.

8.4 Routine Blood and Stool Tests

Specimen (blood, urine, and feces) examination is useful for differential diagnosis of IBS from organic diseases. Calprotectin has been proposed as marker for inflammatory conditions, such as IBD. Dolwani et al. investigated differences in fecal calprotectin value among active Crohn's group, irritable bowel syndrome group, and normal volunteers, and the median calprotectin values were 227 microg/g of stool, 19 microg/g, and 10 microg/g, respectively ($P < 0.0001$). A single stool calprotectin value <60 microg/g of stool is more accurate than the measurement of erythrocyte sedimentation rate or C-reactive protein; the negative predictive value <60 microg/g of stool was 100% compared with 91% each for erythrocyte sedimentation rate > 10 mm and C-reactive protein >6 mg/L in predicting the absence of organic intestinal disease [8]. Fecal occult blood test (FOBT) were widely used in the diagnosis of intestinal inflammation in inflammatory bowel disease (IBD). Fu et al. compared the efficacy of calprotectin and FOBT for discriminating IBD from IBS. Calprotectin ≥50 μg/g yield 76% sensitivity, 93% specificity, 97% PPV, and 53% NPV. FOBT yield 65% sensitivity, 93% specificity, 97% PPV, and 43% NPV [9]. These results suggest that stool calprotectin is more accurate than the measurement of FOBT.

8.5 Celiac Screening

Patients with irritable bowel syndrome (IBS) report abdominal symptoms similar to those in celiac disease. From a systematic review and meta-analysis to estimate prevalence of celiac disease (CD), the prevalence of serologic evidence of celiac disease among IBS patients (endomysial antibodies (EMA) or tissue transglutaminase antibodies (anti-tTG)) is more than threefold higher than among controls without IBS, and the prevalence of biopsy-proved celiac disease in cases meeting diagnostic criteria for IBS was more than fourfold that in controls without IBS [10]. Thus, routine serologic screening for celiac disease is recommended for patients with IBS-D. The prevalence of CD varies from country to country. Although common in Europe and the United States, cases of CD have rarely been encountered in East Asia, especially in Japan [11]. Such tests are not recommended for routine use in East Asia. Non-celiac gluten sensitivity (NCGS) is a syndrome characterized by intestinal and extraintestinal symptoms, related to the ingestion of gluten in subjects who are not affected by CD or wheat allergy. Studies have found that a subset of people with IBS, but without CD, suffer from NCGS and see their IBS symptoms improve or clear up when they eat gluten-free diet. With IBS and gluten sensitivity, there are no screening and diagnostic tests available. An overlap between IBS and NCGS has been detected [12].

8.6 Endoscopy

A colonoscopy or barium enema is useful for differentiating IBS from organic diseases. Colonoscopy may be considered in patients aged >50 years with alarm features [2]. Colonoscopy has a diagnostic value, not only for excluding organic diseases but also for supporting the existence of pathophysiology compatible to IBS due to visceral hypersensitivity to colonoscopic procedures. Kim et al. investigated differences in pain perception during colonoscopy between IBS patients and non-IBS patients and found that the pain scores of IBS patients (52, 34–71) were higher than those of the healthy controls ($P < 0.001$) (22, 12–35). At the pain score level of 31, the sensitivity and specificity were 86.1% and 75.9%, respectively [13].

Mizukami et al. investigated differences in colonic dysmotility during colonoscopy between IBS patients and non-IBS patients and found that colonic dysmotility was more frequent in the IBS group (28.8% vs. 2.0% in controls, $P < 0.001$), especially in cases of IBS with diarrhea (IBS-D) (IBS with constipation (IBS-C) 28.8% vs. IBS-D 60.0% vs. mixed IBS (IBS-M) 5.1%, $P < 0.001$) [14].

Ishihara investigated whether the Rome III criteria can exclude organic colonic lesions prior to the diagnosis of irritable bowel syndrome (IBS). Four thousand one hundred seventy-eight patients received colonoscopy, and organic colonic diseases were found in 10.3% of patients who fulfilled the Rome III criteria and 8.5% of patients who did not fulfill the Rome III criteria. There were no differences, implying that the Rome III criteria cannot exclude organic colonic lesions [15].

Colonoscopy may be considered in patients with alarm symptoms. However, it should be noted that certain percentage of IBS patients lacking alarm features have organic colonic diseases. Gu et al. investigated differences in the prevalence of organic colonic diseases between IBS patients without alarm features and control patients under 50 years of age. Organic colonic lesions were found in 30.3% of the patients with suspected irritable bowel syndrome. Compared with controls, patients with suspected irritable bowel syndrome had higher prevalence of noninflammatory bowel disease and noninfectious colitis and terminal ileitis [16].

In patients with suspected IBS-D, colonoscopy with random mucosal biopsies might be considered if symptoms are not well controlled by antidiarrheal therapy to rule out microscopic colitis. Limsui et al. investigated the prevalence of symptoms of irritable bowel syndrome in a population-based cohort of 131 patients with histologically confirmed microscopic colitis. Of them, 56% of patients met Rome II criteria for irritable bowel syndrome, indicating the symptomatic overlap between these conditions [17].

8.7 Carbohydrate Breath Test

Emerging evidence suggests that small intestinal bacterial overgrowth (SIBO) plays a pathogenic role in IBS. Pimentel et al. investigated the effect of a nonabsorbed oral antibiotic (rifaximin) on the symptoms of the irritable bowel syndrome by a randomized trial. Participants who met enrollment criteria were randomly assigned to receive 400 mg of rifaximin three times daily for 10 days ($n = 43$) or placebo ($n = 44$). Over the 10 weeks of follow-up, rifaximin resulted in greater improvement in IBS symptoms ($P = 0.020$). In addition, rifaximin recipients had a lower bloating score after treatment [18]. Recently, carbohydrate breath test has been used to identify patients with SIBO [19]. There are some methods to diagnose SIBO. Although quantitative jejunal aspirate culture is considered the gold standard for the diagnosis of SIBO, hydrogen breath tests have been popular because of noninvasiveness. The glucose hydrogen breath test is highly specific, but sensitivity is low. The lactulose hydrogen breath test is highly nonspecific. Between 4% and 78% of patients with IBS and 1% and 40% of controls have SIBO; such wide variations in prevalence might result from mainly methods to diagnose SIBO [20]. Thus, so far diagnosing IBS patients with carbohydrate breath test is not recommended.

8.8 Serologic Markers

Several noninvasive diagnostic approaches were investigated for their ability to discriminate IBS from non-IBS disorders. Chromogranins (Cg) and secretogranins (Sg) are proteins ubiquitous in secretory cells of the enteric, endocrine, and immune systems and may reflect activity of these systems. Ohman et al. analyzed CgA, CgB, SgII, SgIII, and calprotectin in fecal samples of 82 IBS patients and 29 healthy controls. IBS patients demonstrated higher levels of fecal CgA ($P = 0.009$), SgII ($P < 0.001$), and SgIII ($P < 0.001$), but lower levels of CgB ($P < 0.001$) compared with controls. SgII had good discriminative validity to positively identify IBS patients [21].

Lembo et al. selected ten serum biomarkers from a potential panel of 140 for their ability to differentiate IBS from non-IBS disease in blood samples from patients with IBS, other gastrointestinal disorders, and healthy volunteers. A predictive modelling tool was developed, and this model was tested in a different cohort of patients. The sensitivity and specificity of the ten-biomarker algorithm for differentiating IBS from non-IBS was 50% and 88%, respectively [22]. A systematic review and a meta-analysis examining various diagnostic criteria in IBS have reported that the best in terms of positive likelihood ratio was fecal calprotectin, intestinal permeability, and Rome I criteria (26.4; 95% CI: 11.4–61.9), and in terms of negative likelihood ratio serum-based biomarkers and psychological markers (0.18; 95% CI: 0.12–0.25) [23]. Combining symptoms with markers appears more effective and may represent the way forward in the diagnosis of IBS.

8.9 Functional MRI

Irritable bowel syndrome (IBS) is associated with exaggerated cerebral response including emotional processing following visceral stimulation. Guleria et al. investigated brain response of male IBS patients following rectal balloon distension as compared to healthy controls using functional magnetic resonance imaging (fMRI). IBS patients showed greater cerebral activations in insula, middle temporal gyrus, and cerebellum in the left hemisphere compared to healthy controls. Neural activation was found in bilateral precuneus/superior parietal lobules in controls but not in patients with IBS. The brain activation differed among IBS-C and IBS-D patients [24]. Although functional MRI is not suitable for daily practice, these scientific and technologic advances will be useful to evolving a new diagnostic tools.

8.10 Psychological Markers

Anxiety, depression, and nongastrointestinal symptoms are often prominent in irritable bowel syndrome. Spiller et al. compared the value of Patient Health Questionnaire 12 SS scores in predicting symptoms and patient behavior in IBS and diverticular disease. The PHQ-12 SS for IBS and symptomatic diverticular disease were significantly higher than healthy volunteers [25]. The use of psychological markers in combination with other biomarkers may help avoid unnecessary diagnostic testing in differentiating IBS from health.

8.11 Diagnostic Algorithm

Based on the statements above, the diagnostic algorithm for IBS (Fig. 8.1) is as follows. In patients with chronic abdominal pain or abdominal discomfort and/or abnormal bowel movement, if any of the alarm symptoms/signs, risk factors, and routine examinations is positive, colonoscopy is recommended. If all of them or colonoscopy is negative, Rome IV criteria is applied. By using Rome IV criteria, we can diagnose relatively fewer heterogenous IBS patients without unnecessary examinations than by using a physician's own criteria. As a result, diagnosis will be IBS or another functional gastrointestinal disorder like functional abdominal pain syndrome, functional constipation, functional diarrhea, functional bloating, unspecified functional bowel disorder, and so on.

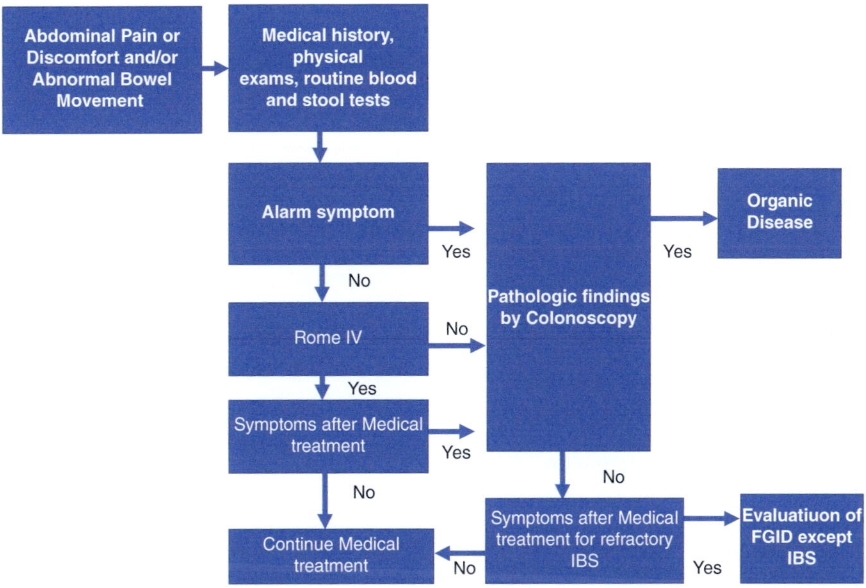

Fig. 8.1 Suggested diagnostic algorithm for IBS. Routine blood examinations are chemical analyses, including plasma glucose and thyroid stimulating hormone, complete blood count, and inflammatory reaction such as (high-sensitive) C-reactive protein. Routine stool tests include fecal calprotectin and occult blood test. Alarm symptoms are fever, arthralgia, bloody in stool or unexpected weight loss more than 3 kg within 6 months, symptoms onset after the age more than 50, past or family history of organic diseases of the colorectum, awakened by GI symptoms, and patient's requirement to have colonic examination. Colonoscopy will be recommended if these factors are positive. Note that positive fecal occult blood, anemia, hypoproteinemia, or positive inflammatory reaction especially requires colonic examination. Depending on the clinical situation, the following detailed examination may be indicated: gastrointestinal mucosal biopsy, upper GI endoscopy, upper GI series, abdominal ultrasonography, fecal ova test, stool bacterial culture, abdominal computed tomography, abdominal magnetic resonance imaging, small intestinal endoscopy, small intestinal fluoroscopy, lactose tolerance test, hydrogen breath test, and so on. If negative clinical examinations and positive Rome IV criteria are found, a diagnosis of IBS is made. If Rome IV for IBS is negative and patients suffer symptoms after medical treatment, patients may be classified into other functional gastrointestinal disorders (FGIDs), including functional abdominal pain, functional bloating, functional constipation, functional diarrhea, or unspecified functional bowel disorder

References

1. Longstreth GF, Thompson WG, Chey WD, Houghton LA, Mearin F. Spiller RC functional bowel disorders. Gastroenterology. 2006;130(5):1480–91.
2. Brandt LJ, Chey WD, Foxx-Orenstein AE, Schiller LR, Schoenfeld PS, Spiegel BM, Talley NJ, Quigley EM. An evidence-based position statement on the management of irritable bowel syndrome. American College of Gastroenterology Task Force on Irritable Bowel Syndrome. Am J Gastroenterol. 2009;104(Suppl 1):S1–S35.
3. Lovell RM, Ford AC. Global prevalence of and risk factors for irritable bowel syndrome: a meta-analysis. Clin Gastroenterol Hepatol. 2012;10:712–21.

4. Lacy BE, Mearin F, Chang L, et al. Bowel disorders. Gastroenterology. 2016;26(150):1393–407.
5. Fukudo S, Kaneko H, Akiho HT. Evidence-based clinical practice guidelines for irritable bowel syndrome. J Gastroenterol. 2015;50(1):11–30.
6. Vanner SJ, Depew WT, Paterson WG, et al. Predictive value of the Rome criteria for diagnosing the irritable bowel syndrome. Am J Med. 1999;94:2912–7.
7. Saito YA, Zimmerman JM, Harmsen WS, et al. Irritable bowel syndrome aggregates strongly in families:a family-based case-control study. Neurogastroenterol Motil. 2008;20:790–7.
8. Dolwani S, Metzner M, Wassell JJ, et al. Diagnostic accuracy of faecal calprotectin estimation in prediction of abnormal small bowel radiology. Aliment Pharmacol Ther. 2004;20:615–21.
9. Fu Y, Wang L, Xie C, et al. Comparison of non-invasive biomarkers faecal BAFF, calprotectin and FOBT in discriminating IBS from IBD and evaluation of intestinal inflammation. Sci Rep. 2017;7(1):2669.
10. Ford AC, Chey WD, Talley NJ, et al. Yield of diagnostic tests for celiac disease in individuals with symptoms suggestive of irritable bowel syndrome: systematic review and meta-analysis. Arch Intern Med. 2009;169:651–8.
11. Fukunaga M, Ishimura N, Fukuyama C, et al. Celiac disease in non-clinical populations of Japan. J Gastroenterol. 2018;53(2):208–14.
12. Catassi C, Alaedini A, Bojarski C, et al. The overlapping area of non-celiac gluten sensitivity (NCGS) and wheat-sensitive irritable bowel syndrome (IBS): an update. Nutrients. 2017;9(11):E1268.
13. Kim ES, Cheon JH, Park JJ, et al. Colonoscopy as an adjunctive method for the diagnosis of irritable bowel syndrome: focus on pain perception. J Gastroenterol Hepatol. 2010;25:1232–8.
14. Mizukami T, Sugimoto S, Masaoka T, et al. Colonic dysmotility and morphological abnormality frequently detected in Japanese patients with irritable bowel syndrome. Intest Res. 2017;15(2):236–43.
15. Ishihara S, Yashima K, Kushiyama Y, et al. Prevalence of organic colonic lesions in patients meeting Rome III criteria for diagnosis of IBS: a prospective multi-center study utilizing colonoscopy. J Gastroenterol. 2012;47:1084–90.
16. Gu HX, Zhang YL, Zhi FC, et al. Organic colonic lesions in 3,332 patients with suspected irritable bowel syndrome and lacking warning signs, a retrospective case—control study. Int J Color Dis. 2011;26:935–40.
17. Limsui D, Pardi DS, Camilleri M, et al. Symptomatic overlap between irritable bowel syndrome and microscopic colitis. Inflamm Bowel Dis. 2007;13:175–81.
18. Pimentel M, Park S, Mirocha J, Kane SV, Kong Y. The effect of a nonabsorbed oral antibiotic (rifaximin) on the symptoms of the irritable bowel syndrome: a randomized trial. Ann Intern Med. 2006;145(8):557–63.
19. Saad RJ, Chey WD. Breath tests for gastrointestinal disease: the real deal or just a lot of hot air? Gastroenterology. 2007;133(6):1763–6.
20. Ghoshal UC, Shukla R, Ghoshal U. Small intestinal bacterial overgrowth and irritable bowel syndrome: a bridge between functional organic dichotomy gut. Liver. 2017;11(2):196–208.
21. Ohman L, Stridsberg M, Isaksson S, et al. Altered levels of fecal chromogranins and secretogranins in IBS: relevance for pathophysiology and symptoms? Am J Gastroenterol. 2012;107:440–7.
22. Lembo AJ, Neri B, Tolley J, et al. Use of serum biomarkers in a diagnostic test for irritable bowel syndrome. Aliment Pharmacol Ther. 2009;29:834–42.
23. Sood R, Gracie DJ, Law GR, Ford AC. Systematic review with meta-analysis: the accuracy of diagnosing irritable bowel syndrome with symptoms, biomarkers and/or psychological markers. Aliment Pharmacol Ther. 2015;42(5):491–503.
24. Guleria A, Karyampudi A, Singh R, et al. Mapping of brain activations to rectal balloon distension stimuli in male patients with irritable bowel syndrome using functional magnetic resonance imaging. J Neurogastroenterol Motil. 2017;23:415–27.
25. Spiller RC, Humes DJ, Campbell E, et al. The Patient Health Questionnaire 12 Somatic Symptom scale as a predictor of symptom severity and consulting behaviour in patients with irritable bowel syndrome and symptomatic diverticular disease. Aliment Pharmacol Ther. 2010;32(6):811–20.

Chapter 9
Differential Diagnosis

Toshimi Chiba

Abstract The Rome IV criteria aids in the diagnosis of irritable bowel syndrome (IBS), as well as in the classification of IBS. Colonoscopy is indicated when alarm symptoms/signs, risk factors, and/or abnormal physical exam findings are present. In this chapter, we describe various conditions that should be considered in the differential diagnosis of IBS, including bile acid diarrhea, celiac disease, food, chronic gastrointestinal infection, inflammatory bowel disease, microscopic colitis, colorectal cancer, drug-induced diarrhea or constipation, amyloidosis, and small intestinal bacterial overgrowth. When Rome IV features for IBS are negative, other functional gastrointestinal disorders, including functional abdominal pain, functional bloating, functional constipation, functional diarrhea, or unspecified functional bowel disorder, should be considered.

Keywords Irritable bowel syndrome · Differential diagnosis · Rome IV criteria · Bile acid · Celiac disease · Food · Gastrointestinal infection · Inflammatory bowel disease · Microscopic colitis · Colorectal Cancer · Amyloidosis · Small intestinal bacterial overgrowth

9.1 Alarm Features

The Rome IV criteria aids in the diagnosis of irritable bowel syndrome (IBS) without the need for invasive procedures and allows clinicians to better utilize resources when evaluating a patient. Alarm symptoms include fever, arthralgia, bloody stool, or unexpected weight loss more than 3 kg within 6 months. Alarm signs include palpable abdominal mass, abdominal fluctuation, or palpable mass and/or blood on digital rectal examination (DRE). Risk factors concerning for non-IBS-related

T. Chiba (✉)
Division of Internal Medicine, Department of Oral Medicine, Iwate Medical University, Morioka, Iwate, Japan
e-mail: toschiba@iwate-med.ac.jp

© The Editor(s) (if applicable) and The Author(s), under exclusive license to Springer Nature Singapore Pte Ltd. 2024

T. Kamiya, S. Fukudo (eds.), *Irritable Bowel Syndrome*,
https://doi.org/10.1007/978-981-97-8410-3_9

disorders include age more than 50 years and past or family history of organic diseases of the colorectum. Routine evaluation includes blood chemical analyses, including plasma glucose and thyroid stimulating hormone, complete blood count, inflammatory reaction such as C-reactive protein, urinalysis, fecal occult blood test, and plain abdominal X-ray. Colonoscopy may be required in the setting of positive fecal occult blood, unexplained anemia, hypoproteinemia, or positive inflammatory markers. Colonoscopy is preferred over barium enema as it allows for mucosal biopsy, particularly when differentiating between microscopic colitis or celiac disease. Additionally, histopathological examination of the gut mucosa could reveal increased mast cells, enterochromaffin cells, and inflammatory cells further guiding a diagnosis away from IBS. Depending on the clinical situation, the following detailed examination might be indicated: gastrointestinal mucosal biopsy, upper gastrointestinal (GI) endoscopy, upper GI series, abdominal ultrasonography, fecal ova test, stool bacterial culture, abdominal computed tomography, abdominal magnetic resonance imaging, small intestinal endoscopy, small intestinal fluoroscopy, lactose tolerance test, and/or hydrogen breath test. Lactose hydrogen breath tests evaluate for lactose malabsorption, such as in patients with lactose intolerance and even small intestinal bacterial overgrowth (SIBO). Ultimately, if the clinical evaluation is negative for the aforementioned features, and Rome IV criteria positive, the diagnosis of IBS can confidently be made [1]. If Rome IV for IBS are negative, patients may be classified into other functional gastrointestinal disorders (FGIDs), including functional abdominal pain, functional bloating, functional constipation, functional diarrhea, or unspecified functional bowel disorder. The diagnostic algorithm in the Japanese IBS Guideline has been shown (Fig. 9.1) [2]. Patients are typically those with chronic abdominal pain or abdominal discomfort and/or abnormal bowel movements. If any alarm signs/symptoms, concerning risk factors, or abnormal exam findings are present, then colonoscopy would be warranted. If there are no concerning signs/symptoms, risk factors, or abnormal evaluation findings, then Rome IV can be utilized alone. The diagnostic algorithm is well indicated for patients with lower GI symptoms for 3 months or more, but not indicated in patients with acute symptoms.

9.2 Differential Diagnosis of IBS

The differential diagnosis of diarrhea-predominant IBS (IBS-D) includes celiac disease, collagenous colitis, Crohn's disease, eosinophilic enteritis, and amyloidosis, whereas chronic intestinal pseudo-obstruction or secondary chronic constipation would be included in a differential diagnoses of constipation-predominant IBS (IBS-C). Drug induced (opioid, anticholinergic agent), endocrine diseases (diabetes, hypothyroidism), neurogenic diseases (diabetic neuropathy, Parkinson's disease), trauma (spinal cord injury, abdominal nerve plexus damage), and amyloidosis could be considered as secondary causes of chronic constipation (Table 9.1).

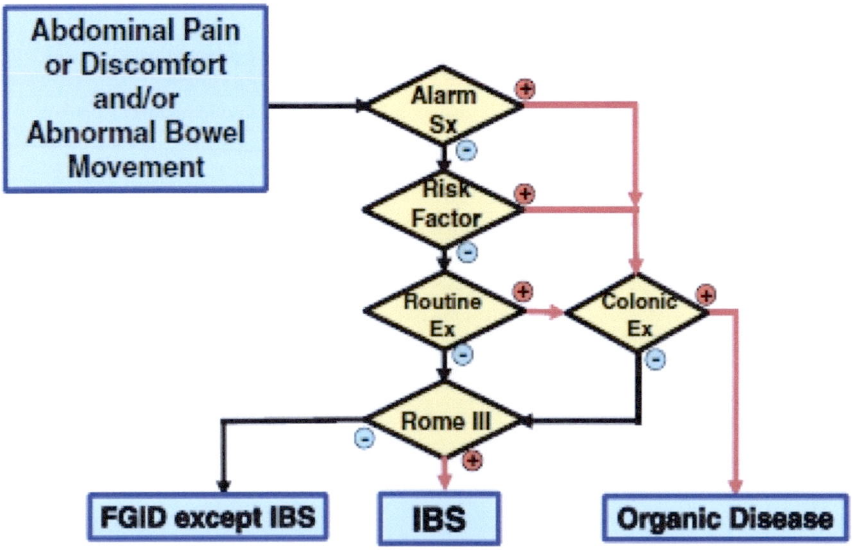

Fig. 9.1 Diagnostic algorithm for IBS (From J Gastroenterol 2021 in reference [2])

9.2.1 Bile Acid Diarrhea

Bile acid diarrhea (BAD) is dysregulated bile acid recycling within the enterohepatic circulation. Unabsorbed bile acids (BA) in the colon cause watery diarrhea by stimulating fluid or sodium secretion, increasing gastrointestinal motility, and stimulating defecation. BAD has been reported in approximately 25–35% of chronic diarrhea patients as well as in IBS-D patients [3, 4]. History of terminal ileal resection, ileal disease, cholecystectomy, radiotherapy, or excess bile acid production, as seen in individuals with a genetic defect that prevents normal feedback inhibition of BA synthesis, are the risk factors of BAD. BA malabsorption is a potentially important factor in the pathophysiology of IBS-D and may be overlooked in clinical practice. A number of diagnostic tests for BAD, including radionuclide and blood tests, can be utilized to identify patients in whom diarrhea is related to excess bile salts in the colon. The selenium homocholic acid taurine (SeHCAT) test utilizes orally administered synthetic 75-selenium-labeled bile acid as an indirect assessment of absorption and fecal excretion of bile acids, and has been reported to have a sensitivity of 89% and specificity of 100% for BAD [5]. Other biomarkers for BAD include measurement of fasting serum fibroblast growth factor 19 (FGF19), a regulatory protein reflecting ileal bile acid transporter reuptake of luminal bile acids. Serum 7a-hydroxy-4-cholesten-3-one (C4) levels reflect hepatic bile synthesis. BAs in a 48-h stool collection were also the biomarker for BAD [6, 7]. SeHCAT test had a higher yield for BAD in patients with IBS-D or FD than FGF19 or C4. Disadvantages of SeHCAT testing include the administration of a radioactive

Table 9.1 Differential diagnosis of IBS

Malabsorption	Bile acid, amyloidosis, lymphangiectasia, chronic pancreatitis, postgastrectomy	
Food	Allergy, celiac disease, eosinophilic enteritis, lactose intolerance, alcohol, high-fat meal	
Endocrine diseases	Hypothyroidism, diabetic neuropathy	
Infectious disease	Amebic dysentery, intestinal tuberculosis	
Inflammatory diseases	Inflammatory bowel disease, ulcerative colitis, Crohn's disease, Behçet's disease, ischemic colitis, microscopic enteritis, collagenous colitis, colonic diverticulosis	
Malignancy	Colon cancer, malignant lymphoma, carcinoid	
Gynecologic disorder	Endometriosis, ovarian tumor, dysmenorrhea	
Psychiatric disorder	Panic disorder, depression	
Chronic constipation	Drug	Opioid, anticholinergic agents, antiparkinson agent, calcium channel blocker
	Endocrine disease	Diabetes, hypothyroidism, hyperparathyroidism, phaeochromocytoma
	Neurogenic diseases	Diabetic neuropathy, Parkinson's disease, shy-Drager syndrome
	Trauma	Spinal cord injury, the abdominal nerve plexus damage
	Pseudo-obstruction	

isotope, the need of dedicated infrastructure, including a gamma camera, and multiple visits to complete the study.

9.2.2 *Celiac Disease*

Celiac disease is a multisystem, autoimmune disorder that occurs in genetically susceptible persons and is triggered by the ingestion of gluten [8]. Gluten is found in wheat, barley, and oat products and leads to small intestinal damage with resultant malabsorption and associated nutritional deficiencies. The estimated prevalence of celiac disease in the general population varies significantly in different regions of the world [9]. Patients with celiac disease commonly report symptoms suggestive of IBS-D, including abdominal pain, discomfort, bloating, and diarrhea. The prevalence of celiac disease in IBS-D has been reported to be more than fourfold in controls without IBS [10]. The symptoms of celiac disease often overlap with IBS, and the gold standard for diagnosis of celiac disease is small bowel biopsy to detect blunted or atrophic villi (including complete destruction of the epithelial surface), crypt hyperplasia, and mononuclear/lymphocytic infiltration into the lamina propria [11]. A number of different serology antibody tests can be used to screen for celiac disease in functional diarrhea and IBS-D, such as IgA anti-tissue transglutaminase antibodies (IgA anti-tTG), IgG anti-tTG, and IgA anti-endomysial antibodies (IgA EMA), as well as IgA and IgG antibodies against deamidated gliadin peptide (IgA/IgG anti-DGP). In one study, 2.1% of patients with IBS-D-related symptoms were found to have positive celiac disease serology (EMA or tTG) compared to 0.8% of controls [12, 13]. Among the tests we evaluated, IgA anti-tTG offered the best combination of sensitivity, specificity, and positive and negative likelihood ratios and has been recognized as the single best serologic test to screen for celiac disease. The sensitivity of serologic tests is reduced in persons who are already on a gluten-free diet. Thus, although IgA EMA performs well, screening for celiac disease in high-risk patients should combine IgA anti-tTG testing with a second test to identify patients with IgA deficiency, or an IgG-based test, such as DGP or tTG [14–16]. Interestingly, patients with IBS-D have been reported to have worse symptoms when eating gluten indicating that non-celiac gluten intolerance should be considered and a gluten-free diet might be recommended to reduce IBS symptoms [17].

9.2.3 Food

Food adverse reactions include food allergy and food intolerance. While food allergies are mediated by immunologic reactions, food intolerance is not and may be due to factors within foods, such as chemical agents (caffeine or tyramine), enzyme deficiency in the host (lactase deficiency), or idiosyncratic responses related to an unknown mechanism [18]. Although patients with IBS self-report food allergies more often than the general population, evidence suggests that true food allergies are relatively uncommon. True food allergies are reported in about 1–4% of adults in the general population, with 50% to 90% of presumed food allergies being food intolerances [19]. In patients with GI symptoms, food allergy was confirmed by elimination diet or rechallenged in only 3.2% of patients, despite 32% of patients with GI symptoms reporting adverse reactions to food [20]. Food triggers are common, with more than half of IBS patients having self-reported food intolerances [21, 22]. The most common food triggers include those with incompletely absorbed carbohydrates (dairy products, beans/lentils, apple, and flour), foods rich in biogenic amines (wine/beer, salami, and cheese), histamine-releasing foods (milk, wine/beer, and pork), and fried or fatty foods [23, 24]. True food allergies are likely rare in IBS patients, and there is little data to support the efficacy of avoiding foods as identified by allergy testing. However, 20% of IBS-D with food hypersensitivity (FH) (cow's milk and/or wheat hypersensitivity) had improved symptom scores when placed on an elimination diet [25].

9.2.4 Chronic Gastrointestinal Infection

Commonly encountered bacterial GI infections include *Salmonella*, *Campylobacter*, *Yersinia*, *Aeromonas*, and *Plesiomonas* which could be detected with an expanded stool culture. It is necessary to exclude *Yersinia enterocolitica* enteritis as part of the differential diagnosis of IBS (Fig. 9.2). *Clostridioides* difficile (*C. difficile*) infection is also one of the more common causes of diarrhea, particularly in a background of recent antibiotic use. Parasites are a more likely cause of chronic diarrhea, especially in developing countries, where the prevalence is high, or in those who have traveled to those countries. The most common causes of parasitic diarrhea are *Giardia*, *Cryptosporidia*, *Cyclospora*, and *Entamoeba histolytica*. *Giardia* is the most common parasite causing chronic diarrhea, with prevalence of 2% in adults and 6%–8% in children in developed countries. *Giardia* infection typically continues 2–6 weeks, and symptoms are similar to IBS-D, including diarrhea, bloating, and abdominal pain. *Giardia* may be detected through the stool ova and parasite test, fecal immunoassays such as the stool enzyme immunoassay, immunochromatography, direct fluorescent antibody, and polymerase chain reaction (PCR) tests [26, 27].

9.2.5 Inflammatory Bowel Disease (IBD)

Inflammatory markers are often utilized in patients with diarrhea to detect IBD (ulcerative colitis and/or Crohn's disease). Symptoms compatible with the diagnosis of IBS are common in IBD patients, and screening for IBD in patients with IBS-D symptoms should be considered. The gold standard for diagnosis of IBD

Fig. 9.2 Colonoscopy finding shows Yersinia enterocolitica enteritis. Colonoscopy revealed redness and swelling of the ileocecal valve. Yersinia enterocolitica was detected with a stool culture

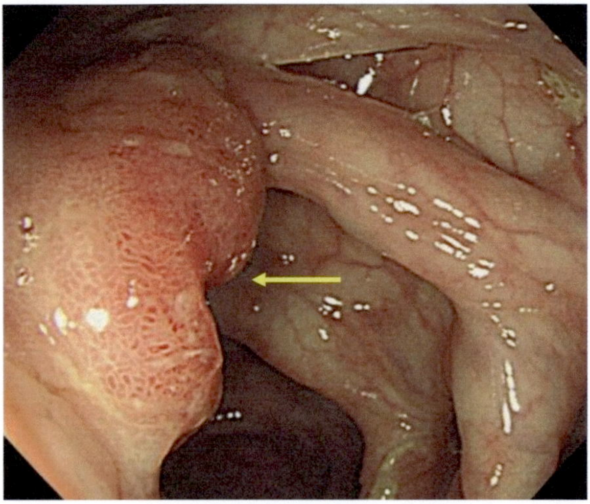

includes colonoscopy and biopsy with evaluation of the small bowel. Colonoscopy revealing small ulcers along the colon may lead to the diagnosis of Crohn's disease in a patient otherwise thought to have IBS-D (Fig. 9.3). A number of blood and stool tests can be used to screen for diseases that cause inflammation in the GI tract, such as erythrocyte sedimentation rate (ESR). Recently, fecal calprotectin (FC), a protein derived from neutrophils, has been found to be a good marker of GI tract inflammation when levels are elevated. The normal FC cutoff is <50 μg/g, with levels of 50–100 μg/g being considered borderline and levels >100 μg/g indicating inflammation [28]. Fecal matrix metalloprotease-9 (MMP-9) concentration was significantly elevated in IBD compared to IBS-D, as IBS-D patients were actually found to have undetectable MMP-9 levels. Fecal MMP-9 may be a novel marker to help in the differential diagnosis of patients with diarrhea and abdominal pain [29]. Fecal lactoferrin (FL) is a protein derived from the secondary granules of neutrophils, and when levels are elevated in stool, it also suggests the presence of inflammation in the GI tract, with a positivity threshold ranging from 4.0 to 7.25 μg/g. As part of routine testing to exclude IBD, however, fecal calprotectin in IBS patients is not effective without the proper clinical presentation (i.e., diarrhea, abdominal pain, and even weight loss) [30].

9.2.6 *Microscopic Colitis*

Microscopic colitis is a diarrheal disease with chronic colonic inflammation, with the gold standard of diagnosis being colorectal biopsy. The pathophysiology of microscopic colitis is not well understood. However, nonsteroidal anti-inflammatory drugs (NSAIDs), proton pump inhibitors (PPI), statins, selective serotonin reuptake

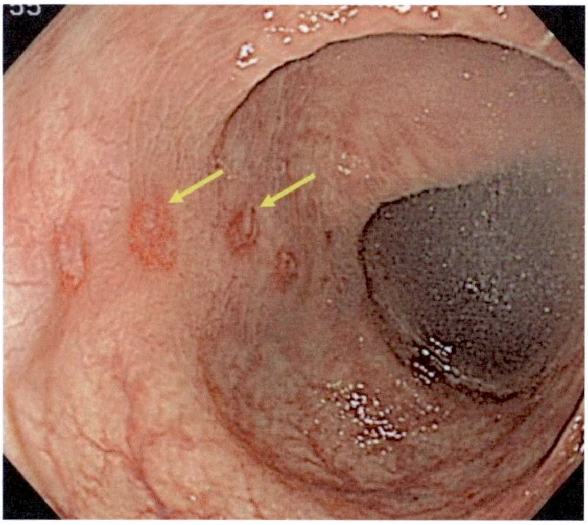

Fig. 9.3 Colonoscopy finding shows Crohn's disease. Arrows indicate small ulcers along the colon. Histopathological findings showed epithelioid granuloma, a finding of Crohn's disease

inhibitors (SSRI), and several other drugs have been implicated as potential causes of microscopic colitis. Microscopic colitis includes collagenous colitis and lymphocytic colitis, which have similar clinical features. The main difference is the presence of a thickened subepithelial collagen band in collagenous colitis. The incidence is estimated at 4.14 per 100,000 person-years for collagenous colitis and 4.85 per 100,000 person-years for lymphocytic colitis and is most common in those over age 60 years [31]. The pooled prevalence of IBS symptoms in patients with microscopic colitis was 33.4%. The prevalence of IBS symptoms in microscopic colitis patients was significantly higher than in healthy controls [32], and a microscopic colitis prevalence of 1.5% in nonconstipated IBS patients has been reported [33]. All of the patients with microscopic colitis were identified in the subgroup with IBS-D, illustrating the importance of colonoscopy and biopsy, particularly in evaluating the differential of IBS-D.

9.2.7 Colorectal Cancer (CRC)

Patients with IBS have a reported increased 10-year risk of being diagnosed with CRC compared with controls. Alarm features are usually defined as vomiting, gastrointestinal bleeding, abdominal mass, dysphagia, unexplained weight loss, and anemia. Only abdominal mass and dark red rectal bleeding were associated with an increased risk of CRC [34]. Colonoscopy is regarded as the gold standard screening test for CRC and should be recommended for all patients ≥50 years of age, regardless of GI-related symptoms. Individuals 50 years or above at average risk for CRC also have the option for CRC screening using fecal occult blood testing [35, 36].

9.2.8 Drug-Induced Diarrhea or Constipation

The diagnosis of iatrogenic diarrhea secondary to drug therapy requires careful history taking and review of prescriptions, over-the-counter medications, and illicit medication/drug use. Unfortunately, the diagnosis of drug-induced diarrhea is made not by serology or lab analysis, but rather by discontinuation of the suspected medication with monitoring for symptom resolution. Some of the more common medications or supplements associated with diarrhea include magnesium-containing supplements and artificial sweeteners, such as sorbitol, which may be found in liquid medications. Enteral feeding is another way in which poorly absorbed substances may enter the alimentary tract and may be associated with diarrhea in some patients. If the drug is essential and cannot be stopped, reducing the dosage or adding a nonspecific antidiarrheal drug may improve symptoms. Common culprits for drug-induced constipation include anticholinergic agents, psychotropic agents (antipsychotic agents, antidepressants), antiparkinson agent, calcium channel blocker, opioids, and diuretics (loop diuretic, aldosterone antagonists) (Table 9.1).

9.2.9 *Amyloidosis*

The classification of amyloidosis includes primary (AL), secondary (AA), dialysis-related (Aβ2MG), senile, and hereditary. Familial amyloid polyneuropathy (FAP) is the most common hereditary amyloidosis and is caused by a mutation in transthyretin (TTR) gene resulting in transthyretin derived (ATTR) amyloidosis. If the gastrointestinal tract is involved, the small intestine is the most commonly affected site. The most common clinical presentations of small bowel amyloidosis are GI bleeding, diarrhea, and dysmotility. One of the main causes of diarrhea is autonomic neuropathy. Other mechanisms include bacterial overgrowth related to dysmotility, ischemia, amyloid infiltration of the lymphatics and villi, bile acid malabsorption, and pancreatic insufficiency. Dysmotility may be secondary to myopathy or neuropathy and is frequently secondary to amyloid deposition within the muscularis propria or autonomic nerves (myenteric plexus). It can present as nausea, vomiting, constipation, diarrhea secondary to rapid intestinal transit, and acute or chronic intestinal pseudo-obstruction [37].

9.2.10 *Small Intestinal Bacterial Overgrowth (SIBO)*

SIBO is a type of functional gastrointestinal disorder presenting with symptoms secondary to maldigestion and malabsorption and is thought to predispose to IBS. The prevalence of SIBO in IBS is 38%, with older age, female sex, and diarrhea predominant symptomatology being the most likely predictors of SIBO. The effectiveness of rifaximin for both SIBO and IBS has been reported, as rifaximin alters gut microbiota to reduce colonic fermentation and improve symptoms. SIBO is not common in IBS but may be relevant to an IBS subgroup, such as postinfectious IBS [38].

9.3 Conclusions

In this chapter, we describe the differential diagnosis of IBS. Proper clinical evaluation of symptom onset character and severity combined with laboratory examination, such as fecal occult blood test, inflammatory markers, peripheral blood cell count, and electrolytes, should be performed for 3 years after the diagnosis of IBS, particularly if resistant to therapy.

References

1. Lacy BE, Mearin F, Chang L, et al. Bowel disorders. Gastroenterology. 2016;150:1393–407. https://doi.org/10.1053/j.gastro.2016.02.031.
2. Fukudo S, Okumura T, Inamori M, et al. Evidence-based clinical practice guidelines for irritable bowel syndrome 2020. J Gastroenterol. 2021;56:193–217. https://doi.org/10.1007/s00535-020-01746-z.
3. Wedlake L, A'Hern R, Russell D, Thomas K, Walters JR, Andreyev HJ. Systematic review: the prevalence of idiopathic bile acid malabsorption as diagnosed by SeHCAT scanning in patients with diarrhoea-predominant irritable bowel syndrome. Aliment Pharmacol Ther. 2009;30:707–17. https://doi.org/10.1111/j.1365-2036.2009.04081.x.
4. Slattery SA, Niaz O, Aziz Q, Ford AC, Farmer AD. Systematic review with meta-analysis: the prevalence of bile acid malabsorption in the irritable bowel syndrome with diarrhoea. Aliment Pharmacol Ther. 2015;42:3–11. https://doi.org/10.1111/apt.13227.
5. Sciarretta G, Vicini G, Fagioli G, Verri A, Ginevra A, Malaguti P. Use of 23-selena-25-homocholyltaurine to detect bile acid malabsorption in patients with ileal dysfunction or diarrhea. Gastroenterology. 1986;91:1–9. https://doi.org/10.1016/0016-5085(86)90431-2.
6. Valentin N, Camilleri M, Altayar O, et al. Biomarkers for bile acid diarrhoea in functional bowel disorder with diarrhoea: a systematic review and meta-analysis. Gut. 2016;65:1951–9. https://doi.org/10.1136/gutjnl-2015-309889.
7. Mottacki N, Simren M, Bajor A. Review article: bile acid diarrhea-pathogenesis, diagnosis and management. Aliment Pharmacol Ther. 2016;43:884–98. https://doi.org/10.1111/apt.13570.
8. Bibbins-Domingo K, Grossman DC, Curry SJ, et al. Screening for celiac disease: US Preventive Services Task Force Recommendation Statement. JAMA. 2017;317:1252–7. https://doi.org/10.1001/jama.2017.1462.
9. Dube C, Rostom A, Sy R, et al. The prevalence of celiac disease in average-risk and at-risk Western European populations: a systematic review. Gastroenterology. 2005;128(Suppl 1):S57–67. https://doi.org/10.1053/j.gastro.2005.02.014.
10. Ford AC, Chey WD, Tally NJ, Malhotra A, Spiegel BMR, Moyayyedi P. Yield of diagnostic tests for celiac disease in individuals with symptoms suggestive of irritable bowel syndrome: systematic review and meta-analysis. Arch Intern Med. 2009;169:651–8. https://doi.org/10.1001/archinternmed.2009.22.
11. Ferguson A, Arranz E, O'Mahony S. Clinical and pathological spectrum of coeliac disease—active, silent, latent, potential. Gut. 1993;34:150–1. https://doi.org/10.1136/gut.34.2.150.
12. Rubio-Tapia A, Kyle RA, Kaplan EL, et al. Increased prevalence and mortality in undiagnosed celiac disease. Gastroenterology. 2009;137:88–93. https://doi.org/10.1053/j.gastro.2009.03.059.
13. West J, Logan RF, Smith CJ, et al. Malignancy and mortality in people with coeliac disease: population based cohort study. BMJ. 2004;329:716–9.
14. Rubio-Tapia A, Hill ID, Semrad C, et al. American college of gastroenterology guidelines update: diagnosis and management of celiac disease. Am J Gastroenterol. 2023;118:59–76. https://doi.org/10.14309/ajg.0000000000002075.
15. Bai JC, Fried M, Corazza GR, et al. World Gastroenterology Organisation global guidelines on celiac disease. J Clin Gastroenterol. 2013;47:121–6. https://doi.org/10.1097/MCG.0b013e31827a6f83.
16. Hill ID, Fasano A, Guandalini S, et al. NASPGHAN clinical report on the diagnosis and treatment of gluten-related disorders. J Pediatr Gastroenterol Nutr. 2016;63:156–65. https://doi.org/10.1097/MPG.0000000000001216.
17. Biesiekierski JR, Newnham ED, Irving PM, et al. Gluten causes gastrointestinal symptoms in subjects without celiac disease: a double-blind randomized placebo-controlled trial. Am J Gastroenterol. 2011;106:508–14. https://doi.org/10.1038/ajg.2010.487.

18. Park MI, Camilleri M. Is there a role of food allergy in irritable bowel syndrome and functional dyspepsia? A systematic review. Neurogastroenterol Motil. 2006;18:595–607. https://doi.org/10.1111/j.1365-2982.2005.00745.x.
19. Eswaran S, Tack J, Chey WD. Food: the forgotten factor in the irritable bowel syndrome. Gastroenterol Clin N Am. 2011;40:141–62. https://doi.org/10.1016/j.gtc.2010.12.012.
20. Bischoff SC, Herrmann A, Manns MP. Prevalence of adverse reactions to food in patients with gastrointestinal disease. Allergy. 1996;51:811–8.
21. Böhn L, Störsrud S, Törnblom H, Bengtsson U, Simrén M. Self-reported food-related gastrointestinal symptoms in IBS are common and associated with more severe symptoms and reduced quality of life. Am J Gastroenterol. 2013;108:634–41. https://doi.org/10.1038/ajg.2013.105.
22. Capili B, Anastasi JK, Chang M. Addressing the role of food in irritable bowel syndrome symptom management. J Nurse Pract. 2016;12:324–9. https://doi.org/10.1016/j.nurpra.2015.12.007.
23. Simrén M, Månsson A, Langkilde AM, et al. Food-related gastrointestinal symptoms in the irritable bowel syndrome. Digestion. 2001;63:108–815. https://doi.org/10.1159/000051878.
24. Chiba T, Mori M, Ikenoue Y, Suzuki K. Food and celiac disease antibodies in irritable bowel syndrome with predominant diarrhea. Med Res Arch. 2022;10(3):1–11. https://doi.org/10.18103/mra.v10i3.2745.
25. Carroccio A, Brusca I, Mansueto P, et al. A cytologic assay for diagnosis of food hypersensitivity in patients with irritable bowel syndrome. Clin Gastroenterol Hepatol. 2010;8:254–60. https://doi.org/10.1016/j.cgh.2009.11.010.
26. Soares R, Tasca T. Giardiasis: an update review on sensitivity and specificity of methods for laboratorial diagnosis. J Microbiol Methods. 2016;129:98–102. https://doi.org/10.1016/j.mimet.2016.08.017.
27. McHardy IH, Wu M, Shimizu-Cohen R, Couturier MR, Humphries RM. Detection of intestinal protozoa in the clinical laboratory. J Clin Microbiol. 2014;52:712–20. https://doi.org/10.1128/JCM.02877-13.
28. Ikhtaire S, Shajib MS, Reinisch W, Khan WI. Fecal calprotectin: its scope and utility in the management of inflammatory bowel disease. J Gastroenterol. 2016;51:434–46. https://doi.org/10.1007/s00535-016-1182-4.
29. Annaházi A, Molnár T, Farkas K, et al. Fecal MMP-9: a new noninvasive differential diagnostic and activity marker in ulcerative colitis. Inflamm Bowel Dis. 2013;19:316–20. https://doi.org/10.1002/ibd.22996.
30. Menees SB, Powell C, Kurlander J, Goel A, Chey WD. A meta-analysis of the utility of C-reactive protein, erythrocyte sedimentation rate, fecal calprotectin, and fecal lactoferrin to exclude inflammatory bowel disease in adults with IBS. Am J Gastroenterol. 2015;110:444–54. https://doi.org/10.1038/ajg.2015.6.
31. Pardi DS. Diagnosis and management of microscopic colitis. Am J Gastroenterol. 2017;112:78–85. https://doi.org/10.1038/ajg.2016.477.
32. Kamp EJ, Kane JS, Ford AC. Irritable bowel syndrome and microscopic colitis: a systematic review and meta-analysis. Clin Gastroenterol Hepatol. 2016;14:659–868. https://doi.org/10.1016/j.cgh.2015.09.031.
33. Chey WD, Nojkov B, Rubenstein JH, Dobhan RR, Greenson JK, Cash BD. The yield of colonoscopy in patients with non-constipated irritable bowel syndrome: results from a prospective, controlled US trial. Am J Gastroenterol. 2010;105:859–65. https://doi.org/10.1038/ajg.2010.55.
34. Ford AC, Veldhuyzen van Zanten SJ, Rodgers CC, et al. Diagnostic utility of alarm features for colorectal cancer: systematic review and meta-analysis. Gut. 2008;57:1545–53. https://doi.org/10.1136/gut.2008.159723.
35. Bibbins-Domingo K, Grossman DC, Curry SJ, et al. US Preventive Services Task Force. Screening for colorectal cancer: US Preventive Services Task Force recommendation statement. JAMA. 2016;315:2564–75. https://doi.org/10.1001/jama.2016.5989.

36. Bacchus CM, Dunfield L, Gorber SC, et al. Canadian Task Force On Preventive Health Care, Recommendations on screening for colorectal cancer in primary care. CMAJ. 2016;188:340–8. https://doi.org/10.1503/cmaj.151125.
37. Bansal R, Syed U, Walfish J, Aron J, Walfish A. Small bowel amyloidosis. Curr Gastroenterol Rep. 2018;20:11. https://doi.org/10.1007/s11894-018-0616-y.
38. Quigley EMM. The spectrum of small intestinal bacterial overgrowth (SIBO). Curr Gastroenterol Rep. 2019;21:3. https://doi.org/10.1007/s11894-019-0671-z.

Chapter 10
Comorbidities

Hideki Mori and Hidekazu Suzuki

Abstract Irritable bowel syndrome (IBS) is known to coexist with gastrointestinal complications such as functional dyspepsia, gastroesophageal reflux disease, and inflammatory bowel disease, as well as extraintestinal complications such as fibromyalgia, chronic fatigue syndrome, and chronic pelvic pain, and psychological disorders including panic disorder and depression. This is easy to understand because IBS is a disease of intestinal motility disorders and visceral hyperalgesia, which may affect the upper gastrointestinal tract, which is a contiguous organ. Furthermore, extra-gastrointestinal complications are associated with visceral hyperalgesia and autonomic nervous system dysfunction, making it easy to understand why they tend to coexist. Because the symptoms of IBS can result in abdominal pain and defecation problems similar to those of inflammatory bowel disease, it is important not to miss the early signs of inflammatory bowel disease or signs of deterioration.

Keywords IBS · Functional dyspepsia · Constipation · Diarrhea · Overlap

10.1 Introduction

Irritable bowel syndrome (IBS) patients are more likely to complain of other intestinal symptoms and besides intestinal symptoms. A greater understanding of what diseases are associated with IBS and the underlying mechanisms is needed.

H. Mori
Division of Gastroenterology and Hepatology, Department of Internal Medicine, Keio University School of Medicine, Tokyo, Japan

H. Suzuki (✉)
Division of Gastroenterology and Hepatology, Department of Internal Medicine, Tokai University School of Medicine, Isehara, Kanagawa, Japan
e-mail: hsuzuki@tokai.ac.jp

© The Editor(s) (if applicable) and The Author(s), under exclusive license to Springer Nature Singapore Pte Ltd. 2024

T. Kamiya, S. Fukudo (eds.), *Irritable Bowel Syndrome*,
https://doi.org/10.1007/978-981-97-8410-3_10

10.1.1 Gastrointestinal Comorbidities

10.1.1.1 Functional Dyspepsia

Functional dyspepsia (FD) is a medical condition that significantly affects patients' daily activities. It is characterized by one or more of the following symptoms: postprandial fullness, early satiation, epigastric pain, and unexplained epigastric pain after routine clinical evaluation [1]. Factors such as gastroduodenal motor and sensory dysfunction, impaired mucosal integrity, low-grade immune activation, and dysregulation of the gut-brain axis have been shown to be related to FD. FD and IBS co-occurrence rates have a wide range of overlap between the two disorders (13–87%) [2]. The frequency of FD overlapping with and without IBS was 24.1% and 7.8%, respectively, among Japanese workers who underwent a routine health check-up, with an odds ratio of 3.78 (95% CI: 2.86–5.00) for FD overlapping with IBS in without IBS [3]. In patients at a university hospital in Korea, the frequency of FD overlapping with and without IBS was 33.9% and 18.1%, respectively, with an odds ratio of 2.32 (95% CI: 1.34–4.04) [4]. In patients at a general gastroenterology outpatient clinic, the frequency of FD overlapping with and without IBS was 31.4% and 18.0%, respectively, with an odds ratio of 2.09 (95% CI: 1.68–2.59) [5]. An Icelandic study of general population revealed that FD overlapped with 61.9% of IBS when using the Rome II criteria [6]. In a questionnaire study of Swedish general population, the frequency of FD overlapping with and without IBS was 87.5% and 21.5%, respectively, with an odds ratio of 25.61(95% CI: 15.32–42.80) [7]. A study conducted by the Mayo Clinic in the United States revealed that the rate of FD overlap with IBS was equivalent to 85.5% for constipation cases and 75.0% for diarrhea cases [8].

Corsetti et al. compared rates of IBS-FD overlap and FD alone to investigate whether coexisting IBS was associated with symptom patterns or pathophysiology in FD [9]. They showed that FD + IBS patients were predominantly female (75% vs. 60%, $p < 0.01$) and likely to experience greater weight loss (5.4 ± 0.6 vs. 3.5 ± 0.4 kg, $p < 0.05$) [9]. Sensitivity to gastric distention and gastric accommodation to a meal were evaluated using a gastric barostat. FD + IBS patients were found to have a lower threshold for first perception (2.9 ± 0.3 vs. 3.8 ± 0.3 mmHg, $p < 0.05$) and discomfort (7.9 ± 0.4 vs. 9.5 ± 0.5 mmHg, $p < 0.05$) and a greater prevalence of hypersensitivity to gastric distention (44% vs. 28%, $p < 0.05$). Furthermore, gastric emptying, accommodation to a meal, and prevalence of *Helicobacter pylori* infection did not significantly differ between the two groups. In other words, their study suggested that visceral hypersensitivity was of particular importance in FD + IBS pathology compared with that of FD alone.

10.1.1.2 Gastroesophageal Reflux Disease

A systematic review analyzed the relationship between gastroesophageal reflux disease (GERD) and IBS [10]. The findings of eight publications suggested that the GERD maximum mean prevalence in patients already diagnosed with IBS was 39.3%, with a weighted mean of 30.3%. The merger rate ranged from 28 to 80%; however, this was attributed to the differences in the diagnosis of GERD. On the other hand, the prevalence of GERD in a non-IBS population was 16.6%. From these results, the review concluded that the rate at which GERD merges with IBS is higher than that of non-IBS. The review also analyzed the rate at which IBS overlapped with GERD. The maximum mean prevalence of IBS in subjects with known GERD was 48.8% with a weighted mean of 60.5%. Depending on the prevalence of IBS (12.1%) and GERD (19.4%) in the community, the calculated rate of IBS in the non-GERD community was only 5.1%.

Most of the studies included in this review had a cross-sectional design, with the exception of one case-control study. In this case-control study, symptomatic assessment and esophageal investigations were performed in 25 consecutive patients with IBS attending a gastroenterological clinic [11]. The frequency of GERD overlapping with and without IBS was 28.0% and 7.0%, respectively, with an odds ratio of 5.44 (95% CI: 1.84–16.09). They also showed that lower esophageal sphincter pressure was significantly less in patients with IBS than in age- and sex-matched controls.

Among 2680 Japanese workers who received a routine health check-up, the frequency of GERD overlapping with and without IBS was 16.0% and 6.4%, respectively, with an odds ratio of GERD overlapping with IBS for without IBS of 2.81 (95% CI: 2.04–3.88) [3].

Similar analysis in the general population have been performed in the United States, South Korea, and Mexico [12]. The frequency of GERD overlapping with IBS was 35.2% (male) and 31.7% (female); 21.2% and 49.6% in the United States, South Korea, and Mexico, respectively; and that of non-IBS was 16.3% (male) and 16.2% (female), 7.2% and 37.7%, respectively, with an odds ratios of overlapping GERD with IBS for non-IBS of 2.81 (95% CI: 1.75–4.52), 2.06 (1.43–2.98), 3.46 (2.18–5.49), and 1.62 (1.04–2.53), respectively [12].

10.1.1.3 Inflammatory Bowel Disease

As for the complications of IBS in inflammatory bowel disease (IBD) in remission, 45.6%, 59.7%, and 57.0% of Crohn's disease (CD) and 46.0%, 38.6%, and 33.0% of ulcerative colitis (UC) have been reported [13–15]. Thus, CD has a greater association with IBS than UC [13–15]. A study conducted in a hospital in Iran compared UC patients and controls recruited from an orthopedic minor trauma outpatient clinic [16]. The results showed that the prevalence of IBS-like symptoms in UC patients in remission and controls was 46.0% and 13.0%, respectively [16]. The odds ratio of IBS overlapping with UC for controls was 5.70 (95% CI: 2.57–12.65).

Simrén et al. showed that the group with IBS-like symptoms (in both UC and CD) had higher levels of anxiety and depression and reduction in well-being than those without IBS-like symptoms [15]. Moreover, anxiety and reduced vitality were found to be independent predictors for IBS-like symptoms in these patients [15].

Because the symptoms of IBS and IBD can be similar, IBS may not simply co-occur with IBD but may, in fact, represent early stages of IBD. A prospective study analyzed the potential of IBS to develop into IBD. García Rodríguez et al., in their study, followed up patients diagnosed with IBS, FD, and controls on average over a 3-year period [17]. The overall incidences of IBD were reported to be 10.3 per 1000 person-years for FD and 2.6 per 1000 person-years for IBS. They found a significantly increased risk of detecting IBD among patients initially diagnosed with IBS (relative risk (RR), 16.3; 95% CI: 6.6–40.7), which was constant during the entire follow-up period. No association was found between FD and IBD.

10.1.2 Extra-Gastrointestinal Physical Comorbidities

Many IBS patients complain of functional symptoms such as headache, noncardiac chest pain, backache, and uncomfortable urination. A systematic review analyzed the relationship between extragastrointestinal physical comorbidities and IBS [18]. The study reported that diseases complicated with IBS were fibromyalgia, chronic fatigue syndrome, chronic pelvic pain, temporomandibular joint disorder, interstitial cystitis, and premenstrual syndrome [18]. The association between IBS and fibromyalgia has been studied more than any other IBS extra-gastrointestinal physical comorbidity. The prevalence of fibromyalgia in the general population was reported to be 2.0% [19]. Fibromyalgia occurs in approximately 32.5% (range, 28%–65%) of IBS patients, and IBS occurs in an estimated 48% (range, 32–77%) of patients with fibromyalgia [18]. The prevalence of chronic fatigue syndrome in the general population was reported to be 0.4% [20]. Compared with the general population, the presence of IBS in patients with chronic fatigue syndrome was reported to a high degree, ranging from 35% to 92% (median, 51%) [18]. A study reported that the presence of chronic fatigue syndrome in IBS was 14% [21]. The prevalence of chronic pelvic pain in the general population was reported to be between 5.7% and 26.6% [22]. Chronic pelvic pain rates in IBS patients were reported to be between 29% and 79% (median, 49.9%) [18]. A study reported that 35% of women with IBS reported chronic pelvic pain [23]. Gallotta et al. performed a cross-sectional analysis regarding the prevalence and risk of temporomandibular joint disorder in patients with IBS [24]. They found that patients with IBS had a higher risk of temporomandibular joint disorder than healthy controls (54.9% vs. 26.3%, odds ratio = 3.41, 95% CI: 1.66–7.01) [24]. Nickel et al. showed that the prevalence of self-reported associated condition diagnosis in interstitial cystitis with and without IBS was 38.6% and 5.2%, respectively [25]. A cross-sectional study revealed that the prevalence of IBS was significantly higher in patients with premenstrual syndrome than in the control group (13.6% vs. 8.1%) [26].

10.1.3 Psychological Comorbidities

A systematic review analyzed more than 20 studies on the overlap between IBS and psychiatric disorders [18]. The analysis revealed that 54–94% of IBS patients meet the criteria for at least one primary psychiatric disorder [18, 27–29]. Most studies reported the prevalence of psychiatric disorders in IBS to be 90% or higher [18, 28–33]. However, when interpreting these statistics, we must consider patients who are present in medical clinics and patients with IBS seen in the community. From this perspective, most IBS patients presenting in medical clinics and approximately 18% of people with IBS seen in the community have one or more psychiatric disorders [18, 28–34]. No single psychiatric disorder is uniquely associated with IBS [18]. However, the psychiatric diagnoses most commonly associated with IBS are major depression, followed by the generalized anxiety disorder [18]. A large-scale survey conducted in Japan showed that the morbidity rates of panic disorder and agoraphobia were significantly higher in IBS than in non-IBS subjects [35]. The odds ratio of panic disorder and agoraphobia overlapping with IBS for non-IBS was calculated as 3.58 (95% CI: 2.23–5.75). Whitehead et al. analyzed the clinical database of healthcare utilization in the United States and compared patients with IBS with age- and gender-matched controls to determine whether IBS patients are at a greater risk for specific comorbid disorders [36]. They showed that the following ten psychiatric diagnoses implied a significant association with IBS: bruxism (stress reaction) (odds ratio 5.93 (95% CI: 3.79–9.27)), attention deficit (odds ratio 3.95 (95% CI: 1.97–7.95)), generalized anxiety (odds ratio 3.76 (95% CI: 2.16–6.56)), anxiety state (odds ratio 3.02 (95% CI: 2.48–3.69)), panic attack (odds ratio 3.00 (95% CI: 2.03–4.46)), stress reaction (odds ratio 2.69 (95% CI: 2.24–3.23)), somatization disorder (odds ratio 2.35 (95% CI: 1.28–4.32)), depression (odds ratio 2.31 (95% CI: 2.01–2.64)), adjustment reaction (odds ratio 2.22 (95% CI: 1.74–2.83)), and substance abuse (odds ratio 1.33 (95% CI: 1.09–1.63)) [36]. Simrén et al. reported that psychologic distress, including anxiety and depression, was associated with the severity of at least one symptom of IBS and a gradual reduction in quality of life [37, 38]. Vanuytsel et al. investigated the effect of mental stress on intestinal permeability using a human stress model [39]. They showed public speech increased intestinal permeability through a significant elevation in cortisol, suggesting the involvement of mast cells [39]. Cytokines and inflammatory reactions also play important roles in the development of IBS [40]. The aggravation of IBS symptoms may exacerbate the psychological burden and anxiety-depression symptoms, exhibiting a close interactive correlation [41] (Fig. 10.1).

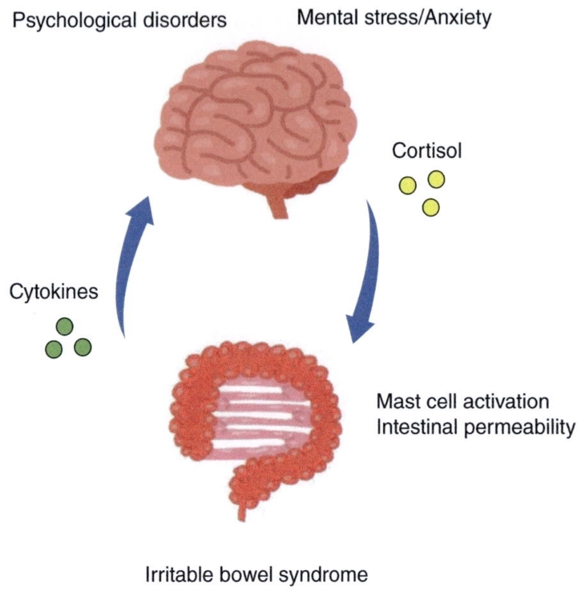

Fig. 10.1 Overlap between IBS and Psychiatric disorders

10.2 Conclusion

FD; GERD; extragastrointestinal physical comorbidities including fibromyalgia, chronic fatigue syndrome, and chronic pelvic pain; and psychological disorders including panic disorder and depression are associated with IBS (Fig. 10.2). These factors can exacerbate IBS symptoms and reduce the patient's quality of life; thus, physicians must pay attention to regions beyond the gastrointestinal tract and consider the most appropriate treatment for IBS comorbidities.

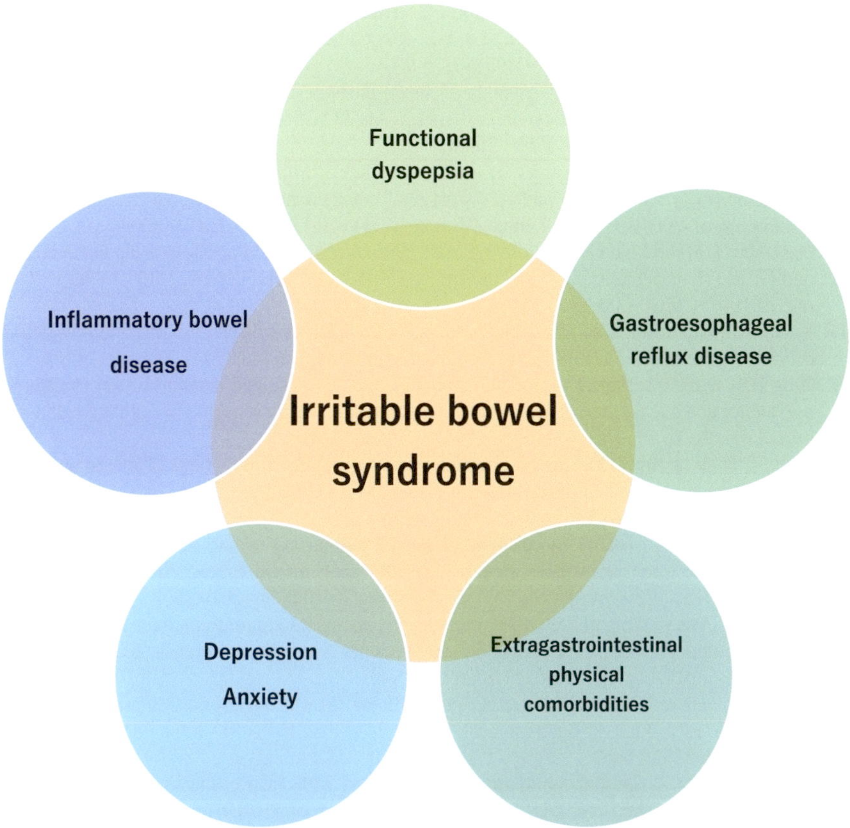

Fig. 10.2 Comorbidities with Irritable Bowel Syndrome (IBS)

References

1. Stanghellini V, et al. Gastroduodenal Disorders. Gastroenterology. 2016;150:1380–92. https://doi.org/10.1053/j.gastro.2016.02.011.
2. Riedl A, et al. Somatic comorbidities of irritable bowel syndrome: a systematic analysis. J Psychosom Res. 2008;64:573–82. https://doi.org/10.1016/j.jpsychores.2008.02.021.
3. Kaji M, et al. Prevalence of overlaps between GERD, FD and IBS and impact on health-related quality of life. J Gastroenterol Hepatol. 2010;25:1151–6. https://doi.org/10.1111/j.1440-1746.2010.06249.x.
4. Lee HJ, et al. Depressive mood and quality of life in functional gastrointestinal disorders: differences between functional dyspepsia, irritable bowel syndrome and overlap syndrome. Gen Hosp Psychiatry. 2010;32:499–502. https://doi.org/10.1016/j.genhosppsych.2010.05.002.
5. Wang A, et al. The clinical overlap between functional dyspepsia and irritable bowel syndrome based on Rome III criteria. BMC Gastroenterol. 2008;8:43. https://doi.org/10.1186/1471-230x-8-43.
6. Olafsdottir LB, Gudjonsson H, Jonsdottir HH, Thjodleifsson B. Natural history of functional dyspepsia: a 10-year population-based study. Digestion. 2010;81:53–61. https://doi.org/10.1159/000243783.

7. Agreus L, Svardsudd K, Nyren O, Tibblin G. Irritable bowel syndrome and dyspepsia in the general population: overlap and lack of stability over time. Gastroenterology. 1995;109:671–80. https://doi.org/10.1016/0016-5085(95)90373-9.
8. Talley NJ, et al. Overlapping upper and lower gastrointestinal symptoms in irritable bowel syndrome patients with constipation or diarrhea. Am J Gastroenterol. 2003;98:2454–9. https://doi.org/10.1111/j.1572-0241.2003.07699.x.
9. Corsetti M, Caenepeel P, Fischler B, Janssens J, Tack J. Impact of coexisting irritable bowel syndrome on symptoms and pathophysiological mechanisms in functional dyspepsia. Am J Gastroenterol. 2004;99:1152–9. https://doi.org/10.1111/j.1572-0241.2004.30040.x.
10. Nastaskin I, Mehdikhani E, Conklin J, Park S, Pimentel M. Studying the overlap between IBS and GERD: a systematic review of the literature. Dig Dis Sci. 2006;51:2113–20. https://doi.org/10.1007/s10620-006-9306-y.
11. Smart HL, Nicholson DA, Atkinson M. Gastro-oesophageal reflux in the irritable bowel syndrome. Gut. 1986;27:1127–31. https://doi.org/10.1136/gut.27.10.1127.
12. Jung HK, et al. Overlap of gastro-oesophageal reflux disease and irritable bowel syndrome: prevalence and risk factors in the general population. Aliment Pharmacol Ther. 2007;26:453–61. https://doi.org/10.1111/j.1365-2036.2007.03366.x.
13. Piche T, et al. Impact of functional bowel symptoms on quality of life and fatigue in quiescent Crohn disease and irritable bowel syndrome. Neurogastroenterol Motil. 2010;22:626–e174. https://doi.org/10.1111/j.1365-2982.2010.01502.x.
14. Keohane J, et al. Irritable bowel syndrome-type symptoms in patients with inflammatory bowel disease: a real association or reflection of occult inflammation? Am J Gastroenterol. 2010;105(1788):1789–94; quiz 1795. https://doi.org/10.1038/ajg.2010.156.
15. Simren M, et al. Quality of life in inflammatory bowel disease in remission: the impact of IBS-like symptoms and associated psychological factors. Am J Gastroenterol. 2002;97:389–96. https://doi.org/10.1111/j.1572-0241.2002.05475.x.
16. Ansari R, et al. Ulcerative colitis and irritable bowel syndrome: relationships with quality of life. Eur J Gastroenterol Hepatol. 2008;20:46–50. https://doi.org/10.1097/MEG.0b013e3282f16a62.
17. Gravina AG, et al. Gastric xanthomatosis associated with gastric intestinal metaplasia in a dyspeptic patient. Dig Liver Dis. 2009;41:765. https://doi.org/10.1016/j.dld.2008.08.003.
18. Whitehead WE, Palsson O, Jones KR. Systematic review of the comorbidity of irritable bowel syndrome with other disorders: what are the causes and implications? Gastroenterology. 2002;122:1140–56. https://doi.org/10.1053/gast.2002.32392.
19. Wolfe F, Ross K, Anderson J, Russell IJ, Hebert L. The prevalence and characteristics of fibromyalgia in the general population. Arthritis Rheum. 1995;38:19–28. https://doi.org/10.1002/art.1780380104.
20. Jason LA, et al. A community-based study of chronic fatigue syndrome. Arch Intern Med. 1999;159:2129–37. https://doi.org/10.1001/archinte.159.18.2129.
21. Jones KR, et al. Comorbid disorders and symptoms in irritable bowel syndrome (IBS) compared to other gastroenterology patients. Gastroenterology. 2001;120:A66. https://doi.org/10.1016/S0016-5085(08)80328-9.
22. Ahangari A. Prevalence of chronic pelvic pain among women: an updated review. Pain Physician. 2014;17:E141–7.
23. Walker EA, Gelfand AN, Gelfand MD, Green C, Katon WJ. Chronic pelvic pain and gynecological symptoms in women with irritable bowel syndrome. J Psychosom Obstet Gynaecol. 1996;17:39–46. https://doi.org/10.3109/01674829609025662.
24. Gallotta S, et al. High risk of temporomandibular disorder in irritable bowel syndrome: is there a correlation with greater illness severity? World J Gastroenterol. 2017;23:103–9. https://doi.org/10.3748/wjg.v23.i1.103.
25. Nickel JC, et al. Interstitial cystitis/painful bladder syndrome and associated medical conditions with an emphasis on irritable bowel syndrome, fibromyalgia and chronic fatigue syndrome. J Urol. 2010;184:1358–63. https://doi.org/10.1016/j.juro.2010.06.005.

26. Bahrami A, et al. The association of trace elements with premenstrual syndrome, dysmenorrhea and irritable bowel syndrome in adolescents. Eur J Obstet Gynecol Reprod Biol. 2019;233:114–9. https://doi.org/10.1016/j.ejogrb.2018.12.017.
27. Irwin C, et al. Comorbidity of posttraumatic stress disorder and irritable bowel syndrome. J Clin Psychiatry. 1996;57:576–8. https://doi.org/10.4088/jcp.v57n1204.
28. Lydiard RB, Fossey MD, Marsh W, Ballenger JC. Prevalence of psychiatric disorders in patients with irritable bowel syndrome. Psychosomatics. 1993;34:229–34. https://doi.org/10.1016/s0033-3182(93)71884-8.
29. Walker EA, Gelfand AN, Gelfand MD, Katon WJ. Psychiatric diagnoses, sexual and physical victimization, and disability in patients with irritable bowel syndrome or inflammatory bowel disease. Psychol Med. 1995;25:1259–67. https://doi.org/10.1017/s0033291700033225.
30. Walker EA, et al. Psychiatric illness and irritable bowel syndrome: a comparison with inflammatory bowel disease. Am J Psychiatry. 1990;147:1656–61. https://doi.org/10.1176/ajp.147.12.1656.
31. Fossey MD, Lydiard RB. Anxiety and the gastrointestinal system. Psychiatr Med. 1990;8:175–86.
32. Liss JL, Alpers D, Woodruff RA Jr. The irritable colon syndrome and psychiatric illness. Dis Nerv Syst. 1973;34:151–7.
33. Woodman CL, et al. The relationship between irritable bowel syndrome and psychiatric illness. A family study. Psychosomatics. 1998;39:45–54. https://doi.org/10.1016/s0033-3182(98)71380-5.
34. Walker EA, Katon WJ, Jemelka RP, Roy-Bryne PP. Comorbidity of gastrointestinal complaints, depression, and anxiety in the Epidemiologic Catchment Area (ECA) Study. Am J Med. 1992;92:26s–30s. https://doi.org/10.1016/0002-9343(92)90133-v.
35. Kumano H, et al. Comorbidity of irritable bowel syndrome, panic disorder, and agoraphobia in a Japanese representative sample. Am J Gastroenterol. 2004;99:370–6. https://doi.org/10.1111/j.1572-0241.2004.04048.x.
36. Whitehead WE, et al. Comorbidity in irritable bowel syndrome. Am J Gastroenterol. 2007;102:2767–76. https://doi.org/10.1111/j.1572-0241.2007.01540.x.
37. Simren M, et al. Cumulative effects of psychologic distress, visceral hypersensitivity, and abnormal transit on patient-reported outcomes in irritable bowel syndrome. Gastroenterology. 2019;157:391–402.e392. https://doi.org/10.1053/j.gastro.2019.04.019.
38. Pohl D, et al. Functional dyspepsia and severity of psychologic symptoms associate with postprandial symptoms in patients with irritable bowel syndrome. Clin Gastroenterol Hepatol. 2018;16:1745–53.e1741. https://doi.org/10.1016/j.cgh.2018.04.034.
39. Vanuytsel T, et al. Psychological stress and corticotropin-releasing hormone increase intestinal permeability in humans by a mast cell-dependent mechanism. Gut. 2014;63:1293–9. https://doi.org/10.1136/gutjnl-2013-305690.
40. Liebregts T, et al. Immune activation in patients with irritable bowel syndrome. Gastroenterology. 2007;132:913–20. https://doi.org/10.1053/j.gastro.2007.01.046.
41. Gao J. Correlation between anxiety-depression status and cytokines in diarrhea-predominant irritable bowel syndrome. Exp Ther Med. 2013;6:93–6. https://doi.org/10.3892/etm.2013.1101.

Part IV
Treatment

Chapter 11
Pharmacotherapy for IBS-D

Yoshiko Fujikawa and Kazunari Tominaga

Abstract Irritable bowel syndrome (IBS) is characterized by chronic and recurrent abdominal pain associated with defecation or a change in bowel habits. These problem are caused by complex and combined physiological factors such as serotonin (5-HT), bile acid, microbiota, low-grade mucosal inflammation, immune activation, intestinal permeability, and psychosocial factors. In accordance with the above pathophysiological factors, antispasmodic drugs, probiotics, loperamide, 5-HT$_3$ receptor antagonists, bile acid sequestrants, and antidepressants have been utilized for pharmacotherapy in patients with diarrhea-dominant IBS (IBS-D). Furthermore, there are many randomized controlled trials that have shown 5-HT$_3$ receptor antagonists (alosetron, ramosetron), a mixed opioid receptor acting drug (eluxadoline), and nonabsorbable antibiotics (rifaximin) are notably effective in improving abdominal pain and stool consistency in patients with IBS-D.

Keywords Enteric nervous system · Irritable bowel syndrome with diarrhea

11.1 Introduction

Irritable bowel syndrome (IBS) is characterized by chronic and recurrent abdominal pain that is associated with defecation or a change in bowel habits in spite of the lack of any macroscopic gastrointestinal changes [1]. The pathogenesis of IBS is primarily due to motility disorders and visceral hypersensitivity of the colon that is associated with the brain-gut axis or gut-brain axis. The gastrointestinal tract is fundamentally innervated by the enteric nervous system (ENS) and the central nervous system (CNS). Interactions between both systems are responsible for controlling digestive tract functions such as motility, secretion, absorption, and blood flow

---

Y. Fujikawa (✉)
Department of Gastroenterology, Higashisumiyoshi Morimoto Hospital, Osaka, Japan

K. Tominaga
Department of Gastroenterology, Osaka Gyoumeikan Hospital, Osaka, Japan

© The Editor(s) (if applicable) and The Author(s), under exclusive license to Springer Nature Singapore Pte Ltd. 2024

T. Kamiya, S. Fukudo (eds.), *Irritable Bowel Syndrome*,
https://doi.org/10.1007/978-981-97-8410-3_11

[2]. Furthermore, various factors ranging from the brain to the digestive tract, such as psychosocial factors (stress, anxiety, depression), microbiota, low-grade mucosal inflammation, immune activation, intestinal permeability, luminal factors including serotonin (5-hydroxytryptamine; 5-HT), bile acid (BA), and short-chain fatty acid (SCFA), have been reported to be associated with gastrointestinal dysfunction [3, 4]. Therefore, treatment for IBS is usually targeted at the predominant or most troublesome symptoms in the patient and primarily associated pathophysiology that might be responsible for the above symptoms. Currently, pharmacotherapy for IBS is divided into peripheral acting drugs such as antispasmodics, probiotics, antibiotics, opioid receptor acting drugs, 5-HT_3 receptor antagonists, and bile acid sequestrants, along with central acting drugs such as tricyclic antidepressants and selective serotonin reuptake inhibitors. In this chapter, we review and introduce the mechanism and pharmaceutical efficacy for agents used for diarrhea-dominant IBS (IBS-D), especially highlighting drugs with regard to their target in order to peripheral action.

11.2 The Roles of ENS and CNS in Physiological Functions of the Gastrointestinal Tract

The ENS is an intrinsic nervous system that has two major plexuses, the myenteric plexus (Auerbach's plexus) and the submucosal plexus (Meissner's plexus). The neural plexus is composed of neurons and enteric glial cells. The myenteric plexus primarily coordinates the gastrointestinal motility, while the submucosal plexus primarily regulates secretion and blood flow. The types of the major neurons are defined as intrinsic primary afferent neurons (IPAN), interneurons, and excitatory or inhibitory motor neurons, all which have been previously characterized [5]. IPANs have cell bodies in the myenteric plexus or in the submucosal plexus, with the processes extending to the muscularis mucosa as well as the processes synapsing with the interneurons. Thus, IPANs are the primary sensors in the gut for luminal distention, chemical content, or 5-HT release from the enterochromaffin cells (ECs), which are detected by the endings of the IPAN. Subsequently, IPANs activate ascending and descending interneurons followed by stimulation of excitatory and inhibitory motor neurons, respectively. Interneurons control motor neurons mediated by neurotransmitters such as encephalin, acetylcholine (ACh), and 5-HT in order to coordinate the timing of contraction and relaxation. Briefly, excitatory motor neurons cause oral muscle contraction by releasing acetylcholine and substance P, while inhibitory motor neurons cause anal muscle relaxation by releasing adenosine triphosphate (ATP)/β nicotinamide adenine dinucleotide, nitric oxide, and vasoactive intestinal peptide (VIP). Thus, this coordination makes it possible to propel the luminal contents in a proximal-distal direction. In addition to the motor reflex, the secretomotor reflexes are also initiated through the IPAN. Submucosal secretomotor neurons stimulate enterocytes that are mediated by the release of ACh and VIP, with the enterocytes then inducing water and electrolyte (Cl^-) secretion.

Although ENS can sense the gut environment and control local peristaltic reflexes independent of the CNS, the CNS is also involved in the motor functions and the sensory information in the gastrointestinal tract through the autonomic nervous system. The parasympathetic efferent pathways, such as vagal and sacral nerves, exert an excitatory effect on the motor and secretomotor functions. On the contrary, the sympathetic efferent pathways inhibit these functions. In contrast, sensory information is transmitted to the CNS by the extrinsic primary afferent neurons (EPAN), which have cell bodies in both the dorsal root ganglia (spinal primary afferent neurons) and the nodose and jugular ganglia (vagal afferent neurons). The vagal afferent neurons transmit non-noxious sensation such as satiety, nausea, bloating response to physiological mechanical distention, or chemical stimulation, while the splanchnic afferent neurons transmit the pain sensation response to noxious stimulation (Fig. 11.1) [5, 6]. Thus, the gastrointestinal functions are physiologically based on this intricate balance of interactions. As a result, if impairment of any of the components associated with the gut environment occurs, this means that physiological conditions cannot be maintained, thereby potentially leading to unfavorable/pathological conditions.

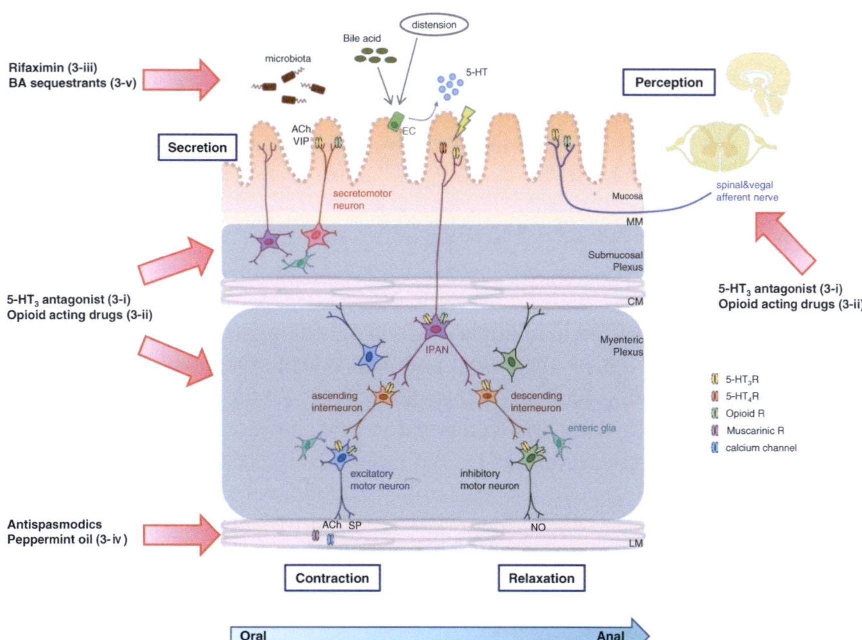

Fig. 11.1 Mechanism of peristaltic reflexes and visceral perception and pharmacological action of IBS-D drugs in the gastrointestinal tract

11.3 Pharmacotherapy for IBS-D

11.3.1 5-HT$_3$ Receptor Antagonists (Alosetron and Ramosetron)

5-HT is an important neurotransmitter in the brain and the ENS, and with 90% of 5-HT in the whole body synthesized, stored, and released by the ECs in the gastrointestinal tract. 5-HT has several roles in gastrointestinal function including peristalsis, secretion, vasodilation, and visceral sensation through activation of intrinsic and extrinsic afferent nerves [7]. It has been reported that abnormalities in 5-HT metabolism has been found to exist in patients with IBS. It has been shown that IBS-D patients have a reduced uptake of 5-HT by platelets and mRNA expression levels of the 5-HT reuptake transporter in the duodenal mucosa [8], in addition to having increased postprandial plasma levels of 5-HT [9]. Due to these abnormal circumstances with regard to the 5-HT contents, this can lead to suffer from chronic diarrhea and abdominal pain in IBS-D patients. Among the various types of 5-HT, both 5-HT$_3$ and 5-HT$_4$ are significantly important for gastrointestinal functions. 5-HT$_3$ receptors are expressed on various cells of the gut, including intrinsic and extrinsic afferent nerves that extend into the mucosa, interneurons, inhibitory and excitatory motor neurons, interstitial cells of Cajal (ICC), smooth muscle, and enterocytes. Although precise mechanisms for the pharmacological action of the 5-HT$_3$ antagonist are unknown, it has been speculated that the 5-HT$_3$ antagonist is involved in inhibiting the activation of IPAN, interneurons, and motor neurons. As a result, propulsive motility and secretion are decreased locally within the gut, thereby leading to alleviation of diarrhea. Furthermore, the 5-HT$_3$ antagonist blocks the visceral pain signal transmission from the gut to the CNS through the 5-HT$_3$ receptors on the EPAN [10].

11.3.1.1 Alosetron

Alosetron has been reported in multiple randomized controlled trials (RCTs) to contribute to adequate relief of abdominal pain and bowel symptoms such as bowel urgency, stool frequency, and stool consistency [11]. When the administration of alosetron (1 mg) twice daily was compared to placebo at 12 weeks, there was a significantly greater proportion of days with satisfactory control of bowel urgency (73% vs. 57%, $p < 0.001$) and IBS global improvement responders (76% vs. 44%, $p < 0.001$), respectively [12]. Furthermore, alosetron (0.5 mg or 1 mg) once daily and 1 mg twice daily were effective in the global improvement of the IBS symptoms as compared to placebo (50.8%, 48% and 42.9% of the patients in the respective treatment group, vs. 30.7% for the placebo). However, there was a gradual increase in the constipation noted in these patients (9%, 16% and 19% patients in the respective treatment groups) [13].

A recent prospective open-label study demonstrated that of 105 fully evaluable patients, approximately half of these patients (45%), met the US Food and Drug Administration (FDA) composite endpoint responder, which was defined as at least a 50% reduction of both abdominal pain intensity and stool consistency during the study evaluation period [14]. However, the use of alosetron was restricted to female IBS-D patients who did not exhibit an adequate response to conventional therapy, in addition to having chronic IBS symptoms (greater than 6 months) due to the risk of adverse events that included severe constipation or ischemic colitis.

11.3.1.2 Ramosetron

Ramosetron is another 5-HT_3 antagonist that has been marketed in Japan, Korea, and Taiwan. A RCT that evaluated the administration of ramosetron (5 μg) once daily in male IBS-D patients showed that the monthly responder rates were significantly better as compared to placebo for improvement in stool consistency (50.8% vs. 19.6%), relief of overall IBS symptoms (31.3% vs. 9.5%), and relief of abdominal pain (32.0% vs. 10.1%) during the first month ($p < 0.001$, respectively) [15]. Subsequently, ramosetron (2.5 μg) was also reported to improve the symptoms of female IBS-D patients [16]. Unlike for alosetron, ischemic colitis as an adverse event was not reported in the ramosetron RCTs. Meta-analysis showed that the pooled risk ratio (RR) for the global IBS symptoms that improved after 5-HT_3 receptor antagonists versus placebo was 1.56 (95% CI: 1.43–1.71), while the pooled RR for the development of constipation with the 5-HT_3 receptor antagonist versus placebo was 3.71 (95% CI: 2.98–4.61) [17]. A network meta-analysis of RCTs showed that both alosetron and ramosetron were more effective for IBS-D treatment as compared to rifaximin and eluxadoline [18].

11.3.2 Drugs Acting on Opioid Receptors (Trimebutine, Loperamide, and Eluxadoline)

Opioid drugs are extensively prescribed for pain treatment. However, long-term use often leads to opioid-induced bowel dysfunction such as constipation and narcotic bowel syndrome, as endogenous opioids and their receptors are expressed in the ENS, ICC, and smooth muscle cells. Opioid receptors are classified into three types of receptors (μ, δ, κ), all of which are G protein-coupled receptors and expressed on myenteric and submucosal neurons in the ENS. In general, opioids affect the entire gastrointestinal tract, which is mediated by the ubiquitously localized μ-receptor. Activation of opioid receptors inhibits the adenylate cyclase and voltage-gated Ca^{2+} channels and activates the K^+ channels. Thus, in the ENS, opioid receptor agonists inhibit the release of neurotransmitter from the myenteric motor neuron, interneurons, and submucosal neurons, thereby causing the inhibition of peristalsis and intestinal secretion [19]. Therefore, drugs that act on opioid receptors, such as trimebutine, loperamide, and eluxadoline, can be used to treat IBS-D.

11.3.2.1 Trimebutine

Trimebutine is an opioid receptor agonist. This drug exerts dual effects on the intestinal motility. For example, a low dose of trimebutine inhibits norepinephrine release from the sympathetic nerve terminal and accelerates motility by preventing the adrenergic inhibition caused by the acetylcholine release. In contrast, a high dose of trimebutine inhibits acetylcholine release from the cholinergic neuron in the myenteric plexus, resulting in suppression of motility [20]. Furthermore, trimebutine has been found to be effective against visceral hyperalgesia induced by inflammation or stress in the rat [21]. Although there have only been a few small size RCTs performed, a meta-analysis demonstrated that trimebutine improved abdominal pain and global symptoms in IBS [22].

11.3.2.2 Loperamide

Loperamide is a peripheral μ-opioid receptor agonist that has been used to treat the antidiarrheal effect in IBS-D patients for many years. However, only a few small-sized RCTs have been able to demonstrate definitive evidence for the treatment efficacy of loperamide in IBS-D patients. These RCTs indicated that loperamide improved both stool frequency and consistency. However, loperamide has not been shown to be effective for abdominal pain and bloating [23].

11.3.2.3 Eluxadoline

Eluxadoline has mixed opioid receptor actions including both the μ-opioid and κ-opioid receptor agonist and the δ-opioid receptor antagonist. This agent was newly approved by the FDA in 2015. The μ-opioid receptor agonist acts by reducing gastrointestinal transit and secretion. However, the δ-opioid receptor antagonist counteracts the excessive inhibition of gastrointestinal motility mediated via the μ-opioid receptor agonistic action [24]. Using a stressed mice model, it was demonstrated that eluxadoline properly regulated the fecal output within control levels over a wide dose range. In contrast, loperamide significantly reduced the fecal output below control levels [25]. Therefore, eluxadoline can normalize bowel function without suppression of gut motility. The role of the κ-opioid receptor agonistic function of eluxadoline remains unclear. However, because the κ-opioid receptor has been shown to be involved in visceral sensation while its agonist (asimadoline) was shown to reduce abdominal pain in patients with IBS-D [26], it was suggested that eluxadoline might be able to improve visceral hyperalgesia.

In two large prospective phase 3 studies (IBS-3001 and IBS-3002), efficacy of eluxadoline (75 and 100 mg twice daily) was evaluated in a total of 2427 patients with IBS-D at 12 weeks (an FDA end-point) and at 26 weeks (a European Medicines Agency end-point). Pooled data indicated that eluxadoline was effective in simultaneously relieving abdominal pain and improving stool consistency as compared to placebo (26.2% and 27.0% with the 75 mg and 100 mg dose, respectively, vs. 16.7% in the placebo, $p < 0.001$, at 12 weeks and 26.7% and 31.0% with the 75 mg and 100 mg dose, respectively, vs, 19.5% placebo, $p < 0.001$, at 26 weeks) [27]. Another post hoc analysis of two phase 3 trials evaluated one-third of the patients who had previously used loperamide. Among the patients that had inadequate control of symptoms after a prior treatment with loperamide, eluxadoline significantly improved the composite symptoms as compared to placebo (26.3% and 27.0% with the 75 mg and 100 mg dose, respectively, vs. 12.7% in the placebo, $p < 0.001$). In contrast, among the patients showing adequate control of symptoms after a prior treatment with loperamide, subsequent treatment with eluxadoline (100 mg) resulted in a significantly greater proportion of responders as compared to placebo (41.8% vs. 25.0%, $p = 0.006$) [28]. Although adverse events such as sphincter of Oddi spasm and pancreatitis were rarely reported in these phase 3 studies, eluxadoline is contraindicated in patients with cholecystectomy and alcohol abuse. In a phase 4 study that excluded patients with a history of pancreatitis, known or suspected biliary duct obstruction, or sphincter of Oddi disease, adverse events were comparable between both the eluxadoline and placebo groups (37.4% vs 35.3%), and there were no cases of sphincter of Oddi spasm or pancreatitis reported [29].

11.3.3 Nonabsorbable Antibiotics (Rifaximin)

It has been shown that some patients with IBS have exhibited alterations in their microbiota profile in the small intestine and colon, along with small intestinal bacterial overgrowth. Changes in gut microbiota can influence the intestinal immune system, bile acid metabolism, and production of SCFA, which leads to an increased intestinal permeability, acceleration of colonic motility, and visceral sensitivity [4].

11.3.3.1 Rifaximin

Rifaximin is an oral nonabsorbable antibiotic that targets the gut and is associated with a low risk of bacterial resistance. The FDA approved rifaximin for the treatment of IBS-D in 2015. Although the mechanisms responsible for the clinical benefits of rifaximin in patients with IBS-D are unknown, it is considered that rifaximin affects the gut microbiota, mucosal inflammation, and intestinal permeability [30]. Two large RCTs (TARGET1 and TARGET2) have examined the efficacy of rifaximin in patients with IBS-D. A 2-week rifaximin treatment (550 mg) three times a day resulted in an adequate relief of global IBS symptoms as compared to placebo during the first 4 weeks after treatment (40.7% vs. 31.7%, $p < 0.001$, combined data from the above two studies). The therapeutic efficacy for the drug persisted for up to 10 weeks after the treatment. In addition, abdominal bloating, abdominal pain, and stool consistency were also remarkably improved [31]. The safety profile for rifaximin use was similar to that found for the placebo, with no reports on any presence of *Clostridium difficile*-associated diarrhea or ischemic colitis. Furthermore, retreatment with rifaximin was effective even in patients with IBS-D who relapsed during the 18-week follow-up period after receiving an initial 2-week treatment with rifaximin. The proportion of responders, which was defined as improvement in both abdominal pain and stool consistency (a primary end point of this study), was greater in the rifaximin-treated group as compared with placebo (38.1% vs. 31.5%, $p = 0.03$). In addition, repeat treatment with rifaximin did not increase the incidence of AEs [32]. Meta-analysis showed that rifaximin was significantly effective as compared to the placebo for global IBS symptom improvement (odds ratio = 1.57; 95% CI = 1.2–2.0, number needed to treat (NNT) = 10.2) [33].

11.3.4 Smooth Muscle Antispasmodics

Antispasmodics inhibit acetylcholine action at muscarinic receptors or via blockade of the calcium channels that are present on the gastrointestinal smooth muscle. Since some of the IBS patients have an abnormal contractility of gastrointestinal smooth muscle and an altered gastrointestinal transit leading to pain and disturbances in bowel habits, antispasmodic drugs have been used to treat these patients for many years. Meta-analysis [34] and Cochrane Reviews [35] have demonstrated that there is evidence that antispasmodics such as cimetropium/dicyclomine, pinaverium, trimebutine, otilonium, hyoscine, and peppermint oil are effective for treating and improving abdominal pain and global symptoms in IBS.

11.3.4.1 Peppermint Oil

Peppermint oil (PO) and its major constituent (menthol) are calcium channel antagonists in the smooth muscle cells. In addition to antispasmodic efficacy, they also have κ-opioid receptor agonism, 5-HT_3 antagonism, anti-inflammatory action, and antinociceptive properties due to the activation of melastatin-related transient receptor potential 8 (TRPM8). It has been reported that a novel formulation of PO, which as designed for sustained release in the small intestine, was able to minimize adverse events such as heartburn and, thus, was effective in patient with IBS-D. A double-blind RCT showed that this novel PO significantly decreased the total IBS symptom score at baseline levels as compared to placebo after 24-h and 4-week treatments (24 hours; −19.6% vs. -10.3%, $p = 0.01$; 4 weeks; −40.0% vs. −25.3%, $p = 0.02$)

[36]. This decrease was especially evident for the visceral perception-related symptoms scores, such as abdominal pain or discomfort, abdominal bloating or distension, pain at evacuation, and urgency of bowel movement [36]. Recently, another meta-analysis of RCTs demonstrated that PO was effective for the global IBS symptoms (RR = 2.39; 95% CI = 1.93–2.97, NNT = 3) and abdominal pain (RR = 1.78; 95% CI = 1.43–2.20, NNT = 4) [37].

11.3.5 Bile Acid Sequestrants

Primary BA such as cholic acid (CA) and chenodeoxycholic acid (CDCA) are synthesized in hepatocytes from cholesterol and then conjugated to glycine or taurine. After eating, conjugated BAs are secreted from the gall bladder into the small intestine, which facilitate the digestion and absorption of fat. When conjugated BAs reach the terminal ileum, over 90% are actively absorbed via the ileal bile acid transporter (IBAT) and returned to the liver by the portal circulation. In the colon, bacteria will change the primary BAs that escape the ileal uptake into secondly BAs, such as deoxycholic acid (DCA), litocholic acid (LCA), and ursodeoxycholic acid (UDCA), with these residual secondary BAs excreted into the fecal material.

In the colon, luminal BAs can activate the transmembrane G protein-coupled receptor 5 (TGR5) on EC cells and stimulate secretion of 5-HT that then activates 5-HT4 receptors on IPAN. Activated IPAN releases calcitonin gene-related peptide which stimulates ascending and descending interneurons that cause the peristaltic reflex. Furthermore, activated TGR5 on the enterocytes can also induce chloride secretion via the cAMP/PKA pathway-dependent activation of the cystic fibrosis transmembrane conductance regulator (CFTR) channel [38]. Thus, BAs that modulate colonic transit are mediated by two mechanisms: secretory and prokinetic. In contrast, increased delivery of BAs into the colon causes diarrhea. In fact, the total fecal BAs and the primary BAs have been shown to be correlated with stool number and can affect both the stool form and colonic motility [39]. Approximately 25% of patients with IBS-D were shown to have BA malabsorption based on a 75SeHCAT retention test [40]. These patients have an increase of fecal BA excretion, especially of the primary BAs and serum C4, which suggests that there is a compensatory increase in the hepatic synthesis of BAs [39, 41, 42].

Unfortunately, to date, there have been no RCTs that have examined BA sequestrants in IBS. However, some BA sequestrants are known to improve IBS symptoms. For example, colestipol treatment for 8 weeks improved IBS symptom severity scores and reduced stool frequency [42]. Furthermore, colesevelam sequestered luminal BAs into the stool, thereby reducing the bowel movement and improving stool consistency [43].

11.4 Conclusions

IBS is a symptom-based disease for which suitable biomarkers for evaluation of diagnosis and treatment have yet to be established. Since the generation of IBS-D symptoms is based on the physiological gastrointestinal function, treatments with strongly acting drugs are commonly suspected to cause AEs such as constipation and ischemic colitis. However, there has been a recent increase in detailed data on potential pharmacological treatments for patients with IBS-D, due to the gradual clarification of the IBS pathogenesis and the completion of highly specific RCTs. Even so, not all of these patients are necessarily satisfied with the current treatments, a factor which is likely related to the presence of the heterogeneity of the IBS pathogenesis on a case by case basis. Therefore, we expect there will be additional progress with regard to therapeutic options when potent drugs such as histamine type 1 antagonists and NK2 antagonists are introduced as treatments in the future.

References

1. Lacy BE, Mearin F, Chang L, et al. Bowel disorders. Gastroenterology. 2016;150:1393–407.
2. Goyal RK, Hirano I. The enteric nervous system. N Engl J Med. 1996;334:1106–15.
3. Tominaga K, Fujikawa Y, Tanaka F, et al. Pharmacological treatment for functional dyspepsia and irritable bowel syndrome: current standards and promising therapies. J Gen Fam Med. 2015;16:242–51.
4. Camilleri M, Ford AC. Irritable bowel syndrome: pathophysiology and current therapeutic approaches. Handb Exp Pharmacol. 2017;239:75–113.
5. Furness JB. The enteric nervous system and neurogastroenterology. Nat Rev Gastroenterol Hepatol. 2012;9:286–94.
6. Furness JB, Jones C, Nurgali K, et al. Intrinsic primary afferent neurons and nerve circuits within the intestine. Prog Neurobiol. 2004;72:143–64.
7. Gershon MD, Tack J. The serotonin signaling system: from basic understanding to drug development for functional GI disorders. Gastroenterology. 2007;132:397–414.
8. Foley S, Garsed K, Singh G, et al. Impaired uptake of serotonin by platelets from patients with irritable bowel syndrome correlates with duodenal immune activation. Gastroenterology. 2011;140:1434–43.
9. Houghton LA, Atkinson W, Whitaker RP, et al. Increased platelet depleted plasma 5-hydroxytryptamine concentration following meal ingestion in symptomatic female subjects with diarrhoea predominant irritable bowel syndrome. Gut. 2003;52:663–70.
10. Mawe GM, Hoffman JM. Serotonin signalling in the gut—functions, dysfunctions and therapeutic targets. Nat Rev Gastroenterol Hepatol. 2013;10:473–86.
11. Brenner DM, Sayuk GS. Current US Food and Drug Administration—approved pharmacologic therapies for the treatment of irritable bowel syndrome with diarrhea. Adv Ther. 2020;37:83–96.
12. Lembo T, Wright RA, Bagby B, et al. Alosetron controls bowel urgency and provides global symptom improvement in women with diarrhea-predominant irritable bowel syndrome. Am J Gastroenterol. 2001;96:2662–70.
13. Krause R, Ameen V, Gordon SH, et al. A randomized, double-blind, placebo-controlled study to assess efficacy and safety of 0.5 mg and 1 mg alosetron in women with severe diarrhea-predominant IBS. Am J Gastroenterol. 2007;102:1709–19.

14. Lacy BE, Nicandro JP, Chuang E, et al. Alosetron use in clinical practice: significant improvement in irritable bowel syndrome symptoms evaluated using the US Food and Drug Administration composite endpoint. Ther Adv Gastroenterol. 2018;11:1–11.
15. Fukudo S, Ida M, Akiho H, et al. Effect of ramosetron on stool consistency in male patients with irritable bowel syndrome with diarrhea. Clin Gastroenterol Hepatol. 2014;12:953–9.
16. Fukudo S, Kinoshita Y, Okumura T, et al. Ramosetron reduces symptoms of irritable bowel syndrome with diarrhea and improves quality of life in women. Gastroenterology. 2016;150:358–66.
17. Zheng Y, Yu T, Tang Y, et al. Efficacy and safety of 5-hydroxytryptamine 3 receptor antagonists in irritable bowel syndrome: a systematic review and meta-analysis of randomized controlled trials. PLoS One. 2017;12:e0172846.
18. Black CJ, Burr NE, Camilleri M, et al. Efficacy of pharmacological therapies in patients with IBS with diarrhoea or mixed stool pattern: systematic review and network meta-analysis. Gut. 2020;69:74–82.
19. Galligan JJ, Sternini C. Insights into the role of opioid receptors in the gi tract: experimental evidence and therapeutic relevance. Handb Exp Pharmacol. 2017;239:363–78.
20. Taniyama K, Sano I, Nakayama S, et al. Dual effect of trimebutine on contractility of the Guinea pig ileum via the opioid receptors. Gastroenterology. 1991;101:1579–87.
21. Lacheze C, Coelho AM, Fioramonti J, et al. Influence of trimebutine on inflammation- and stress-induced hyperalgesia to rectal distension in rats. J Pharm Pharmacol. 1998;50:921–8.
22. Poynard T, Regimbeau C, Benhamou Y. Meta-analysis of smooth muscle relaxants in the treatment of irritable bowel syndrome. Aliment Pharmacol Ther. 2001;15:355–61.
23. Ford AC, Moayyedi P, Lacy BE, et al. American College of Gastroenterology monograph on the management of irritable bowel syndrome and chronic idiopathic constipation. Am J Gastroenterol. 2014;109(Suppl):S2–S26.
24. Lacy BE. Emerging treatments in neurogastroenterology: eluxadoline—a new therapeutic option for diarrhea-predominant IBS. Neurogastroenterol Motil. 2016;28:26–35.
25. Wade PR, Palmer JM, McKenney S, et al. Modulation of gastrointestinal function by MuDelta, a mixed μ opioid receptor agonist/μ opioid receptor antagonist. Br J Pharmacol. 2012;167:1111–25.
26. Camilleri M. Novel pharmacology: asimadoline, a kappa-opioid agonist, and visceral sensation. Neurogastroenterol Motil. 2008;20:971–9.
27. Lembo AJ, Lacy BE, Zuckerman MJ, et al. Eluxadoline for irritable bowel syndrome with diarrhea. N Engl J Med. 2016;374:242–53.
28. Lacy BE, Chey WD, Cash BD, et al. Eluxadoline efficacy in IBS-D patients who report prior Loperamide use. Am J Gastroenterol. 2017;112:924–32.
29. Brenner DM, Sayuk GS, Gutman CR, et al. Efficacy and safety of eluxadoline in patients with irritable bowel syndrome with diarrhea who report inadequate symptom control with loperamide: RELIEF phase 4 study. Am J Gastroenterol. 2019;114:1502–11.
30. Chey WD, Shah ED, DuPont HL. Mechanism of action and therapeutic benefit of rifaximin in patients with irritable bowel syndrome: a narrative review. Ther Adv Gastroenterol. 2020;13:1–16.
31. Pimentel M, Lembo A, Chey WD, et al. Rifaximin therapy for patients with irritable bowel syndrome without constipation. N Engl J Med. 2011;364:22–32.
32. Lembo A, Pimentel M, Rao SS, et al. Repeat treatment with rifaximin is safe and effective in patients with diarrhea-predominant irritable bowel syndrome. Gastroenterology. 2016;151:1113–21.
33. Menees SB, Maneerattannaporn M, Kim HM, et al. The efficacy and safety of rifaximin for the irritable bowel syndrome: a systematic review and meta-analysis. Am J Gastroenterol. 2012;107:28–35.
34. Ford AC, Talley NJ, Spiegel BM, et al. Effect of fibre, antispasmodics, and peppermint oil in the treatment of irritable bowel syndrome: systematic review and meta-analysis. BMJ. 2008;337:a2313.

35. Ruepert L, Quartero AO, de Wit NJ, et al. Bulking agents, antispasmodics and antidepressants for the treatment of irritable bowel syndrome. Cochrane Database Syst Rev. 2011;8:CD003460.
36. Cash BD, Epstein MS, Shah SM. A novel delivery system of peppermint oil is an effective therapy for irritable bowel syndrome symptoms. Dig Dis Sci. 2016;61:560–71.
37. Alammar N, Wang L, Saberi B, et al. The impact of peppermint oil on the irritable bowel syndrome: a meta-analysis of the pooled clinical data. BMC Complement Altern Med. 2019;19:21.
38. Bunnett NW. Neuro-humoral signalling by bile acids and the TGR5 receptor in the gastrointestinal tract. J Physiol. 2014;592:2943–50.
39. Shin A, Camilleri M, Vijayvargiya P, et al. Bowel functions, fecal unconjugated primary and secondary bile acids, and colonic transit in patients with irritable bowel syndrome. Clin Gastroenterol Hepatol. 2013;11:1270–5.
40. Aziz I, Mumtaz S, Bholah H, et al. High prevalence of idiopathic bile acid diarrhea among patients with diarrhea-predominant irritable bowel syndrome based on Rome III criteria. Clin Gastroenterol Hepatol. 2015;13:1650–5.
41. Wong BS, Camilleri M, Carlson P, et al. Increased bile acid biosynthesis is associated with irritable bowel syndrome with diarrhea. Clin Gastroenterol Hepatol. 2012;10:1009–15.
42. Bajor A, Törnblom H, Rudling M, et al. Increased colonic bile acid exposure: a relevant factor for symptoms and treatment in IBS. Gut. 2015;64:84–92.
43. Camilleri M, Acosta A, Busciglio I, et al. Effect of colesevelam on faecal bile acids and bowel functions in diarrhoea-predominant irritable bowel syndrome. Aliment Pharmacol Ther. 2015;41:438–48.

Chapter 12
Pharmacotherapy for Irritable Bowel Syndrome with Constipation

Masahiko Inamori

Abstract This chapter outlines the drug treatment of constipated irritable bowel syndrome, especially laxatives, mucosal epithelial function-altering drugs, bile acid transporter inhibitors, and 5-hydroxytryptamine receptor 4 agonists.

Keywords Irritable bowel syndrome · Constipation · Laxative · Lubiprostone · Linaclotide · Elobixibat · Tegaserod

12.1 Introduction

Many drugs are used in pharmacotherapy for the treatment of irritable bowel syndrome with constipation (IBS-C). Many improve the form of the stool and increase the frequency of bowel movements. In addition, patients with IBS-C need to be treated for gastrointestinal symptoms, such as abdominal pain and bloating. Table 12.1 lists various currently used drugs. There is a wide variety of drugs, and the evidence of their treatment with IBS-C is shown in Table 12.2. In addition, adverse events caused by these drugs are shown in Table 12.3. The following sections summarize and discuss the main drugs used for the treatment of IBS-C.

12.2 Laxative

Laxatives are broadly classified into nonirritating laxatives and osmotic laxatives. Osmotic laxatives are described in many reviews and guidelines [1–11] and are widely used in the treatment of IBS-C worldwide. There is no large-scale

M. Inamori (✉)
Department of Medical Education, Yokohama City University School of Medicine, Yokohama, Kanagawa, Japan
e-mail: inamorim@med.yokohama-cu.ac.jp

© The Editor(s) (if applicable) and The Author(s), under exclusive license to Springer Nature Singapore Pte Ltd. 2024

T. Kamiya, S. Fukudo (eds.), *Irritable Bowel Syndrome*,
https://doi.org/10.1007/978-981-97-8410-3_12

Table 12.1 Existing pharmacological therapy for IBS-C

Laxative
Osmotic
Magnesium oxide
Magnesium sulfate
Polyethylene glycol (PEG)
Lactulose
Stimulants
Senna
Rhubarb
Bisacodyl
Picosulfate
Mucosal epithelial function altering drugs
Chloride channel activators
Lubiprostone
Guanylate cyclase receptor activators
Linaclotide
Plecanatide
Sodium/hydrogen exchanger 3 inhibitor
Tenapanor
Bile acid transporter inhibitors
Elobixibat
5-HT 4 receptor agonist
Prucalopride
Mosapride

Table 12.2 Evidence of pharmacological therapy for IBS-C and chronic constipation

Treatment drug	Action sequence	Evidence quality
Magnesium oxide	Laxative osmotic	Low [1–11]
Magnesium sulfate	Laxative osmotic	Moderate [12–15]
Polyethylene glycol (PEG)	Laxative osmotic	Moderate [16–20]
Lactulose	Laxative osmotic	Moderate [18]
Senna	Laxative stimulants	Low [1, 6, 7, 9–11, 14, 21–23]
Rhubarb	Laxative stimulants	Low [1, 6, 7, 9–11, 14, 21–23]
Bisacodyl	Laxative stimulants	High [24, 25]
Picosulfate	Laxative stimulants	High [26–29]
Lubiprostone	Chloride channel activators	High [30–36]
Linaclotide	Guanylate cyclase receptor	High [37–43]
Plecanatide	Guanylate cyclase receptor activators	High [43]
Tenapanor	Sodium/hydrogen exchanger 3 inhibitor	High [43]
Elobixibat	Bile acid transporter inhibitors	High [44–48]
Tegaserod	5-HT 4 receptor agonist	High [52, 53]
Renzapride	5-HT 4 receptor agonist	High [54–57]
Prucalopride	5-HT 4 receptor agonist	High [58, 59]
Velusetrag	5-HT 4 receptor agonist	High [60]
Naronapride	5-HT 4 receptor agonist	High [61]
YKP10811	5-HT 4 receptor agonist	High [62]
Cisapride	5-HT 4 receptor agonist	High [63, 64]
Mosapride	5-HT 4 receptor agonist	Moderate [65, 66]

Table 12.3 Major adverse events of pharmacological therapy for patients with IBS-C and chronic constipation

Treatment drug	Adverse events
Magnesium oxide	Hypermagnesemia
Senna	Development of tolerance, colon pigmentation known as (pseudo-)melanosis coli and abuse
Lubiprostone	Nausea
Tegaserod	Cardiovascular events
Cisapride	QT prolongation, ventricular arrhythmia

randomized controlled trial (RCT) for magnesium oxide, the most widely used laxative in Japan, in patients with IBS-C and patients with chronic constipation. For magnesium sulfate, there is no RCT for patients with IBS; however, an RCT has shown the efficacy of magnesium sulfate in the treatment of constipation [12].

Magnesium oxide has been reported to cause hypermagnesemia when administered to patients with renal dysfunction [13]. According to the "Guidelines for Safe

Pharmaceutical Therapy for the Elderly 2015" [14] and safety information on pharmaceuticals and medical devices [15], care must be taken with the use of magnesium oxide.

The effectiveness of polyethylene glycol has been reported in a systematic review in patients with nonorganic constipation, functional constipation, and fecal impaction and in elderly patients with chronic constipation [16–18]. An RCT of patients with IBS-C showed improvements in rectal perception, symptoms, and constipation [19, 20].

There is no RCT for lactulose in patients with IBS-C, but the efficacy of lactulose has been reported in a systematic review [18] on elderly patients with chronic constipation.

Simulative laxatives are classified into anthraquinones and diphenylmethanes. Typical anthraquinone laxatives include senna and rhubarb, which are commonly used in Japan.

There are no placebo-controlled RCTs in patients with IBS-C and adults with chronic constipation regarding anthraquinone simulative laxatives, but there are many reviews and guidelines [1, 6, 7, 9–11, 21, 22]. It is widely used in the treatment of IBS-C in Japan.

Recently, the adverse effects of anthraquinone laxatives have gained attention, for which long-term administration has not been shown to be safe. It is recommended to be used on demand to avoid inducing habits owing to repeated use and abuse [14, 22, 23].

Diphenylmethane drugs include bisacodyl and picosulfate. There is no RCT for bisacodyl in patients with IBS-C, but an RCT [24, 25] has shown the efficacy of bisacodyl in the treatment of constipation. For picosulfate, there is no RCT in patients with IBS-C, but an RCT has shown the efficacy of picosulfate for the treatment of constipation [26, 27]. An RCT comparing both drugs has also been reported, and the efficacy of both drugs was showed on patients with constipation [28]. Due to concerns about the safety of the prolonged use of stimulant laxatives, a systematic review of bisacodyl and picosulfate studies in patients with constipation has been conducted, and safety up to 4 weeks has been reported [29].

12.3 Mucosal Epithelial Function-Altering Drugs

Mucosal epithelial function-altering drugs were developed relatively recently. To date, lubiprostone and linaclotide have been used as therapies [30].

Lubiprostone is scarcely absorbed into the body and activates chloride channel protein-2 channels present on intestinal mucosal epithelial cells to promote the secretion of Cl ions into the intestinal lumen. As a result, water secretion into the intestinal tract is increased, stool softening and intestinal transport are promoted, and constipation is reduced. Phase II [31, 32] and Phase III [33, 34] RCTs that show the efficacy of lubiprostone in patients with IBS-C have been reported. A meta-analysis of these RCTs shows that lubiprostone is effective for the reduction of IBS symptoms such as abdominal pain, abdominal discomfort, and abdominal distention [35]. The side effects are mainly mild diarrhea and nausea, and the drug is safe and tolerable for long-term use [36].

Linaclotide is hardly absorbed by the body, acts on the guanylate cyclase C (GC-C) receptor, activates the cystic fibrosis transmembrane conductance regulator via cGMP, and promotes the secretion of Cl ions into the intestinal lumen. As a result, water secretion into the intestinal tract is increased, stool softening and intestinal transport are promoted, and constipation is reduced. In addition, cGMP reduces visceral hypersensitivity via the suppression of submucosal afferent sensory nerves. At 12 weeks, a 30% reduction in abdominal pain and one or more spontaneous defecations without any feeling of residual stool are reported [37]. The response rates were approximately 20% in the placebo group and 34% in the linaclotide group [38]. Efficacy has also been reported in Europe [39], China [40], and Japan [41]. However, Fukudo et al. [41] showed a significantly higher overall improvement of IBS symptoms in the placebo group (33.7%) than in the linaclotide group (17.5%). Additionally, the effect was maintained for a longer period in the placebo group than in the linaclotide group.

A meta-analysis published in 2018 for GC-C receptor agonists showed that linaclotide is more effective than a placebo, with an odds ratio of 2.43 and confidence interval of 1.43–3.98 [42]. A systematic review network meta-analysis published in 2018 also reports that four mucosal epithelial function-altering drugs (lubiprostone, linaclotide, plecanatide, and tenapanor) are effective in the treatment of patients with IBS-C [43].

12.4 Bile Acid Transporter Inhibitors

Bile acids are steroid compounds that are biosynthesized from cholesterol in the liver, many of which are conjugated to glycine or taurine, secreted as the main component of bile, and temporarily stored in the gallbladder. Bile acids are then secreted into the intestine with the consumption of food, where it mixes with the pancreatic juice to activate lipase, forming micelles with dietary lipids and promoting lipid absorption. In addition, bile acids play a role in the regulation of cholesterol metabolism via bile acid reabsorption from the intestinal tract and through the conversion of cholesterol to bile acids in the liver. Bile acids secreted into the intestinal tract are modified by intestinal bacteria by deconjugation and dehydroxylation, and some are converted from primary bile acids (such as cholic acid and chenodeoxycholic acid) to secondary bile acids (such as deoxycholic acid and lithocholic acid). Approximately 95% of the bile acids secreted into the small intestine are reabsorbed by the ileal bile acid transporter (IBAT) present in the terminal ileum. These return to the liver via the portal vein and are secreted as bile again in the enterohepatic circulation. On the other hand, the remaining 5% of bile acids are excreted in the stool.

Bile acids act on transmembrane G protein-coupled receptor 5 (TGR5), which is present in colonic and intestinal epithelial cells. Bile acids activate the cystic fibrosis transmembrane conductance regulator via cAMP and stimulate the secretion of Cl ions into the intestinal tract. Bile acids also release serotonin via TGR5 on enterochromaffin cells, which acts on intrinsic sensory nerves in the submucosal layer, causing the peristaltic reflex. In other words, bile acids exert the effects of water secretion and peristalsis [44]. These effects can cause diarrhea due to the damage to the enterohepatic circulation (such as biliary obstruction/obstructive jaundice, cholecystectomy, ileum resection, and changes in the intestinal flora).

There have been attempts to use the effects of bile acids to treat chronic constipation, for example, the RCT of Rao et al. [45] in women with IBS-C. The administration of chenodeoxycholic acid, a kind of bile acid, for 4 days promotes intestinal motility in a dose-dependent manner, increases the number of bowel movements, and improves stool shape and intestinal transit time compared to the placebo. However, approximately half of the patients experience abdominal pain as a side effect, probably owing to increased intestinal peristalsis.

Elobixibat is a low-molecular-weight compound developed based on a compound discovered in the search for a drug for the treatment of dyslipidemia. Elobixibat inhibits IBAT expression in epithelial cells in the terminal ileum and suppresses bile acid reabsorption, thereby increasing the amount of bile acids flowing into the lumen of the large intestine. Elobixibat also affects the enterohepatic circulation, promoting bile acid synthesis in the liver and increasing the amount of endogenous bile acids. The development of elobixibat as a chronic constipation treatment started in April 2012.

A placebo-controlled, randomized, double-blind, multicenter, parallel-group Japanese Phase II study has been conducted on 163 patients with chronic constipation [46]. A primary dose of elobixibat (5, 10, or 15 mg) or placebo was administered orally once daily for 14 days before breakfast, and the change in the number of spontaneous bowel movements from the first week to the second week of administration was the primary endpoint of efficacy. They discovered that the 10-mg and 15-mg groups show a significant increase in the number of spontaneous bowel movements compared to the placebo group.

A placebo-controlled, randomized, double-blind, comparative Japanese Phase III study has been conducted on 132 Japanese patients with chronic constipation [47]. Elobixibat (10 mg) or placebo was orally administered once a day for 14 days, and the change in the number of spontaneous defecations from the first week to the second week of administration was the primary endpoint. They discovered that the elobixibat group shows an increase in the number of spontaneous bowel movements compared to the placebo. In addition, statistically significant improvements with the administration of elobixibat were observed in the secondary endpoints, such as the change in the number of complete spontaneous defecations, the time to the first spontaneous defecation, and stool hardness.

A Japanese long-term treatment study was a 52-week, open-label, Phase III clinical study of 340 Japanese patients with chronic constipation [47]. The efficacy and safety of the long-term administration of elobixibat were evaluated. Elobixibat was orally administered at a dose of 10 mg once daily for 7 days, after which it was administered once daily according to symptoms, in a range of 5, 10, and 15 mg, for 52 weeks. As a result, an increase in the number of complete spontaneous defecations was observed compared to the first week of administration and was maintained until week 52. In addition, there was a tendency for satisfaction with defecation to increase as the treatment period increased. In the score of the Japanese version of the Patient Assessment of Constipation Quality of Life Questionnaire [48], a significant decrease was observed as the treatment period increased.

The major side effects in all studies were gastrointestinal disorders, such as abdominal pain and diarrhea, but no serious side effects were observed. Based on these trials, elobixibat was approved in Japan in January 2018. The drug is administered orally at a dose of 10 mg once a day before meals, and the dose can be adjusted as needed (maximum dose: 15 mg/day).

Elobixibat is a drug with a new mechanism of action for the treatment of chronic constipation and has been approved after clinical trials. The results of conventional bile acid research reveal some interesting issues, such as the effects of elobixibat on intestinal bacteria. This will be one of the interesting drugs for the treatment of IBS-C in the future.

12.5 5-Hydroxytryptamine Receptor 4 Agonist

Tegaserod, which has been shown to be effective in an RCT for the treatment of IBS-C [49–51] and in a systematic review for the treatment of IBS-C and chronic constipation [52], is widely used for the treatment of IBS-C. The US Food and Drug Administration discontinued this product in 2007 because of an increase in the frequency of cardiovascular events. However, a large number of case-control studies reported no such event [53].

An RCT [54–56] and a systematic review [57] have reported the use of renzapride for the treatment of IBS-C. The RCT showed the benefit, especially in women, on improved fecal transit time, but a systematic review involving 2528 patients showed no benefit of renzapride.

The efficacy of prucalopride has been reported in a systematic review of 11 RCTs on patients with chronic constipation [58], but no effect was shown in large-scale RCTs [59]. It is licensed in the USA for the treatment of chronic constipation.

The use of velusetrag [60], naronapride [61], and YKP10811 [62] for the treatment of chronic constipation, and their efficacies have been reported in RCTs. None of these can be used in Japan.

Cisapride has been shown to be effective in a systematic review for chronic constipation and IBS-C [63] and in an RCT for IBS-C [64]. Owing to the adverse events of QT prolongation and ventricular arrhythmia, it was discontinued in 1999 and cannot be used at this time.

Mosapride is used mainly in Japan and other Asian countries. It is reported to improve colorectal motility in patients with IBS-C [65], and an RCT [66] has shown its efficacy in combination with probiotics in patients with IBS. It can be used in patients with chronic gastritis in Japan, but not in patients with IBS-C or chronic constipation.

12.6 Conclusion

This article outlines the drug treatment options for IBS-C. New drugs for patients with IBS-C and chronic constipation will be developed in the near future. It is expected that some studies will focus on chronic constipation alone; however, this article indicates that a treatment for IBS-C can be developed based on the close relationship between IBS-C and chronic constipation. In addition, the treatment of IBS-C cannot be completed using drugs that only cause changes in stool shape, stool frequency, and digestive symptoms. We believe that approaches based on brain-intestinal correlation and intestinal flora will become important in the future.

GI motility modifier, bulking polymer, and herbal medicine: see Chap. 13.
Antidepressant, anxiolytics, and psychotherapy: see Chap. 14.
Probiotics and antibiotics: see Chap. 16.

References

1. Tack J, Fried M, Houghton LA, Spicak J, Fisher G. Systematic review: the efficacy of treatments for irritable bowel syndrome—a European perspective. Aliment Pharmacol Ther. 2006;24:183–205.
2. Videlock EJ. Irritable bowel syndrome: current approach to symptoms, evaluation, and treatment. Gastroenterol Clin N Am. 2007;36:665–85.
3. Khan S. Diagnosis and management of IBS. Nat Rev Gastroenterol Hepatol. 2010;7:565–81.
4. Saad RJ. Recent developments in the therapy of irritable bowel syndrome. Expert Opin Investig Drugs. 2008;17:117–30.
5. Camilleri M. Current medical treatments of dyspepsia and irritable bowel syndrome. Gastroenterol Clin N Am. 2010;39:481–93.
6. Spiller R, Aziz Q, Creed F, Emmanuel A, Houghton L, Hungin P, Jones R, Kumar D, Rubin G, Trudgill N, Whorwell P. Clinical Services Committee of the British Society of Gastroenterology. Guidelines on the irritable bowel syndrome: mechanisms and practical management. Gut. 2007;56:1770–98.
7. Gwee KA, Bak YT, Ghoshal UC, Gonlachanvit S, Lee OY, Fock KM, Chua AS, Lu CL, Goh KL, Kositchaiwat C, Makharia G, Park HJ, Chang FY, Fukudo S, Choi MG, Bhatia S, Ke M, Hou X, Hongo M, Asian Neurogastroenterology and Motility Association. Asian consensus on irritable bowel syndrome. J Gastroenterol Hepatol. 2010;25:1189–205.
8. Wilkins T, Pepitone C, Alex B, Schade RR. Diagnosis and management of IBS in adults. Am Fam Physician. 2012;86:419–26.
9. Jadallah KA, Kullab SM, Sanders DS. Constipation-predominant irritable bowel syndrome: a review of current and emerging drug therapies. World J Gastroenterol. 2014;20:8898–909.

10. Fukudo S, Kaneko H, Akiho H, Inamori M, Endo Y, Okumura T, Kanazawa M, Kamiya T, Sato K, Chiba T, Furuta K, Yamato S, Arakawa T, Fujiyama Y, Azuma T, Fujimoto K, Mine T, Miura S, Kinoshita Y, Sugano K, Shimosegawa T. Evidence-based clinical practice guidelines for irritable bowel syndrome. J Gastroenterol. 2015;50:11–30.
11. Krarup AL, Engsbro ALØ, Fassov J, Fynne L, Christensen AB, Bytzer P. Danish national guideline: diagnosis and treatment of irritable bowel syndrome. Dan Med J. 2017;64:pii: C5382.
12. Dupont C, Campagne A, Constant F. Efficacy and safety of a magnesium sulfate-rich natural mineral water for patients with functional constipation. Clin Gastroenterol Hepatol. 2014;12:1280–7.
13. Nyberg C, Hendel J, Nielsen OH. The safety of osmotically acting cathartics in colonic cleansing. Nat Rev Gastroenterol Hepatol. 2010;7:557–64.
14. Safe Medication Guidelines for the Elderly 2015, The Japan Gerontological Society, MEDICAL VIEW CO.,LTD. Tokyo, 2015.
15. Safety Information on Drugs and Medical Devices No328. 2015/11/28 https://www.pmda.go.jp/files/000208517.pdf#page=3 (final access 2019/7/29).
16. Belsey JD, Geraint M, Dixon TA. Systematic review and meta-analysis: polyethylene glycol in adults with non-organic constipation. Int J Clin Pract. 2010;64:944–55.
17. Mínguez M, López Higueras A, Júdez J. Use of polyethylene glycol in functional constipation and fecal impaction. Rev Esp Enferm Dig. 2016;108:790–806.
18. Fleming V, Wade WE. A review of laxative therapies for treatment of chronic constipation in older adults. Am J Geriatr Pharmacother. 2010;8:514–50.
19. Chapman RW, Stanghellini V, Geraint M, Halphen M. Randomized clinical trial: macrogol/PEG 3350 plus electrolytes for treatment of patients with constipation associated with irritable bowel syndrome. Am J Gastroenterol. 2013;108:1508–15.
20. Awad RA, Camacho S. A randomized, double-blind, placebo-controlled trial of polyethylene glycol effects on fasting and postprandial rectal sensitivity and symptoms in hypersensitive constipation-predominant irritable bowel syndrome. Color Dis. 2010;12:1131–8.
21. Ulbricht C, Conquer J, Costa D, Hamilton W, Higdon ER, Isaac R, Rusie E, Rychlik I, Serrano JM, Tanguay-Colucci S, Theeman M, Varghese M. An evidence-based systematic review of senna (Cassia senna) by the Natural Standard Research Collaboration. J Diet Suppl. 2011;8:189–238.
22. Wald A. Is chronic use of stimulant laxatives harmful to the colon? J Clin Gastroenterol. 2003;36:386–9.
23. Alsalimy N, Madi L, Awaisu A. Efficacy and safety of laxatives for chronic constipation in long-term care settings: a systematic review. J Clin Pharm Ther. 2018;43:595–605.
24. Kamm MA, Mueller-Lissner S, Wald A, Richter E, Swallow R, Gessner U. Oral bisacodyl is effective and well-tolerated in patients with chronic constipation. Clin Gastroenterol Hepatol. 2011;9:577–83.
25. Kienzle-Horn S, Vix JM, Schuijt C, Peil H, Jordan CC, Kamm MA. Efficacy and safety of bisacodyl in the acute treatment of constipation: a double-blind, randomized, placebo-controlled study. Aliment Pharmacol Ther. 2006;23:1479–88.
26. Wulkow R, Vix JM, Schuijt C, et al. Randomised, placebo-controlled, double-blind study to investigate the efficacy and safety of the acute use of sodium picosulphate in patients with chronic constipation. Int J Clin Pract. 2007;61:944–50.
27. Mueller-Lissner S, Kamm MA, Wald A, et al. Multicenter, 4-week, double-blind, randomized, placebo-controlled trial of sodium picosulfate in patients with chronic constipation. Am J Gastroenterol. 2010;105:897–903.
28. Kienzle-Horn S, Vix JM, Schuijt C, Peil H, Jordan CC, Kamm MA. Comparison of bisacodyl and sodium picosulphate in the treatment of chronic constipation. Curr Med Res Opin. 2007;23:691–9.
29. Noergaard M, Traerup Andersen J, Jimenez-Solem E, Bring CM. Long term treatment with stimulant laxatives—clinical evidence for effectiveness and safety? Scand J Gastroenterol. 2019;54:27–34.

30. Simrén M, et al. New treatments and therapeutic targets for IBS and other functional bowel disorders. Nat Rev Gastroenterol Hepatol. 2018;15:589–605.
31. Johanson JF, et al. Clinical trial: phase 2 study of lubiprostone for irritable bowel syndrome with constipation. Aliment Pharmacol Ther. 2008;27:685–96.
32. Fukudo S, et al. Efficacy and safety of oral lubiprostone in constipated patients with or without irritable bowel syndrome: a randomized, placebo-controlled and dose-finding study. Neurogastroenterol Motil. 2011;23:544-e205.
33. Drossman DA, et al. Clinical trial: lubiprostone in patients with constipation-associated irritable bowel syndrome-results of two randomized, placebo-controlled studies. Aliment Pharmacol Ther. 2009;29:329–41.
34. Chang L, et al. Effects of baseline abdominal pain and bloating on response to lubiprostone in patients with irritable bowel syndrome with constipation. Aliment Pharmacol Ther. 2016;44:1114–22.
35. Li F, et al. Lubiprostone is effective in the treatment of chronic idiopathic constipation and irritable bowel syndrome: a systematic review and meta-analysis of randomized controlled trials. Mayo Clin Proc. 2016;91:456–68.
36. Chey WD, et al. Safety and patient outcomes with lubiprostone for up to 52 weeks in patients with irritable bowel syndrome with constipation. Aliment Pharmacol Ther. 2012;35:587–99.
37. Chey WD, et al. Linaclotide for irritable bowel syndrome with constipation: a 26-week, randomized, double-blind, placebo-controlled trial to evaluate efficacy and safety. Am J Gastroenterol. 2012;107:1702–12.
38. Rao S, et al. A 12-week, randomized, controlled trial with a 4-week randomized withdrawal period to evaluate the efficacy and safety of linaclotide in irritable bowel syndrome with constipation. Am J Gastroenterol. 2012;107:1714–24.
39. Quigley EM, et al. Randomised clinical trials: linaclotide phase 3 studies in IBS-C– a prespecified further analysis based on European Medicines Agency-specified endpoints. Aliment Pharmacol Ther. 2013;37:49–61.
40. Yang Y, et al. Linaclotide in irritable bowel syndrome with constipation: a phase 3 randomized trial in China and other regions. J Gastroenterol Hepatol. 2018;33:980–9.
41. Fukudo S, et al. A randomized controlled and long-term linaclotide study of irritable bowel syndrome with constipation patients in Japan. Neurogastroenterol Motil. 2018;30:e13444.
42. Shah ED, et al. Efficacy and tolerability of guanylate cyclase-C agonists for irritable bowel syndrome with constipation and chronic idiopathic constipation: a systematic review and meta-analysis. Am J Gastroenterol. 2018;113:329–38.
43. Black CJ, et al. Efficacy of secretagogues in patients with irritable bowel syndrome with constipation: systematic review and network meta-analysis. Gastroenterology. 2018;155:1753–63.
44. Bunnett NW. Neuro-humoral signalling by bile acids and the TGR5 receptor in the gastrointestinal tract. J Physiol. 2014;592:2943–50.
45. Rao AS, et al. Chenodeoxycholate in females with irritable bowel syndrome-constipation: a pharmacodynamic and pharmacogenetic analysis. Gastroenterology. 2010;139:1549–58.
46. Nakajima A, et al. Determining an optimal clinical dose of elobixibat, a novel inhibitor of the ileal bile acid transporter, in Japanese patients with chronic constipation: a phase II, multicenter, double-blind, placebo-controlled randomized clinical trial. J Gastroenterol. 2018;53:525–34.
47. Nakajima A, et al. Safety and efficacy of elobixibat for chronic constipation: results from a randomised, double-blind, placebo-controlled, phase 3 trial and an open-label, single-arm, phase 3 trial. Lancet Gastroenterol Hepatol. 2018;3:537–47.
48. Nomura H, et al. Validity and reliability of the Japanese version of the patient assessment of constipation quality of life questionnaire. J Gastroenterol. 2014;49:667–73.
49. Müller-Lissner SA, Fumagalli I, Bardhan KD, et al. Tegaserod, a 5-HT(4) receptor partial agonist, relieves symptoms in irritable bowel syndrome patients with abdominal pain, bloating and constipation. Aliment Pharmacol Ther. 2001;15:1655–66.

50. Novick J, Miner P, Krause R, et al. A randomized, double-blind, placebo-controlled trial of tegaserod in female patients suffering from irritable bowel syndrome with constipation. Aliment Pharmacol Ther. 2002;16:1877–88.
51. Tack J, Muller-Lissner S, Bytzer P, Corinaldesi R, Chang L, Viegas A, Schnekenbuehl S, Dunger-Baldauf C, Rueegg P. A randomised controlled trial assessing the efficacy and safety of repeated tegaserod therapy in women with irritable bowel syndrome with constipation. Gut. 2005;54:1707–13.
52. Evans BW, Clark WK, Moore DJ, Whorwell PJ. Tegaserod for the treatment of irritable bowel syndrome and chronic constipation. Cochrane Database Syst Rev. 2007;4:ID:CD003960.
53. Anderson JL, May HT, Bair TL, et al. Lack of association of tegaserod with adverse cardiovascular outcomes in a matched case-control study. J Cardiovasc Pharmacol Ther. 2009;14:170–5.
54. George AM, Meyers NL, Hickling RI. Clinical trial: renzapride therapy for constipation-predominant irritable bowel syndrome: multicentre, randomized, placebo-controlled, double-blind study in primary healthcare setting. Aliment Pharmacol Ther. 2008;27:830–7.
55. Camilleri M, McKinzie S, Fox J, et al. Effect of renzapride on transit in constipation-predominant irritable bowel syndrome. Clin Gastroenterol Hepatol. 2004;2:895–904.
56. Lembo AJ, Cremonini F, Meyers N, et al. Clinical trial: renzapride treatment of women with irritable bowel syndrome and constipation: a double-blind, randomized, placebo-controlled, study. Aliment Pharmacol Ther. 2010;31:979–90.
57. Mozaffari S, Nikfar S, Abdollahi M. Efficacy and tolerability of renzapride in irritable bowel syndrome: a meta-analysis of randomized, controlled clinical trials including 2528 patients. Arch Med Sci. 2014;10:10–8.
58. Shin A, Camilleri M, Kolar G, Erwin P, West CP, Murad MH. Systematic review with meta-analysis: highly selective 5-HT4 agonists (prucalopride, velusetrag or naronapride) in chronic constipation. Aliment Pharmacol Ther. 2014;39:239–53.
59. Piessevaux H, Corazziari E, Rey E, Simren M, Wiechowska-Kozlowska A, Kerstens R, et al. A randomized, double-blind, placebo-controlled trial to evaluate the efficacy, safety, and tolerability of long-term treatment with prucalopride. Neurogastroenterol Motil. 2015;27:805–15.
60. Goldberg M, Li YP, Johanson JF, Mangel AW, Kitt M, Beattie DT, et al. Clinical trial: the efficacy and tolerability of velusetrag, a selective 5-HT4 agonist with high intrinsic activity, in chronic idiopathic constipation—a 4-week, randomized, double-blind, placebo-controlled, dose-response study. Aliment Pharmacol Ther. 2010;32:1102–12.
61. Palme M, Milner PG, Ellis DJ, Marmon T, Canafax DM. 905 A novel gastrointestinal prokinetic, ATI-7505, increased spontaneous bowel movements (Sbms) in a phase II, randomized, placebo-controlled study of patients with chronic idiopathic constipation (CIC). Gastroenterology. 2010;138:S-128–S-9.
62. Shin A, Acosta A, Camilleri M, Boldingh A, Burton D, Ryks M, et al. A randomized trial of 5-hydroxytryptamine4-receptoragonist, YKP10811, on colonic transit and bowel function in functional constipation. Clin Gastroenterol Hepatol. 2015;13:701–8.
63. Aboumarzouk OM, Agarwal T, Antakia R, Shariff U, Nelson RL. Cisapride for intestinal constipation. Cochrane Database Syst Rev. 2011;1:ID:CD007780.
64. Van Outryve M, Milo R, Toussaint J, et al. "Prokinetic" treatment of constipation-predominant irritable bowel syndrome: a placebo-controlled study of cisapride. J Clin Gastroenterol. 1991;13:49–57.
65. Kanazawa M, Watanabe S, Tana C, Komuro H, Aoki M, Fukudo S. Effect of 5-HT4 receptor agonist mosapride citrate on rectosigmoid sensorimotor function in patients with irritable bowel syndrome. Neurogastroenterol Motil. 2011;23:754–e332.
66. Choi CH, Kwon JG, Kim SK, Myung SJ, Park KS, Sohn CI, Rhee PL, Lee KJ, Lee OY, Jung HK, Jee SR, Jeen YT, Choi MG, Choi SC, Huh KC, Park H. Efficacy of combination therapy with probiotics and mosapride in patients with IBS without diarrhea: a randomized, double-blind, placebo-controlled, multicenter, phase II trial. Neurogastroenterol Motil. 2015;27:705–16.

Chapter 13
GI Motility Modifier, Bulking Polymer, and Herbal Medicine

Ken Sato

Abstract Gastrointestinal dysmotility is one of the important pathophysiology in IBS. Trimebutine maleate is the most popular and has been commonly used for IBS to control abdominal pain after bowel habits. Trimebutine has dual action for GI motilities, so effective for not only constipation-predominant type but also diarrhea-predominant type of IBS. In some guidelines and reviews, the use of trimebutine is generally recommended.

Polycarbophil calcium as a bulking polymer improves the symptoms either diarrhea or constipation. The efficacy of polycarbophil calcium has been proven in placebo-controlled RCTs.

About dietary fiber for the efficacy of IBS, a systematic review and meta-analysis were investigated, the effectiveness of soluble fiber for IBS was proved, but the effectiveness of an insoluble fiber for IBS was limited.

The evidence for herbal treatment, most of which is conducted by traditional Chinese medicine. Overall, the evidence level of these studies is low quality. In Japan, traditional Japanese medicines (Kampo agents) have been used for treating IBS, but the study of efficacy for IBS is limited. Keishi-ka-shakuyaku-to significantly improved abdominal pain of diarrhea-predominant IBS in RCT of Japan. High levels of RCTs are needed to investigate the efficacy of herbal medicine.

Keyword Irritable bowel syndrome · GI motility modifier · Trimebutine · Eluxadoline · Bulking polymer · Polycarbophil calcium · Herbal medicine · Kampo agents

---

K. Sato (✉)
Department of Gastroenterology, Hematology and Clinical Immunology, Hirosaki University School of Medicine, Hirosaki, Japan
e-mail: kenjirou@hirosaki-u.ac.jp

© The Editor(s) (if applicable) and The Author(s), under exclusive license to Springer Nature Singapore Pte Ltd. 2024

T. Kamiya, S. Fukudo (eds.), *Irritable Bowel Syndrome*,
https://doi.org/10.1007/978-981-97-8410-3_13

13.1 GI Motility Modifier

Gastrointestinal dysmotility is one of the important pathophysiology in IBS. Gastrointestinal motility modifiers have been used for IBS and effective in treating IBS. Specifically, trimebutine maleate is the most popular and has been commonly used for IBS to control abdominal pain after bowel habits. The action of trimebutine on the gastrointestinal tract are mediated via an agonist effect on peripheral μ, κ, and δ opiate receptors and release of gastrointestinal peptide such as motilin and modulation of the release of other peptides, including vasoactive intestinal peptide, gastrin, and glucagon. Trimebutine accelerates premature phase III of the migrating motor complex in the intestine and modulates the contractile activity of the colon [1].

Trimebutine attenuated intestinal motility mainly through inhibition of L-type Ca2+ channels at higher concentrations. At lower concentrations of trimebutine, however depolarization of membrane potentials by reducing outward BKca currents could be a dominant signal to enhance the contractions of colonic muscles [2] (Fig. 13.1).

By these mechanisms, trimebutine is effective for not only constipation-predominant type but also diarrhea-predominant type of IBS.

In some guidelines and reviews, the use of trimebutine is generally recommended [3, 4]. Japanese version of guideline for IBS [5], thought weak recommendation, trimebutine was also recommended.

The efficacy of trimebutine in IBS patients was investigated in several RCTs and meta-analyses conducted overseas. In these studies, trimebutine improved abdominal pain and the other gastrointestinal symptoms of IBS, moreover defecation frequency and stool consistency [6].

The other agent of GI motility modifier, dopamine D2 blocking agent, there were only a small RCT and meta-analysis. The use of domperidone in IBS patients showed the beneficial effect on gastrointestinal symptoms. There has no study that

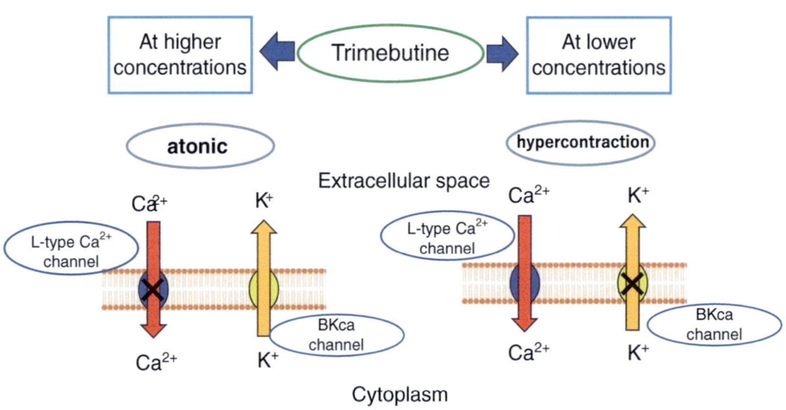

Fig. 13.1 Trimebutine has the concentration-dependent dual actions on GI smooth muscle cells by the ionic currents through the L-type Ca2+ channel and BKca channel

investigated about metoclopramide, and its extrapyramidal side effects have been recognized [3, 7]. There is no clinical evidence about the efficacy of neostigmine and itopride for IBS patients.

Recently a new oral agent with mixed opioid effects, μ and κ opioid receptor agonist and δ opioid receptor antagonist, was appeared. A new agent eluxadoline affects only the nerve system of the intestine, not the central nerve system. The significant effects for IBS-D compared with placebo in several RCTs was indicated [8–10]. The RCT of the efficacy of eluxadoline for 2427 cases of IBS-D indicated significant improvement of abdominal pain and stool forms [9].

13.2 Bulking Polymer and Dietary Fiber

Dietary fiber improves the symptoms of IBS. A soluble fiber (psyllium, ispaghula, etc.) becomes a gel-like stool and enables stool movement easier. On the other hand, insoluble fibers (cone, white bran, etc.) absorb water and expand itself; it makes stools increase the volume. An increased stool stimulates bowel movements. In a Japanese version of the guideline for IBS [5], the use of bulking polymer and dietary fiber were strongly recommended for IBS.

A bulking polymer as an agent of treating IBS is polycarbophil calcium. Polycarbophil calcium is a polyacrylic resin that is hydrophilic but insoluble in water, and it functions as a soluble fiber by maintaining water in the gastrointestinal tract and by stimulating the transport of bowel contents. This mechanism improves the symptoms either diarrhea or constipation [11].

Polycarbophil calcium releases a calcium in the stomach under strong acidity, and then it shows water absorption power depending on ph. The higher pH, the more water it can absorb.

The efficacy of polycarbophil calcium has been proven in placebo-controlled RCTs as well as large-scale clinical trials conducted in Japan [12]. In 26 IBS patients (14 diarrhea-predominant type, 12 constipation-predominant type), polycarbophil calcium is effective for improving colonic transit, bowel movement, stool form, and abdominal pain in both type of IBS, after 8 weeks of administration of 3 g/day. More specifically, in diarrhea-predominant type, the mean colonic transit time increased, bowel movements decreased in frequency, the stool form scale score decreased, and the abdominal pain appeared to be diminished after treatment ($p < 0.05$). On the other hand, in constipation-predominant type, the mean colonic transit time decreased, bowel movements increased in frequency, the stool form scale score increased, and the abdominal pain appeared to be diminished after treatment ($p < 0.05$). The study indicated that polycarbophil calcium has dual actions for improving the symptoms for each type of IBS [13] (Table 13.1).

About the studies of dietary fiber for the efficacy of IBS, a systematic review and meta-analysis in these days, the effectiveness of soluble fiber for IBS was proven, but the effectiveness of an insoluble fiber for IBS was limited [14]. A study comparing the efficacy of soluble fiber (psyllium Plantago psyllium, ispaghula, and polycarbophil

Table 13.1 Calcium polycarbophil improves colonic transit, bowel movements, stool form and abdominal pain in both diarrhea-predominant and constipation-predominant type of IBS

	Diarrhea-predominant IBS			Constipation-predominant IBS		
	Baseline	8w	*p* value	Baseline	8w	*p* value
Mean colonic transit time (h)	2.1 ± 3.3	9.4 ± 10.5	0.02	51.2 ± 28.0	34.6 ± 30.0	0.01
Average bowel movements (week)	22.5 ± 6.3	9.5 ± 3.5	<0.001	2.1 ± 0.4	4.0 ± 1.9	0.004
Bristol Stool Form Scale	4.3 ± 0.7	3.8 ± 0.4	0.04	1.9 ± 0.4	3.3 ± 0.7	<0.001
Abdominal pain	1.7 ± 0.5	0.6 ± 0.7	<0.001	1.4 ± 0.5	0.9 ± 0.8	0.02

Table 13.2 Soluble fibers (psyllium) significantly improved abdominal pain and discomfort connected with IBS after 1 or 2 months intake

	Responders	RR (95% SI)
Treatment		
Month 1		
Psyllium	45/79 (57%)	1.60 (1.13–2.26)*
Bran	31/77 (40%)	1.13 (0.81–1.58)
Placebo	27/78 (35%)	NA
Month 2		
Psyllium	39/66 (59%)	1.44(1.02–2.06)*
Bran	32/63 (51%)	1.22 (0.86–1.72)
Placebo	27/66 (41%)	NA
Month 3		
Psyllium	25/54 (46%)	1.36 (0.90–2.04)
Bran	31/54 (57%)	1.70 (1.12–2.57)*
Placebo	18/56 (32%)	NA

*$P < 0.05$ vs. placebo

calcium) and insoluble fiber (cone and wheat bran) in IBS patients revealed that soluble fiber significantly improved IBS general symptoms (RR 1.55, 95% CI 1.35–1.78) and constipation (RR 1.6, 95%CI 1.1–2.14), but insoluble fiber was ineffective and even worsened general symptoms and abdominal pain of IBS in some patients [15]. The placebo-controlled RCT study of 275 IBS patients indicated that soluble fibers (psyllium) significantly improved abdominal pain and discomfort connected with IBS after 1 or 2 months intake; on the other hand, insoluble fiber(bran) did not significantly improve the symptoms of IBS compared with control [16] (Table 13.2).

13.3 Herbal Medicine

The most evidence for herbal treatment is conducted by traditional Chinese medicine. But overall, the evidence level of these studies is low quality. In Japan, traditional Japanese medicines (Kampo agents) have been used for treating IBS, but the study of efficacy for IBS is limited.

One systematic review of 72 RCTs by using traditional Chinese medicine concluded that traditional Chinese medicine combined with Western medicine improved IBS symptoms compared with Western medicine alone (RR 1.21, 95% CI 1.18–1.24). However, comparison of each medicines were indirect, and selected RCTs were methodologically low quality [17].

Other RCTs indicated that various types of herbal medicine were effective for IBS. For example, two types of mixed herbal medicine, STW5 (bitter candytuft, chamomile flower, peppermint leaves, caraway fruit, licorice root, lemon balm leaves, celandine herbs, angelica root, milk thistle fruit) and STW5-II(bitter candytuft, chamomile flower, peppermint leaves, caraway fruit, licorice root, lemon balm leaves), were the medicine given to 208 IBS patients for 4 weeks; the symptoms of IBS significantly improved (STW5 RR 1.68 (1.13–2.51), STW5-IIRR 1.90 (1.30–2.78)) [18]. Chinese herbal medicine (*Artemesiae capillaris herba*, *Codonopsis pilosulae radix*, *Coicis lachrymal-jobi semen*, schisandra fruit, etc.) were given to 116 IBS patients for 16 weeks; the symptoms of IBS significantly improved (RR 2.63(1.44–4.78) [19]. The 3-month administration of a Tibetan herbal formula (padma lax) improved IBS symptoms significantly (RR 7.24(2.37–22.12) [20]. Though the efficacy of herbal medicines was indicated in these studies, high levels of RCTs are needed to investigate the efficacy of herbal medicine.

On the other hand, the efficacy of traditional Japanese herbal medicine for IBS symptoms has been reported. Mainly, Keishi-ka-shakuyaku-to, Hange-shashin-to, and Dai-kenchu-to have been investigated.

A multicenter, placebo-controlled study was conducted for 232 IBS patients, after a 4-week administration of Keishi-ka-shakuyaku-to which indicated the tendency to reduce abdominal pain of IBS, and in a diarrhea-predominant group, significant improvement of abdominal pain was indicated [21] (Fig. 13.2). It is supposed that the mechanism of improving the symptoms of IBS by Keishi-ka-shakuyaku-to is by modifying the GI motility and antispastic effect of the colon.

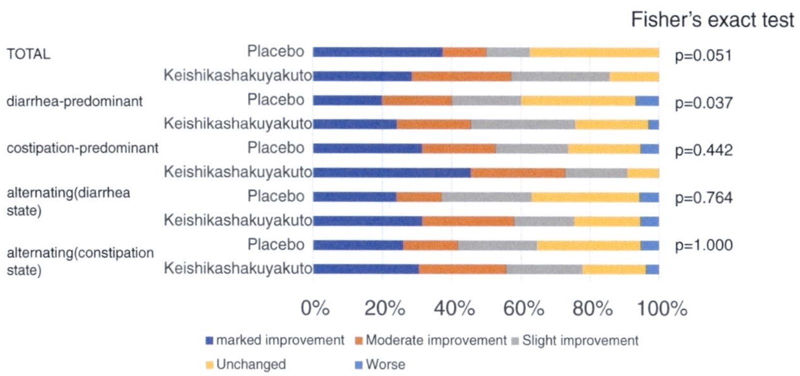

Fig. 13.2 Keishi-ka-shakuyaku-to significantly improved the abdominal pain of the diarrhea-predominant IBS

Several studies reported that Hange-shashin-to improves the symptoms of diarrhea-predominant IBS. Hange-shashin-to has the effect of reducing the prostaglandin E2 and promoting water absorption in the large intestine [22].

It is supposed that Dai-kenchu-to is effective for constipation-predominant IBS. It has become clear that Dai-kenchu-to stimulates the colonic contraction via TRPV1 (transient receptor potential cation channel subfamily V member 1) receptor, acetylcholine receptor, and 5-HT3 receptor [23].

It is supposed that Keishi-ka-shakuyaku-to, Hange-shashin-to, and Dai-kenchu-to are effective for IBS. It is necessary to choose the appropriate herbal medicine in consideration of the type of IBS.

References

1. Delvaut M, Wingate D. Trimebutine: mechanism of action, effects on gastrointestinal function and clinical results. J Int Med Res. 1997;25:225–46.
2. Lee HT, Kim BJ. Trimebutine as a modulator of gastrointestinal motility. Arch Pharm Res. 2011;34:861–4.
3. Tack J. Systemic review: the efficacy of treatments for irritable bowel syndrome: a European perspective. Aliment Pharmacol Ther. 2006;24:183–205.
4. Heading R. Systemic review: the safety and tolerability of pharmacological agents for treatment of irritable bowel syndrome: a European perspective. Aliment Pharmacol Ther. 2006;24:207–36.
5. Fukudo S, Kaneko H, et al. Evidence-based clinical practice guidelines for irritable bowel syndrome. J Gastroenterol. 2015;50:11–30.
6. Ruepert L, Quartero AO, et al. Bulking agents, antispasmodics and antidepressants for the treatment of irritable bowel syndrome. Cochrane Database Syst Rev. 2011;8:CD003460.
7. Talley NJ. Evaluation of drug treatment in irritable bowel syndrome. Br J Clin Pharmacol. 2003;56:362–9.
8. Dove LS, Lembo A, et al. Eluxadolin benefits patients with irritable bowel syndrome with diarrhea in a phase 2 study. Gastroenterology. 2013;145:329–38.
9. Lembo AJ, Lacy BE, et al. Eluxadolin for irritable bowel syndrome with diarrhea. N Engl J Med. 2016;374:242–53.
10. Brenner DM, Sayuk GS, et al. Efficacy and safety of Eluxadolin in patients with irritable bowel syndrome with diarrhea who report inadequate symptom control with loperamide: RELIEF phase 4 study. Am J Gastroenterol. 2019;114:1502–11.
11. Toskes PP, Connery KI, et al. Calcium polycarbophil compared with placebo in irritable bowel syndrome. Aliment Pharmacol Ther. 1993;7:87–92.
12. Masamune K, Miwa T, et al. Phase III trial of calcium polycarbophil in patients with irritable bowel syndrome. Double-blind randomized, controlled trial comparing trimebutine maleate. Yakuri-to-chiryou. 1998;26:967–96. (Japanese)
13. Chiba T, Kudara N, et al. Colonic transit, bowel movements, stool form, and abdominal pain in irritable bowel syndrome by treatment with calcium polycarbophil. Hepato-Gastroenterology. 2005;52:1416–20.
14. Moayyedi P, Quigley EM, et al. The effect of fiber supplementation on irritable bowel syndrome a systematic review and meta-analysis. Am J Gastroenterol. 2014;109:1367–74.
15. Bijkerk CJ, Muris JW, et al. Systematic review: the role of different type of fibre in the treatment of irritable bowel syndrome. Aliment Pharmacol Ther. 2004;19:245–51.
16. Bijkerk CJ, de Wit NJ, et al. Soluble or insoluble fibre in irritable bowel syndrome in primary care? Randomised placebo-controlled trial. BMJ. 2009;339:b3154.

17. Li CY, Ain Mohd Tahir N, et al. A systematic review of integrated traditional Chinese and Western medicine for managing irritable bowel syndrome. Am J Clin Med. 2015;43(3):385–406.
18. Madisch A, Holtmann G, et al. Treatment of irritable bowel syndrome with herbal preparations: results of a double-blind, randomized, placebo-controlled, multi-Centre trial. Aliment Pharmacol Ther. 2004;19:271–9.
19. Bensoussan A, Tally NJ, et al. Treatment of irritable bowel syndrome with Chinese herbal medicine: a randomized, controlled trial. JAMA. 1998;280:1585–9.
20. Sallon S, Ben-Arye E, et al. A novel treatment for constipation-predominant irritable bowel syndrome using Padma lax, a Tibetan herbal formula. Digestion. 2002;65:161–71.
21. Sasaki D, et al. Clinical efficacy of Keishikashakuyakuto in patients with irritable bowel syndrome: a multicenter collaborative randomaized controlled study. Rinsho to Kenkyu (The Japanese Journal of Clinical and Experimental Medicine). 1998;75:1136–52.
22. Kase Y, Hayakawa T, et al. The effect of Hange-shashin-to on the content of prostaglandin E2 and water absorption in the large intestine of rats. Biol Pharm Bull. 1997;20:954–7.
23. Kikuchi D, Shibata C, et al. Intragastric Dai-kenchu-to, a Japanese herbal medicine, stimulates colonic motility via ransient receptor potential cation channel subfamily V member 1 in dogs. Tohoku J Exp Med. 2013;230:197–204.

Chapter 14
Antidepressant, Anxiolytics, and Psychotherapy

Motoyori Kanazawa and Shin Fukudo

Abstract Dysfunction in the brain-gut axis is the biologic basis for irritable bowel syndrome (IBS). Psychiatric conditions including depression, anxiety, and somatization often coexist in IBS. Antidepressants, anxiolytics, and/or psychotherapy can be considered when patients have failed to respond to standard medical treatments. Previous clinical trials revealed that tricyclic antidepressants (TCAs), selective serotonin reuptake inhibitors (SSRIs), cognitive behavioral therapy (CBT), relaxation training, hypnotherapy, and psychodynamic therapy are probably effective treatments for IBS. Further studies are warranted to confirm augmentative effect of combining psychological therapies with antidepressants for refractory patients with IBS.

Keywords Irritable bowel syndrome (IBS) · Brain-gut axis · Antidepressants · Anxiolytics · Psychotherapy · Meta-analysis · Clinical practice guideline

14.1 Introduction

With the publication of Rome IV in 2016 [1], the functional gastrointestinal disorders (FGIDs) including irritable bowel syndrome (IBS) have been redefined as disorders of brain-gut interaction, characterized by any combination of gastrointestinal (GI) motility disturbance, visceral hypersensitivity, altered mucosal and immune function, altered gut microbiota, and altered central nervous system (CNS) processing. Dysfunction in this brain-gut axis (the bidirectional neurohormonal communication between GI tract and CNS) is the biologic basis for these disorders and symptoms. Psychiatric conditions including depression, anxiety, and somatization often coexist in IBS [2]. The influence of psychological disorders in the pathology

M. Kanazawa (✉) · S. Fukudo
Department of Behavioral Medicine, Tohoku University Graduate School of Medicine, Sendai, Miyagi, Japan
e-mail: motoyori.kanazawa.d4@tohoku.ac.jp; shin.fukudo.c6@tohoku.ac.jp

© The Editor(s) (if applicable) and The Author(s), under exclusive license to Springer Nature Singapore Pte Ltd. 2024

T. Kamiya, S. Fukudo (eds.), *Irritable Bowel Syndrome*,
https://doi.org/10.1007/978-981-97-8410-3_14

of IBS increases as the severity of IBS increases [3]. A cohort study revealed that depressive or anxiety disorder is a risk factor for the development of IBS [4]. On the contrary, IBS status also increases the incidence of depressive or anxiety disorders [5].

Antidepressants can be considered when IBS symptoms are moderate to severe, when patients have failed to respond to standard medical treatments. For IBS patients with anxiety, antidepressants with anxiolytic action are also indicated, and antianxiety drugs for a short duration may be helpful for relieving anxiety [6]. In some cases, psychotherapy will be added to manage psychosocial stress and negative emotion [6]. This chapter highlights the value and utility of antidepressants, anxiolytics, and psychotherapy in treating patients with IBS.

14.2 Antidepressants

The brain-gut axis is partially regulated by noradrenergic, serotonergic, and dopaminergic neurotransmitter systems. It is particularly relevant that gut motor function and/or visceral pain are/is affected by agents which modify these transmitters. Thus, antidepressants will have effects not only on psychiatric symptoms but also on chronic GI symptoms. Several antidepressants such as tricyclic antidepressants (TCAs) and SSRIs are often prescribed in IBS. The rationale includes (1) treatment of psychiatric comorbidity (e.g., depression and anxiety disorders) associated with IBS, (2) alteration of GI physiology (e.g., visceral sensitivity, motility, and secretion), or (3) reduction of central pain perception arising from afferent signals in the gut [6]. Recent meta-analyses by Ford AC et al. [7] have suggested that some of antidepressants are effective treatments for IBS. However, whether the benefit of antidepressants arises from the treatment of coexistent depression is controversial [7, 8].

Most of clinical practice guidelines for IBS recommended that antidepressants are effective in treating IBS [8–11]. Tricyclic antidepressants (TCAs) or selective serotonin reuptake inhibitors (SSRIs) are recommended for some patients with IBS, bearing in mind the side effects. By contrast, there is no clear evidence of serotonin noradrenaline reuptake inhibitors (SNRIs) and noradrenergic and specific serotonergic antidepressant (NaSSA) to date [7]. Thus, antidepressants should be used in patients who fail to benefit from standard drug therapy, after considering the advantages and disadvantages of antidepressants in individual patients.

14.2.1 Tricyclic Antidepressants (TCAs)

There are 12 randomized clinical trials (RCTs) compared TCAs with placebo. The doses of TCA trials were considerably lower than those used for mood disorders. The number needed to treat (NNT) with TCAs was 4.5 (95% CI 3.5–7) [7]. Six trials reported on overall adverse events with TCAs versus placebo. There were no serious adverse events but was a significantly higher rate of adverse events (RR = 1.59; 95% CI 1.23–2.06). Drowsiness and dry mouth were more common in patients randomized to TCAs than those receiving placebo. In clinical practice, the use of low-starting doses with a gradual increase to a dose associated with a beneficial effect, while minimizing adverse events, is recommended [8]. The efficacy of antidepressants according to predominant stool pattern reported by the patient has also not been well studied. TCAs prolong orocecal and whole gut transit times [12]. Therefore, it would seem biologically plausible that TCAs would be more effective in IBS with diarrhea.

Interestingly, one of TCAs, amitriptyline, has been shown to alter the activation of limbic brain regions in response to an auditory stressor combined with rectal painful distention [13]. There are data demonstrating the efficacy of TCAs in other painful functional disorders, such as fibromyalgia and chronic headache [14]. Although evidence for any effect of antidepressants on visceral hypersensitivity in the GI tract is limited, TCAs would be expected to reduce abdominal pain in patients with IBS.

14.2.2 Selective Serotonin Reuptake Inhibitors (SSRIs)

There were seven trials comparing SSRIs with placebo. In a meta-analysis SSRIs improved general physical condition, while tricyclic antidepressants (TCAs) improved abdominal pain and IBS severity score [7]. In treatment trials of SSRIs for IBS, the doses used were almost identical to those used to treat depression. The NNT with SSRIs was 5 (95% CI 3–16.5) [7].

SSRIs decrease orocecal transit time [12] and would have greater benefit in IBS with constipation.

14.2.3 Serotonin and Norepinephrine Reuptake Inhibitors (SNRIs)

While theoretically there may be an advantage of SNRIs over TCAs and SSRIs for the treatment of IBS symptoms, clinical trial evidence for such superiority is currently not available. In an open-label study, duloxetine significantly improved the severity of abdominal pain, QOL, stool consistency, inconvenience at work or home, and anxiety [15]. Although some of the strongest evidence for the pain modifying effects of antidepressants in chronic painful disorders comes from high-quality RCTs of duloxetine and milnacipran [14], neither of which have been investigated in IBS trials so far.

14.2.4 Tetracyclic Antidepressants and Noradrenergic and Specific Serotonergic Antidepressant (NaSSA)

In a small RCT study for IBS, the administration of the tetracyclic antidepressant mianserin significantly improved abdominal symptoms and social dysfunction, compared with a placebo [16]. However, further RCT studies using a large sample size are warranted to confirm the effects of mianserin and NaSSA such as mirtazapine.

14.3 Anxiolytics

Anxiolytic medications (benzodiazepines or azapirones) have sometimes been prescribed for patients with IBS because of the frequent comorbidity of anxiety disorders with IBS [2] and many recognize that acute psychological distress can make bowel symptoms worse [3]. It has been reported that flutazolam was more effective for IBS than a placebo in a double-blind study [17]. In addition, the rates of improvement of abdominal bloating, diarrhea, anxiety, and tension were higher with flutazolam than with diazepam [18]. In another double-blind study, the combined use of chlordiazepoxide and amitriptyline was more effective than antispasmodics, dietary fiber, or a placebo [19]. In a multicenter double-blind study, the combined use of the antispasmodic octatropine and diazepam significantly improved abdominal pain and discomfort from baseline, but not compared with placebo [20]. However, the regular use of benzodiazepine anxiolytics and sedatives is discouraged due to the risk of habituation and potential for dependency.

Apart from benzodiazepines, tandospirone citrate is a partial agonist of the 5-hydroxytryptamine 1A (5-HT1A) receptor and has also demonstrated neuropharmacological properties that may contribute to its efficacy in the treatment of anxiety. One study demonstrated that the combination of tandospirone and an antispasmodic agent, pinaverium, was associated with a significantly increased overall response rate in IBS patients with diarrhea [21].

The efficacy of a single anxiolytic has seldom been investigated worldwide to date because of issues associated with drug dependency at the recommended dose. Anxiolytics are weakly recommended only for high anxious patients with IBS for a short period of time [10].

14.4 Psychotherapy

Psychotherapy can be considered when IBS symptoms are intractable, when patients have failed to respond to pharmacological treatment, or when there is evidence that stress or psychological factors are contributing to GI symptom exacerbations. There was evidence to suggest that psychotherapies overall can be effective for the management of IBS symptoms [7]. When all psychotherapies, including hypnotherapy, were considered, the NNT was 4 [7]. In addition, adverse events data were poorly reported among trials of psychotherapies. Psychological or behavioral treatments appear to be effective in the management of IBS. Nevertheless, psychological treatment trials have methodological limitations because of the inability to blind patients or the investigators as to treatment assignment, and the difficulty of coming up with a placebo treatment that is credible but also not effective to patients. The patient's understanding of the rationale for psychological treatment and their motivation to undertake such treatment is critical to a successful outcome [8]. Thus, psychotherapy is recommended for IBS patients who do not respond to standard pharmacological treatment although it is recognized that availability can be a problem in clinical practice [10].

14.4.1 Cognitive Behavioral Therapy (CBT)

CBT is based on the assumption that IBS symptoms are a response to stressful life events or daily hassles, producing maladaptive behavior and inappropriate symptom attributions: (1) symptoms are acquired (learned) and reflect specific skills deficits in domains of cognitive and behavioral functioning, and (2) teaching and rehearsing skills for modifying maladaptive behaviors and thinking patterns can remediate these deficits which, in turn, relieves symptoms [22]. Treatment involves identifying the triggers for symptom exacerbation, understanding the patient's response to symptoms, and teaching more adaptive ways of responding. Specific technical components of CBT protocols typically include (a) the provision of information about stress and its relationship to IBS; (b) self-monitoring of antecedent and consequent events associated with IBS flare ups; (c) problem-solving strategies around stressors that aggravate symptoms; (d) muscle relaxation exercises for cultivating lower physiologic arousal and increased sense of mastery over symptoms; and/or (e) cognitive restructuring for modifying faulty threat appraisals that underlie physiologic and emotional reactivity [22]. The NNT with CBT was 4 (95% CI 3–9) [7]. A large randomized-controlled trial found that standard ten weekly sessions of CBT improves IBS symptoms by reducing comorbid psychological distress, but that these therapeutic gains are not dependent on or mediated by changes in patients' overall level of psychological distress [22].

Recent multicenter randomized-controlled trial revealed that only a four-session, primarily home-based version of CBT produced substantial and generally enduring IBS symptom improvement that was comparable to "gold standard" clinic-based CBT administered weekly over 10 weeks and was generally better than control education [23]. Such self-administered or minimal contact CBT for IBS may become widespread in the near future because of simple and cost-effective psychological treatment.

14.4.2 Relaxation Training

Relaxation techniques are generally elements of other types of psychological therapies, such as CBT. This treatment is useful when stress causes exacerbation of symptoms, which can be relieved by progressive muscle relaxation, biofeedback [24], and transcendental or yoga meditations [25], although it is unclear how much of the benefit is the result of the nonspecific factor of increased attention from a therapist [26]. Clinical trial results with relaxation training were inconsistent and may depend on the techniques that were used. The NNT with overall relaxation training was 6 (95% CI 3–60) [7].

14.4.3 Hypnotherapy

The first controlled trial assessing the value of gut-directed hypnotherapy in patients with IBS refractory to other treatments was reported in 1984 [27]. In this study hypnotherapy focused toward control of gut function to help reduce symptoms was shown to produce a significantly greater improvement over a 3-month period than supportive therapy combined with the administration of a placebo drug, regardless of IBS subtype. Furthermore, the beneficial effects appear to be sustained over time, with patients reporting continued relief from symptoms for at least 5 years. There is evidence to suggest that in patients with IBS, hypnotherapy may normalize rectal sensitivity [28], reduce colonic phasic contractions [29], and reverse the patients' negative thoughts about their condition [30]. The NNT with hypnotherapy was 5 (95% CI 3.5–10) [7].

Autogenic training (AT) is considered to be one of the self-induced hypnotherapies [31]. It has been demonstrated that AT is more effective in the general improvement of IBS compared with the supportive nutritional education (Fig. 14.1) [31].

14.4.4 Psychodynamic Therapy

Psychodynamic therapy attempts to provide the patient with insights into why symptoms developed in the context of difficulties or changes in key relationships [32]. This helps patients to understand relationship between emotions, and bowel symptoms may become clearer [33]. It has been reported that psychodynamic therapy was more effective in reducing IBS symptom severity than control therapy [34]. The improvement was still observed after 1 year. The NNT with psychodynamic therapy was 4 (95% CI 2–20) [7].

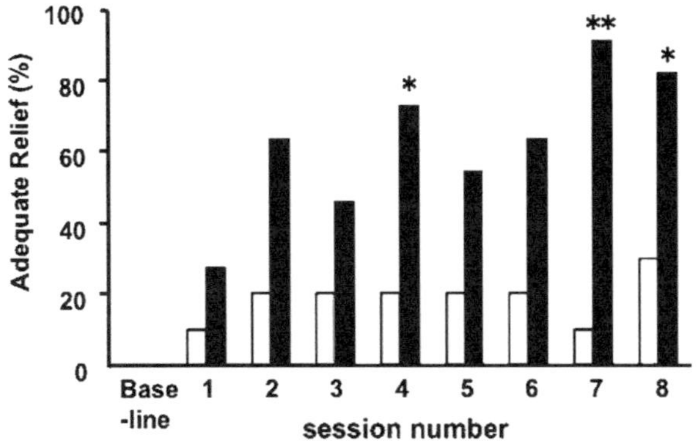

Fig. 14.1 Effect of autogenic training (AT) in patients with IBS (Shinozaki et al. 2010 [31] with permission). AT-induced changes in adequate relief (%). Open bar, control group ($n = 10$); closed bar, AT group ($n = 11$). *$p < 0.05$, **$p < 0.001$ vs. control group. Baseline means before the first session. The open and closed bars indicate the proportion of adequate relief (AR)

14.4.5 Mindfulness-Based Stress Reduction (MBSR)

Mindfulness training may also hold promise for IBS patients who remain highly symptomatic in spite of the best efforts of conventional medical treatment. This is a method of cultivating awareness of feelings or thoughts without processing them, another form of cognitive behavioral management. MRBS involves the cultivation of a state characterized by an attentive and nonjudgmental metacognitive monitoring of moment-by-moment cognition, emotion, perception, and sensation without fixation on thoughts of the past and future [35]. It has been reported that the 8-week intervention led to reduced IBS severity in those who received MBSR, and the therapeutic effect was still observed at a 3-month follow-up [36].

14.5 Conclusions

In summary, TCAs, SSRIs, CBT, relaxation training, hypnotherapy, and psychodynamic therapy are probably effective treatments for IBS. Adverse effects are more common with antidepressants, particularly TCAs. Anxiolytics may also be effective for IBS patients with anxiety but should be prescribed for a short period of time due to the risk of potential for dependency. The choice of psychological treatment will depend on what type of therapy is available in the residential area and on patient preference. Some patients may refuse to take psychological treatment because they perceive (1) that they are being treated for a psychiatric problem, (2) that the medication may be addicting or "mind altering," or (3) they do not think the doctor accepts the symptoms as "real." These issues need to be properly addressed and clarified when they occur. The patient's understanding of the rationale for psychological treatment and their motivation and expectations to undertake such treatment is critical to a successful outcome [8]. Therefore, the physician has an important role in clearly communicating why referral for psychological treatment is recommended. Further studies are warranted to confirm augmentative effect of combining psychological therapies with antidepressants for refractory patients with IBS.

References

1. Drossman DA. Functional gastrointestinal disorders: history, pathophysiology, clinical features, and Rome IV. Gastroenterology. 2016;150:1262–79.
2. Whitehead WE, Palsson O, Jones KR. Systematic review of the comorbidity of irritable bowel syndrome with other disorders: what are the causes and implications? Gastroenterology. 2002;122:1140–56.
3. Drossman DA. Do psychosocial factors define symptom severity and patient status in irritable bowel syndrome? Am J Med. 1999;107:41S–50S.
4. Sibelli A, Chalder T, Everitt H, Workman P, Windgassen S, Moss-Morris R. A systematic review with meta-analysis of the role of anxiety and depression in irritable bowel syndrome onset. Psychol Med. 2016;46:3065–80.
5. Yeh HW, Chien WC, Chung CH, Hu JM, Tzeng NS. Risk of psychiatric disorders in irritable bowel syndrome-a nationwide, population-based, cohort study. Int J Clin Pract. 2018;72:e13212.
6. Drossman DA, Tack J, Ford AC, Szigethy E, Törnblom H, Van Oudenhove L. Neuromodulators for functional gastrointestinal disorders (disorders of gut-brain interaction): a Rome Foundation Working Team Report. Gastroenterology. 2018;154:1140–71.
7. Ford AC, Lacy BE, Harris LA, Quigley EMM, Moayyedi P. Effect of antidepressants and psychological therapies in irritable bowel syndrome: an updated systematic review and meta-analysis. Am J Gastroenterol. 2019;114:21–39.
8. Drossman DA, Camilleri M, Mayer EA, Whitehead WE. AGA technical review on irritable bowel syndrome. Gastroenterology. 2002;123:2108–31.
9. Spiller R, Aziz Q, Creed F, Emmanuel A, Houghton L, Hungin P, Jones R, Kumar D, Rubin G, Trudgill N, Whorwell P, Clinical Services Committee of The British Society of Gastroenterology. Guidelines on the irritable bowel syndrome: mechanisms and practical management. Gut. 2007;56:1770–98.
10. Fukudo S, Kaneko H, Akiho H, Inamori M, Endo Y, Okumura T, Kanazawa M, Kamiya T, Sato K, Chiba T, Furuta K, Yamato S, Arakawa T, Fujiyama Y, Azuma T, Fujimoto K, Mine T, Miura S, Kinoshita Y, Sugano K, Shimosegawa T. Evidence-based clinical practice guidelines for irritable bowel syndrome. J Gastroenterol. 2015;50:11–30.
11. Moayyedi P, Andrews CN, MacQueen G, Korownyk C, Marsiglio M, Graff L, Kvern B, Lazarescu A, Liu L, Paterson WG, Sidani S, Vanner S. Canadian Association of Gastroenterology Clinical Practice Guideline for the Management of Irritable Bowel Syndrome (IBS). J Can Assoc Gastroenterol. 2019;2:6–29.
12. Gorard DA, Libby GW, Farthing MJ. Influence of antidepressants on whole gut orocaecal transit times in health and irritable bowel syndrome. Aliment Pharmacol Ther. 1994;8:159–66.
13. Morgan V, Pickens D, Gautam S, Kessler R, Mertz H. Amitriptyline reduces rectal pain related activation of the anterior cingulate cortex in patients with irritable bowel syndrome. Gut. 2005;54:601–7.
14. Dharmshaktu P, Tayal V, Kalra BS. Efficacy of antidepressants as analgesics: a review. J Clin Pharmacol. 2012;52:6–17.

15. Brennan BP, Fogarty KV, Roberts JL, Reynolds KA, Pope HG Jr, Hudson JI. Duloxetine in the treatment of irritable bowel syndrome: an open-label pilot study. Hum Psychopharmacol. 2009;24:423–8.
16. Tanum L, Malt UF. A new pharmacologic treatment of functional gastrointestinal disorder. A double-blind placebo-controlled study with mianserin. Scand J Gastroenterol. 1996;31:318–25.
17. Kawano T, Nakayama T, Yamazoe A, et al. Double-blind, randomized placebo-controlled trial of MS-4101(flutazolam) on patients with irritable bowel syndrome. Yakuri-to-chiryo. 1978;6:1769–89. (in Japanese)
18. Miyoshi A, Sugata F, Kawakami K, et al. Double-blind, randomized, multicenter placebo-controlled trial of MS-4101 (flutazolam) on patients with irritable bowel syndrome and the other functional disorders. Igaku-no-ayumi. 1981;119:106–25. (in Japanese)
19. Nigam P, Kapoor KK, Rastog CK, Kumar A, Gupta AK. Different therapeutic regimens in irritable bowel syndrome. J Assoc Physicians India. 1984;32:1041–4.
20. Pace F, Maurano A, Ciacci C, Savarino V, Attili A, Iaquinto G, Magni E, Porro GB. Octatropine methyl bromide and diazepam combination (Valpinax) in patients with irritable bowel syndrome: a multicentre, randomized, placebo-controlled trial. Eur Rev Med Pharmacol Sci. 2010;14:155–62.
21. Lan L, Chen YL, Zhang H, Jia BL, Chu YJ, Wang J, Tang SX, Xia GD. Efficacy of tandospirone in patients with irritable bowel syndrome-diarrhea and anxiety. World J Gastroenterol. 2014;20:11422–8.
22. Lackner JM, Jaccard J, Krasner SS, Katz LA, Gudleski GD, Blanchard EB. How does cognitive behavior therapy for irritable bowel syndrome work? A mediational analysis of a randomized clinical trial. Gastroenterology. 2007;133:433–44.
23. Lackner JM, Jaccard J, Keefer L, Brenner DM, Firth RS, Gudleski GD, et al. Improvement in gastrointestinal symptoms after cognitive behavior therapy for refractory irritable bowel syndrome. Gastroenterology. 2018;155:47–57.
24. Blanchard EB, Greene B, Scharff L, Schwarz-McMorris SP. Relaxation training as a treatment for irritable bowel syndrome. Biofeedback Self Regul. 1993;18(3):125–32.
25. Kuttner L, Chambers CT, Hardial J, Israel DM, Jacobson K, Evans K. A randomized trial of yoga for adolescents with irritable bowel syndrome. Pain Res Manag. 2006;11:217–23.
26. Blanchard EB, Schwarz SP, Neff DF, Gerardi MA. Prediction of outcome from the self-regulatory treatment of irritable bowel syndrome. Behav Res Ther. 1988;26:187–90.
27. Whorwell PJ, Prior A, Faragher EB. Controlled trial of hypnotherapy in the treatment of severe refractory irritable-bowel syndrome. Lancet. 1984;2:1232–4.
28. Lea R, Houghton LA, Calvert EL, Larder S, Gonsalkorale WM, Whelan V, Randles J, Cooper P, Cruickshanks P, Miller V, Whorwell PJ. Gut-focused hypnotherapy normalizes disordered rectal sensitivity in patients with irritable bowel syndrome. Aliment Pharmacol Ther. 2003;17:635–42.
29. Whorwell PJ, Houghton LA, Taylor EE, Maxton DG. Physiological effects of emotion: assessment via hypnosis. Lancet. 1992;340:69–72.
30. Gonsalkorale WM, Toner BB, Whorwell PJ. Cognitive change in patients undergoing hypnotherapy for irritable bowel syndrome. J Psychosom Res. 2004;56:271–8.
31. Shinozaki M, Kanazawa M, Kano M, Endo Y, Nakaya N, Hongo M, Fukudo S. Effect of autogenic training on general improvement in patients with irritable bowel syndrome: a randomized controlled trial. Appl Psychophysiol Biofeedback. 2010;35:189–98.
32. Svedlund J, Sjodin I, Ottosson JO, Dotevall G. Controlled study of psychotherapy in irritable bowel syndrome. Lancet. 1983;2:589–92.
33. Guthrie E. Brief psychotherapy with patients with refractory irritable bowel syndrome. Br J Psychother. 1991;8:175–88.
34. Hyphantis T, Guthrie E, Tomenson B, Creed F. Psychodynamic interpersonal therapy and improvement in interpersonal difficulties in people with severe irritable bowel syndrome. Pain. 2009;145:196–203.

35. Garland EL, Gaylord SA, Palsson O, Faurot K, Douglas Mann J, Whitehead WE. Therapeutic mechanisms of a mindfulness-based treatment for IBS: effects on visceral sensitivity, catastrophizing, and affective processing of pain sensations. J Behav Med. 2012;35:591–602.
36. Gaylord SA, Palsson OS, Garland EL, Faurot KR, Coble RS, Mann JD, Frey W, Leniek K, Whitehead WE. Mindfulness training reduces the severity of irritable bowel syndrome in women: results of a randomized controlled trial. Am J Gastroenterol. 2011;106:1678–88.

Chapter 15
Diet and Behavioral Modification for Irritable Bowel Syndrome in Japan

Yusuke Okuyama and Yoshiyuki Watanabe

Abstract Dietary habit may be associated with the prevalence of IBS. Furthermore, certain food components, such as caffeine, fat, spicy food, milk and dairy products, and insoluble fiber, are probably associated with exacerbation of symptoms with IBS. For patients with refractory IBS symptoms, cognitive behavioral therapy (CBT) have been found to be beneficial. In Japan, interoceptive exposure-based CBT program (CBT-IE) with complementary video materials and group cognitive behavioral therapy (GCBT) for moderate to severe IBS have been investigated by experienced and well-trained behavioral specialists.

Keywords Dietary habit · Food component · Psychological treatments · Interoceptive exposure-based CBT program

15.1 Main Text

15.1.1 Association Between Dietary Habit and Prevalence of IBS

Irritable bowel syndrome (IBS) is classified as a functional disorder, and the diagnosis depends on several symptoms, which were characterized by abdominal discomfort and alterations in bowel habits. Unsuitable intake of dietary components may cause and exacerbate their symptoms. In general guidelines for the management of IBS, dietary advice is one of important items.

Y. Okuyama (✉)
Department of Gastroenterology, Japanese Red Cross Kyoto Daiichi Hospital, Kyoto, Japan
e-mail: yusuke-okuyama@kyoto1.jrc.or.jp

Y. Watanabe
Department of Nursing, Faculty of Health and Medical Sciences, Kyoto University of Advanced Science, Kyoto, Japan
e-mail: watanabe@koto.kpu-m.ac.jp

© The Editor(s) (if applicable) and The Author(s), under exclusive license to Springer Nature Singapore Pte Ltd. 2024

T. Kamiya, S. Fukudo (eds.), *Irritable Bowel Syndrome*,
https://doi.org/10.1007/978-981-97-8410-3_15

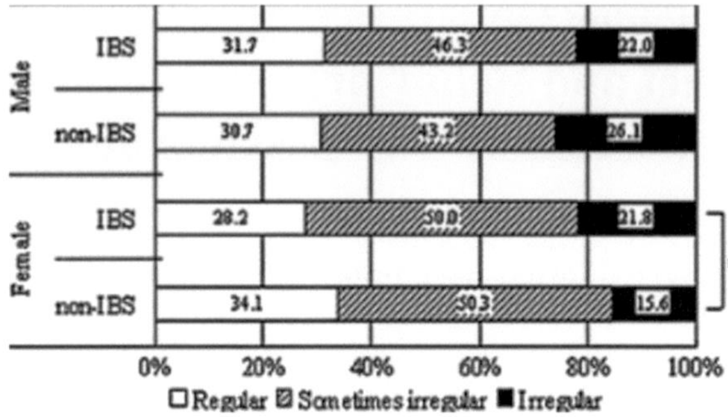

Fig. 15.1 Mealtime in the IBS group and the non-IBS group among nursing and medical school students. $*p = 0.013$, χ^2 test. This contents were quoted from the published paper by Okami et al.

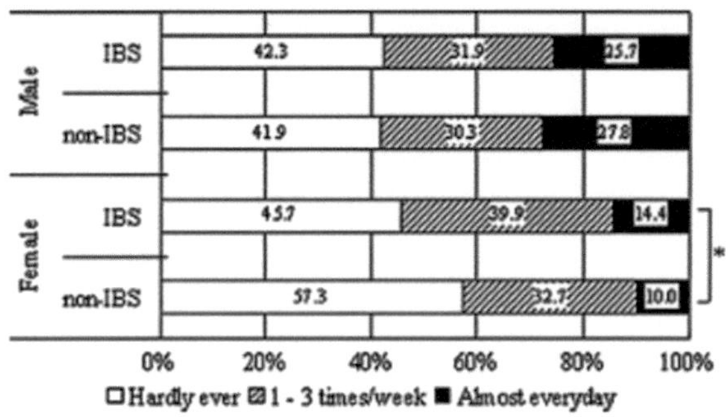

Fig. 15.2 Skipping meals in the IBS group and the non-IBS group among nursing and medical school students. $*p = 0.001$, χ^2 test. This contents were quoted from the published paper by Okami et al.

As for dietary habits, the higher intake of fluid with meals were positively associated with IBS [1]. Furthermore, regular or irregular meals may also be associated with the prevalence of IBS. By the way, it has been reported that females with irregular meal pattern had a 30% greater risk of having IBS, compared with those with regular meal pattern [2]. Then, we also investigated the relationship between IBS prevalence and dietary habits in nursing and medical students in Japan [3]. In this study, females in the IBS group had more irregular meals and skipped meals more frequently than the non-IBS group ($p = 0.013$, $p = 0.001$) (Figs. 15.1 and 15.2). Additionally, in males, the rate of missing meals every day was 29.2% in the IBS-C (constipation-predominant type) subgroup and 26.2% in the IBS-D (diarrhea-predominant type) subgroup (figure not shown). Therefore, "eating regularly" and "not skipping meals" might be associated with the reduction in prevalence of IBS.

15.1.2 Association between Components of Food and Abdominal Symptoms

In this part, we summarize that several components of food, such as caffeine, fat, spicy food, milk and dairy products, and insoluble fiber, may cause and exacerbate symptoms with IBS, referring to past literatures in the world, as described below.

Firstly, we focused on caffeine products. They increase colon motor activity and stimulate colon activity. Several case-control studies showed that patients with IBS do not drink more coffee and tea than patients without IBS [4]. Eliminating caffeine is one of the most reliable means of improving IBS symptoms. Secondly, we attended on fat. Several studies evaluated that the infusion of fat into intestine caused IBS symptoms, through the impairments in gut motility, gas trapping, luminal distension, and bloating [5]. More patients with IBS than control reported high-fat-induced IBS symptoms appeared in IBS than in control [6, 7].

Next, there are observational studies to support the contention that common spices, such as red Chili used in cooking, may alter IBS symptoms. There are a number of studies showing that patients with IBS are more susceptible to spicy foods, in particular, red Chili. Capsaicin, which is the active component in red Chili, have been shown to hasten gut motility and cause a burning sensation [8].

Then, we focused on milk and dairy products, which trigger gastrointestinal symptoms, including abdominal cramping, bloating, flatulence, and diarrhea, due to lactose malabsorption. More than one-third of patients with IBS have symptoms after the ingestion of lactose products [9]. Low-lactose diet have affected the IBS symptom scores positively in several clinical studies [10, 11]. At last, we attended on fiber. It is considered that a high-fiber diet is desirable for the standard of care with IBS patients [12, 13]. Data from a meta-analysis indicate that soluble fiber, such as ispaghula, psyllium, can improve bowel regularity and seem to improve IBS symptoms, but insoluble fiber, such as wheat bran, is no better than placebo [14]. In Japan, fiber supplements may also be recommended to increase fiber intake since it is difficult to consume enough fiber in the diet. Fiber supplements should be started at a low dose and increased slowly over several weeks to reduce the symptoms of excessive intestinal gas, which can occur in some people when beginning fiber therapy.

Throughout the text, there are currently few available evidence-based items for diet practice in IBS, as very few randomized, controlled trials exist in Japan. Regular dietary habit is required for all IBS patients. On the other hand, the diet that relieves symptoms will not be the same for each patient. Eliminating food component, which causes abdominal symptoms, are required for each particular patient. In the future, effective and universal diet therapy for IBS will be expected to establish in Japan.

15.1.3 Behavioral Modification for Irritable Bowel Syndrome

Irritable bowel syndrome (IBS) is a common chronic functional gastrointestinal disorder that affects about 14% of the Japanese population [15]. Several experts in the field now focus on the pathophysiology of IBS as a "disorder of brain-gut" rather than a functional condition [16]. Psychological treatment are considered an important treatment for patients with moderate to severe symptoms or those with comorbid psychological factors that have not responded to initial pharmacological treatments, as the first and second steps of the clinical guideline issued by the Japanese Society of Gastroenterology(GSGE) [17].

Cognitive behavioral therapy (CBT) combines behavioral therapy and cognitive therapy. Behavioral therapy helps patients weaken the connections between troublesome situations and habitual reactions to them. On the other hand, cognitive therapy teaches how certain thinking patterns cause symptoms. CBT had significantly improved symptoms in patients with moderate to severe IBS in comparison with education or self-administered therapy [18].

In Japan, specific psychotherapies are also recommended in the clinical guideline issued by the JSGE as the third step of IBS treatment that has been refractory to the other steps [19]. However, CBT for IBS is available only in specific centers in Japan, and the evidence of its efficacy has not been established, although evidence for CBT has been growing in the world [20–22].

Among the several CBT programs for IBS, interoceptive exposure-based CBT program (CBT-IE) for IBS were reported by Craske et al. [23]. CBT-IE for IBS includes exposure to abdominal sensations in addition to psychoeducation, self-monitoring, cognitive restructuring, attention training, and in vivo exposure, which are often used in traditional CBT.

Patients are exposed to self-induced abdominal sensations, such as tightening abdominal muscles, consuming avoided foods to reduce anxiety in response to abdominal disturbance in IBS.

In Japan, Oe et al. had developed a Japanese version of the cognitive behavioral therapy protocol according to the CBT-IE [23] and have been practicing on IBS patients. Their target is not only the disappearance of symptoms but also the improving the quality of life.

Kawanishi et al. had started multicenter randomized controlled trial in order to confirm the effect of CBT-IE with complementary video materials for moderate to severe IBS patients from 2019 [24]. The CBT-IE with complementary video intervention consists of ten weekly sessions, shown at Table 15.1. Each session consists of two parts: one part is viewing 3- to 13-min videos at home, and the other part is 30-min face-to-face therapy session with a licensed therapist at the hospital.

Kikuchi et al. also have started randomized controlled trial in order to confirm the effect of group cognitive behavioral therapy (GCBT) for moderate to severe IBS patients from 2020 [25]. The intervention consists of ten weekly 90-min sessions with homework and one booster session after 4 weeks. GCBT will be delivered face to face in groups of up to four participants and one or two therapists. The simple contents of the intervention are included in Table 15.2.

We expect that in these two randomized controlled studies, CBT might be effective for the refractory IBS patients.

IBS involves dysregulation of the brain-gut axis and psychological process. Despite the benefits of CBT for refractory IBS, very few patients have access to this approach. Not only in Japan but also in the world, future efforts should focus on CBT for the refractory IBS.

Table 15.1 Contents of each session of CBT-IE with complementary video materials by Kawanishi H et al.

Session number	Contents of intervention	Handouts	Play time of video
1	Education about IBS and psychological stress on digestive functioning, awareness-raising	Personal IBS profile	12′ 16″
		Monitoring IBS distress	
2	Education about the role of conditioning in IBS, attentional training	Monitoring IBS distress	6′ 44″
		Guide for attentional training	
		Common IBS symptom appraisal list	
3	Attentional training, cognitive restructuring for IBS sensations risk estimates	Monitoring IBS distress	9′ 31″
		Common IBS symptom appraisal list	
4	Cognitive restructuring for symptoms of	Monitoring IBS distress	9′ 05″
	IBS, valence estimates, hierarchy	Deliberate exposure hierarchy	
5	Cognitive restructuring, interoceptive exposure assessment, in vivo exposure	Monitoring IBS distress	11′ 36″
		Interoceptive exposure exercise	
		Interoceptive exposure FAQ	
		Guide for IBS and in vivo exposure	
		In vivo exposure instructions	
		Deliberate exposure record	
6–9	Conduct of interoceptive exposure, in vivo exposure	Monitoring IBS distress	5′ 40″
		Interoceptive exposure instructions	3′ 32″
		Interoceptive exposure record	3′ 43″ 3′ 35″
10	Interoceptive exposure, in vivo exposure, summary of the all sessions, relapse prevention	Monitoring IBS distress	77 44″
		Relapse prevention map	
		Dealing with setbacks	
		List of positive accomplishments	

Table 15.2 Group cognitive behavioral therapy (GCBT) programmed by Kikuch et al.

a. Explanation of a psychological model of IBS
b. the role of awareness of IBS-related stimuli
c. Explanation of the role of negative thoughts in exacerbating IBS
d. Explanation of how IBS-related avoidance and control behaviours maintain the fear and awareness of IBS symptoms
e. Interoceptive exposure to reduce fear of the sensations
f. Exposure to feared/avoided situations in which IBS sensations are expected
g. Education for how to handle relapse

Acknowledgments We thank Dr. Yukiko Okami, Dr. Shino Kikuchi, and Dr. Hitomi Kawanishi for the quoting their published figures and tables to complete this work.

References

1. Khayyatzadeh SS, Kazemi-Bajestani SMR, Mirmousavi SJ, Heshmati M, Khoshmohabbat S, Ferns GA, et al. Dietary behaviors in relation to prevalence of irritable bowel syndrome in adolescent girls. J Gastroenterol Hepatol. 2018;33(2):404–10.
2. Zaribaf F, Keshteli AH, Esmaillzadeh A, Saneei P, Feizi A, Daghaghzadeh H, et al. Empirically derived dietary habits are associated with irritable bowel syndrome. Eur J Clin Nutr. 2018;72(11):1537–47.
3. Okami Y, Kato T, Nin G, Harada K, Aoi W, Wada S, et al. Lifestyle and psychological factors related to irritable bowel syndrome in nursing and medical school students. J Gastroenterol. 2011;46(12):1403–10.
4. Simren M, Mansson A, Langkilde AM, Svedlund J, Abrahamsson H, Bengtsson U, et al. Food-related gastrointestinal symptoms in the irritable bowel syndrome. Digestion. 2001;63(2):108–15.
5. Caldarella MP, Milano A, Laterza F, Sacco F, Balatsinou C, Lapenna D, et al. Visceral sensitivity and symptoms in patients with constipation- or diarrhea-predominant irritable bowel syndrome (IBS): effect of a low-fat intraduodenal infusion. Am J Gastroenterol. 2005;100(2):383–9.
6. Faresjo A, Johansson S, Faresjo T, Roos S, Hallert C. Sex differences in dietary coping with gastrointestinal symptoms. Eur J Gastroenterol Hepatol. 2010;22(3):327–33.
7. Serra J, Salvioli B, Azpiroz F, Malagelada JR. Lipid-induced intestinal gas retention in irritable bowel syndrome. Gastroenterology. 2002;123(3):700–6.
8. Gonlachanvit S, Fongkam P, Wittayalertpanya S, Kullavanijaya P. Red chili induces rectal hypersensitivity in healthy humans: possible role of 5HT-3 receptors on capsaicin-sensitive visceral nociceptive pathways. Aliment Pharmacol Ther. 2007;26(4):617–25.
9. Mullin GE. Food allergy and irritable bowel syndrome. JAMA. 1991;265(13):1736.
10. Bohmer CJ, Tuynman HA. The clinical relevance of lactose malabsorption in irritable bowel syndrome. Eur J Gastroenterol Hepatol. 1996;8(10):1013–6.
11. Bohmer CJ, Tuynman HA. The effect of a lactose-restricted diet in patients with a positive lactose tolerance test, earlier diagnosed as irritable bowel syndrome: a 5-year follow-up study. Eur J Gastroenterol Hepatol. 2001;13(8):941–4.
12. Mertz HR. Irritable bowel syndrome. N Engl J Med. 2003;349(22):2136–46.
13. Thompson WG. The treatment of irritable bowel syndrome. Aliment Pharmacol Ther. 2002;16(8):1395–406.

14. Ford AC, Talley NJ, Spiegel BM, Foxx-Orenstein AE, Schiller L, Quigley EM, et al. Effect of fibre, antispasmodics, and peppermint oil in the treatment of irritable bowel syndrome: systematic review and meta-analysis. BMJ. 2008;337:a2313.
15. Kanazawa M, Endo Y, Whitehead WE, Kano M, Hongo M, Fukudo S. Patients and nonconsulters with irritable bowel syndrome reporting a parental history of bowel problems have more impaired psychological distress. Dig Dis Sci. 2004;49(6):1046–53.
16. Mearin F, Lacy BE, Chang L, Chey WD, Lembo AJ, Simren M, et al. Bowel Disorders. Gastroenterology. 2016;150:1393–407.
17. Simren M, Tornblom H, Palsson OS, Whitehead WE. Management of the multiple symptoms of irritable bowel syndrome. Lancet Gastroenterol Hepatol. 2017;2(2):112–22.
18. Lackner JM, Jaccard J. IBS outcome study research group. Factors associated with efficacy of cognitive behavior therapy vs education for patients with irritable bowel syndrome. Clin Gastroenterol Hepatol. 2019;17(8):1500–8.
19. Fukudo S, Kaneko H, Akiho H, Inamori M, Endo Y, Okumura T, et al. Evidence-based clinical practice guidelines for irritable bowel syndrome. J Gastroenterol. 2015;50(1):11–30.
20. Kennedy T, Jones R, Darnley S, Seed P, Wessely S, Chalder T. Cognitive behaviour therapy in addition to antispasmodic treatment for irritable bowel syndrome in primary care: randomised controlled trial. BMJ. 2005;331(7514):435.
21. Drossman DA, Toner BB, Whitehead WE, Diamant NE, Dalton CB, Duncan S, et al. Cognitive-behavioral therapy versus education and desipramine versus placebo for moderate to severe functional bowel disorders. Gastroenterology. 2003;125(1):19–31.
22. Lackner JM, Jaccard J, Keefer L, Brenner DM, Firth RS, Gudleski GD, et al. Improvement in gastrointestinal symptoms after cognitive behavior therapy for refractory irritable bowel syndrome. Gastroenterology. 2018;155(1):47–57.
23. Craske MG, Wolitzky-Taylor KB, Labus J, Wu S, Frese M, Mayer EA, et al. A cognitive-behavioral treatment for irritable bowel syndrome using interoceptive exposure to visceral sensations. Behav Res Ther. 2011;49(6–7):413–21.
24. Kawanishi H, Sekiguchi A, Funaba M, Fujii Y, Yoshiuchi K, Kikuchi H, et al. Cognitive behavioral therapy with interoceptive exposure and complementary video materials for irritable bowel syndrome (IBS): protocol for a multicenter randomized controlled trial in Japan. Biopsychosoc Med. 2019;13:14.
25. Kikuchi S, Oe Y, Sasaki Y, Ishii H, Ito Y, Horikoshi M, et al. Group cognitive behavioural therapy (GCBT) versus treatment as usual (TAU) in the treatment of irritable bowel syndrome (IBS): a study protocol for a randomized controlled trial. BMC Gastroenterol. 2020;20(1):29.

Chapter 16
Probiotics and Antibiotics

Takeshi Kamiya

Abstract Probiotics are defined as live microorganisms which exert health benefits to the host. There have been many high-quality systematic reviews, meta analyses, and randomized controlled trials to investigate the effectiveness of probiotics in the treatment of IBS. However, the results of them were somewhat inconsistent. These discrepancies in results may be attributable to methodological differences among trials, such as the type pf probiotic used, duration of treatment, and endpoint. Overall, probiotics are considered beneficial for IBS and recommended to use because of their relatively low cost and safety.

There are a few studies investigating the utility of prebiotics or synbiotics, a combination of probiotics and prebiotics, in the treatment of IBS. Some nonabsorbable antibiotics such as rifaximin and neomycin are recommended as a treatment for IBS based on moderate evidence. The potential for prebiotics, synbiotics, and antibiotics are worth further exploration.

Keywords Irritable bowel syndrome · Treatment · Probiotics · Prebiotics · Synbiotics · Antibiotics

16.1 Introduction

Gut microbiota plays an important role in the health of the host. It also possesses immune modulatory capacity. A disturbance in the balance of normal intestinal microflora or the host response to this has been shown to play a pathological role in several diseases. Irritable bowel syndrome (IBS) is a highly prevalent functional bowel disease without the presence of organic disease [1]. Although the pathogenesis of IBS is complicated, altered gut microbiota [2–4], small intestinal bacterial

T. Kamiya (✉)
Department of Medical Innovation, Nagoya City University Graduate School of Medical Sciences, Nagoya, Japan
e-mail: kamitake@med.nagoya-cu.ac.jp

© The Editor(s) (if applicable) and The Author(s), under exclusive license to Springer Nature Singapore Pte Ltd. 2024

T. Kamiya, S. Fukudo (eds.), *Irritable Bowel Syndrome*,
https://doi.org/10.1007/978-981-97-8410-3_16

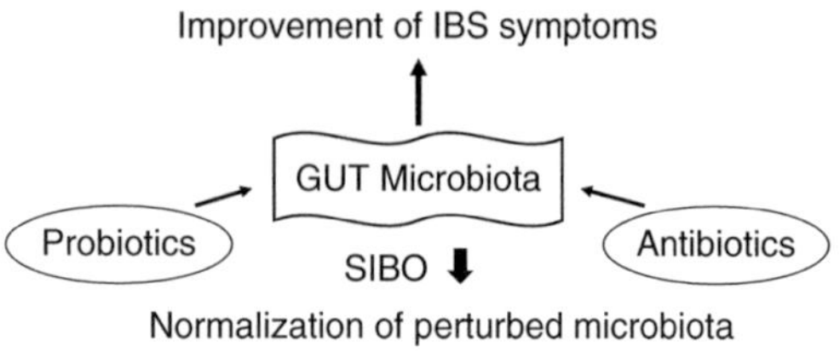

Fig. 16.1 The potential role of gut microbiota in IBS symptoms and putative modulators of gut microbiota

overgrowth (SIBO) [5, 6], and altered gut mucosal immune function are thought to cause IBS symptoms. Since the exact mechanisms of IBS symptoms are not well understood, IBS treatment should focus on symptomatic relief. Therefore, gut dysbiosis as the therapeutic target in IBS seems desirable. Probiotics, prebiotics, and antibiotics are used to readjust the gut flora (Fig. 16.1). This article summarizes the probiotics, prebiotics, and antibiotics used for the treatment of IBS.

16.2 Probiotics

Probiotics are defined [7, 8] as live or attenuated microorganisms, which on ingestion in adequate concentration, confer health benefits to the host. Probiotics have been used for the treatment of acute intestinal infections such as antibiotic-associated diarrhea, *Clostridium difficile* infection, and traveler's diarrhea. Some clinical studies have shown the therapeutic effects of probiotics for the treatment of inflammatory bowel disease, including ulcerative colitis and Crohn's disease, or the prevention of allergic diseases such as atopic dermatitis and asthma. Several high-quality systematic reviews and meta-analyses [9–13] have suggested that treatment with various probiotic bacteria can improve IBS symptoms.

Bifidobacteria, *Lactobacilli*, and *Saccharomyces* are commonly used as a commensal bacteria with probiotic activity. Many placebo-controlled trials have investigated several *Bifidobacteria* spp. including *B. bifidum*, *B. infantis*, and *B. lactis*. Treatment with of *B. bifidum* for 4 weeks have been shown [14] to significantly improve the global assessment of IBS symptoms, bowel discomfort, distension/bloating, urgency, and quality of life (QOL) in patients with IBS. *B. animalis* has been shown [15] to have a beneficial effect on the health-related QOL score, bloating, and stool frequency in patients with constipation predominant IBS (IBS-C). Furthermore, treatment with *B. infantis* for 4 or 8 weeks has been shown [16, 17] to improve most of the IBS symptoms such as abdominal pain/discomfort and bloating. However, in a previous study [18], treatment with *B. infantis* for 8 weeks did not result in significant improvements in individual IBS symptoms. In another study [19], oral administration of *B. lactis* was effective in abdominal distension and gastrointestinal transit in female patients with IBS-C. In a systematic review [13], *Bifidobacteria* did not show statistically significant efficacy compared with placebo, although it showed a beneficial with regard to global IBS symptoms or abdominal pain score. Moreover, treatment with *L. plantarum* alleviated pain and flatulence in patients with IBS after 12 months of treatment in a previous study [20]. In another study [21], treatment with *L. plantarum* improved all IBS symptoms. However, Ligaarden et al. [22] reported that treatment with *L. plantarum* might have an unfavorable effect on symptoms in patients with IBS. Furthermore, in a previous study [23], *L. casei* Shirota administrated twice daily did not significantly improve individual symptom scores after 8 weeks of treatment; however, the patients who received it showed an improvement in discomfort and flatulence scores 8 weeks after treatment (i.e., 16 weeks). In an animal study [24], *L. reuteri* showed marked inhibitory effects on visceral pain induced by colorectal distension. Tiequn et al. performed a meta-analysis [25] on the therapeutic effects of *Lactobacilli* in the treatment of IBS. The relative risk for clinical improvement with *Lactobacillus* treatment was 7.69 (17.62 for adults and 3.71 for children) in an analysis of six randomized clinical trials (RCTs). The authors concluded that *Lactobacillus* treatment was associated with a significantly higher rate of treatment responders in the overall population with IBS compared with placebo. However, another systematic review [13] of eight trials showed that *Lactobacillus* treatment had no clear benefit over placebo in terms of global IBS symptoms and symptom persistence. The risk ratio of symptoms persistence with active *L. plantarum* DSM 9843 therapy was significantly lower than that with control therapy.

A few studies that examined the efficacy of *Saccharomyces* yeast strains in patients with IBS have shown significant improvement in IBS symptoms. In a previous study [26], *S. cerevisiae* reduced abdominal pain/discomfort scores in 179 patients with IBS after 4 weeks of treatment; however, no significant improvement was observed in other IBS symptoms. In another study [27] for treatment with *S. cerevisiae*, a similar improvement in abdominal pain/discomfort was observed only in patients with IBS-C. A meta-analysis [28] of two studies supports previous data that *S. cerevisiae* significantly improves abdominal pain/discomfort and bloating in patients with global IBS, IBS-C, and diarrhea-predominant IBS (IBS-D). A statistically significant reduction in the symptom score of patients with IBS-D was observed after 30 days of treatment with *S. boulardii* in a study [29].

In terms of a multispecies probiotic supplement, the efficacy of VSL#3, a probiotic formulation containing eight different species of several *Bifidobacterium*, *Lactobacillus*, and *Streptococcus* strains, was investigated in some trials. In one study [30], the flatulence score and colonic transit time improved significantly after 4 and 8 weeks of VSL#3 treatment in patients with IBS compared with placebo. In a systematic review [4], overall, the efficacy of VSL#3 was similar to that of placebo in four clinical studies of patients with IBS although VSL#3 has shown a beneficial trend over placebo. In another study [31], treatment with SCM-III, a probiotic formulation containing *L. acidophilus*, *L. helveticus*, and *Bifidobacterium* sp., was "effective" or "very effective" in >80% of patients with IBS. Furthermore, in one study [32], I.31., a combination of two *L. plantarum* strains and *Pediococcus acidilactici*, was better than placebo in improving IBS-related QOL in patients with IBS and diarrhea. However, several clinical studies on other multispecies probiotics in patients with IBS have reported inconsistent results. Some studies comparing multispecies probiotics and placebo have demonstrated a significant improvement in adequate or global IBS symptoms relief, while other studies have not. A systematic review [13] on combinations of probiotics has suggested a significant improvement in IBS symptom scores compared with the control. Hungin et al. [11] reported that specific probiotics help relieve the overall symptom burden in some patients with IBS. Overall, probiotics appeared to have beneficial effects on global IBS symptoms considering their relatively low cost and safety; however, it was impossible to draw definitive conclusions about their efficacy.

The mechanisms of action of treatment with probiotics have not been completely elucidated and are probably multifactorial; the following mechanisms [33] have been demonstrated (Fig. 16.2):

1. Competitive exclusion of pathogenic bacteria and prevention of their invasion in the human body
2. Inhibition of pathogenic bacterial overgrowth and normalization of perturbed intestinal microbiota
3. Enhancement of intestinal epithelial barrier function
4. Modulation of the immune system

Probiotic bacteria eliminate pathogenic bacteria by producing antimicrobial substances and compete with pathogenic bacteria for binding sites and nutritional sources. IBS has been significantly associated with SIBO, which often causes symptoms particularly bloating. Probiotics have been suggested to inhibit pathogenic bacterial overgrowth and normalize the intestinal microbiota.

Accumulated evidences [5, 6] has shown that SIBO alters microbiota host interaction and that mucosal inflammation is associated with IBS symptoms. Intestinal microbiota is an important factor affecting low-grade mucosal inflammation and function. Disturbed commensal flora may increase permeability by altering tight junction protein expression and function and promoting pro-inflammatory cytokines. Mucosal inflammation may result in impaired epithelial barrier function. Alterations in the microbiota may also influence the development and function of

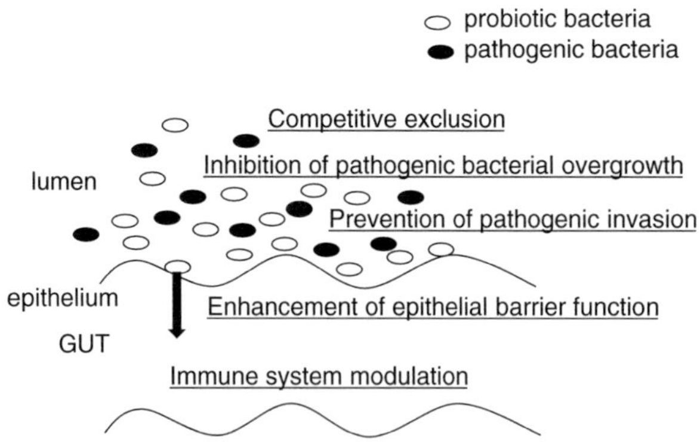

Fig. 16.2 The mechanisms of action of probiotics

the central and enteric nervous system. Dysbiosis is thought to be a potential pathogenic mechanism of IBS.

Probiotics have been suggested to improve the cytokine profile [17] and enhance mucosal barrier function. In addition, some probiotic bacteria secrete short-chain fatty acids (SCFAs) [33] and neurotransmitters. Signaling from the gut microbiota to the brain is mediated by several microbially derived molecules such as SCFAs and secondary bile acids. The expression of neurotransmitters is associated with receptors such as opioids and cannabinoids, which reduce visceral pain. Therefore, the beneficial effects of probiotics are thought to be mediated by modulation of the immune response and the brain-gut axis. Further studies are needed to elucidate the precise mechanisms of action of probiotics.

16.3 Prebiotics and Synbiotics

Prebiotics are nondigestible food ingredients that have beneficial effects on the host [34]. Prebiotics promote the growth and/or function of commensal microorganisms in the small intestine or colon. Galacto-oligosaccharides (GOS), oligofructose/fructo-oligosaccharides (FOS), and inulin, which are plant storage carbohydrates in vegetables, cereals, and fruits, are associated with prebiotic activity. However, only a few studies are currently investigating the utility of prebiotics in the treatment of IBS, although the use of prebiotics is recommended. Recent reviews [13] have summarized several RCTs for investigating the efficacy and safety of probiotics. Silk et al. performed a 12-week parallel crossover trial [35] comparing the efficacy of low-dose (3.5 g/day) prebiotic trans-GOS, high-dose (7 g/day) prebiotic trans GOS, and placebo (7 g/day) after 4 weeks of treatment; low-dose prebiotic treatment significantly changed the stool consistency and improved flatulence, bloating, the composite score of symptoms, and subjective global assessment (SGA) score, while high-dose prebiotic treatment significantly improved the SGA and anxiety scores. Based on these results, the authors suggested the potential for prebiotics in the treatment of IBS. In their other randomized double-blind study [36], regular consumption of B-GOS 2.75 g/day reduced the scores for bloating and flatulence. However, three RCTs [37, 38] demonstrated no therapeutic effect of FOS. The potential for prebiotics as a therapeutic agent in IBS is worth further exploration; however, its effectiveness in the treatment of IBS is inconclusive.

Synbiotics are a combination of prebiotics and probiotics in a single formulation (Fig. 16.3). The prebiotics in the symbiotic mixture promote the growth and survival of probiotic bacteria and stimulate the activity of the endogenous organisms in the host. Several RCTs and open-label clinical studies have investigated the efficacy of synbiotics in IBS, which have shown mixed results. Min et al. [39] investigated whether a composite yogurt enriched with acacia dietary fiber and high-dose *B. lactis* had additive therapeutic effects in 130 patients with IBS. Improvements in bowel habit satisfaction and overall IBS symptoms from baseline were significantly higher in the test group than in the control group. This study suggests that composite yogurt

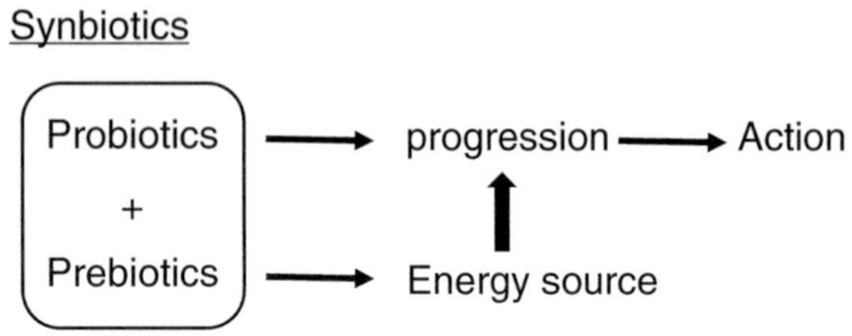

Fig. 16.3 The relationship between probiotics, prebiotics, and synbiotics

containing acacia fiber and *B. lactis* has greater therapeutic effects than in standard yogurt in patients with IBS. A recent RCT [40] objectively assessed the additive effects of polydextrose and a probiotic in 163 patients with IBS-C compared with the probiotic alone. The addition of polydextrose to sterilized *L. helveticus* did not show significant benefits in patients with IBS-C. However, daily consumption of a sterilized probiotic containing *L. helveticus* with or without polydextrose for a week alleviated constipation-related symptoms and objectively reduced both fecal pH and intestinal transit time. One systematic review [13] demonstrated that there were no statistically significant effects of synbiotics in reducing IBS symptoms. In addition, the superiority of synbiotics to either probiotics or prebiotics has not been demonstrated.

16.4 Antibiotics

The American College of Gastroenterology guidelines [41] strongly recommended using of nonsystemic antibiotics such as rifaximin and neomycin for the treatment of IBS based on moderate evidence. These nonsystemic antibiotics are used for IBS mainly in the USA. Rifaximin is a nonsystemic, broad-spectrum antibiotic that acts against gastrointestinal aerobic and anaerobic gram-positive and gram-negative bacteria. Rifaximin has a relatively low risk of bacterial resistance due to its low systemic absorption. The Food and Drug Agency (FDA) had initially approved it for the treatment of traveler's diarrhea and hepatic encephalopathy. Rifaximin was also approved for the treatment of IBS-D in 2017. Eradication of SIBO and normalization of intestinal microbiota have been proposed to account for the main mechanisms of the clinical efficacy of rifaximin in patients with IBS-D.

Several studies have demonstrated the efficacy of rifaximin in patients with IBS-D. The patients were administrated 550 mg of rifaximin thrice daily for 2 weeks in all studies. Pimentel et al. [42] conducted two identically designed RCTs (TARGET 1 and TARGET 2) and demonstrated the significant effect of rifaximin on global IBS symptoms in both studies. Moreover, two open-label trials have been conducted. In one trial [43], the patients received open-label rifaximin and were followed up for 4 weeks to assess abdominal pain and stool consistency response. Patients with recurrence were randomly assigned to receive two 2-week courses of double-blind rifaximin or placebo, 10 weeks part. A significantly higher percentage of patients treated with rifaximin were observed to have abdominal pain after the first and second double-blind repeat treatment in one study. Another study [44] examined the use of lactulose breath testing (LBT) in predicting response to rifaximin therapy. This study showed that a positive baseline LBT result predicted a higher likelihood of response to rifaximin in patients with IBS-D. A meta-analysis of five studies revealed that rifaximin was more efficacious than placebo for improving global IBS symptom scores in patients with IBS. In addition, repeat treatment with rifaximin was effective in patients with relapsing IBS-D symptoms. Furthermore, one trial [45] showed that neomycin was effective in 35% patients than 11% patients receiving the placebo. Another study of the same group [46] indicated neomycin-treated IBS patients with SIBO experienced a 48% improvement in IBS symptoms. However, treatment with neomycin is thought to produce rapid resistance. In Japan, the use of antibiotics in patients with IBS was not recommended in the previous guidelines. The FDA approved the administration of rifaximin in patients with IBS in 2017, and it is approved for the treatment of hepatic encephalopathy under the Japanese health insurance system. Therefore, nonabsorbable antibiotics are recommended weekly for the treatment of IBS according to the Japanese revised guidelines.

References

1. Lacy BE, Mearin F, Chang L, Chey WD, Lembo AJ, Simren M, Spiller R. Bowel disorder. Gastroenterology. 2016;150:1393–407.
2. Kassinen A, Krogius-Kurikka L, Makivuokko H, Rinttila T, Paulin L, Corander J, Malinen E, Apajalanti J, Palva A. The fecal microbiota of irritable bowel syndrome patients differs significantly from that of healthy subjects. Gastroenterology. 2007;133:24–33.
3. Tana C, Umesaki Y, Imaoka A, Handa T, Kanazawa M, Fukudo S. Altered profiles of intestinal microbiota and organic acids may be the origin of symptoms in irritable bowel syndrome. Neurogastroenterol Motil. 2010;22:512–9.
4. Harris LA, Baffy N. Modulation of the gut microbiota: a focus on treatments for irritable bowel syndrome. Postgrad Med. 2017;129:872–88.
5. Lin HC. Small intestinal bacterial overgrowth: a framework for understanding irritable bowel syndrome. JAMA. 2004;292:852–8.
6. Ghoshal UC, Ghoshal U. Small intestinal bacterial overgrowth and other intestinal disorders. Gastroenterol Clin N Am. 2017;46:103–20.
7. Fuller R. Probiotics in human medicine. Gut. 1991;32:439–42.
8. Hill C, Guarner F, Reid G, Gibson GR, Merenstein DJ, Pot B, Morelli L, Canani RB, Flint HJ, Salminen S, Calder PC, Sanders ME. Expert consensus document. The international scientific association for probiotics and prebiotics consensus statement on the scope and appropriate use of the term probiotics. Nat Rev Gastroenterol Hepatol. 2014;11:506–14.
9. Brenner DM, Moeller MJ, Chey WD, Schoenfeld PS. The utility of probiotics in the treatment of irritable bowel syndrome: a systematic review. Am J Gastroenterol. 2009;104:1033–49.
10. Moayyedi P, Ford AC, Talley NJ, Cremonini F, Foxx-Orenstein AE, Brandt LJ, Quigley EM. The efficacy of probiotics in the treatment of irritable bowel syndrome: a systematic review. Gut. 2010;59:325–32.
11. Hungin APS, Mitchell CR, Whorwell P, Mulligan C, Cole O, Agreus L, Fracasso P, Lionis C, Mendive J, Philippart de Foy JM, Seifert B, Wensaas KA, Winchester C, de Wit N. Systematic

review: probiotics in the management of lower gastrointestinal symptoms – an updated evidence-based international consensus. Aliment Pharmacol Ther. 2018;47:1054–70.
12. Barbara G, Cremon C, Azpiroz F. Probiotics in irritable bowel syndrome: where are we? Neurogastroenterol Motil. 2018;30:e13513.
13. Ford AC, Harris LA, Lacy BE, Quigley EMM, Moayyedi P. Systematic review with meta-analysis: the efficacy of prebiotics, probiotics, synbiotics and antibiotics in irritable bowel syndrome. Aliment Pharmacol Ther. 2018;48:1044–60.
14. Gugliemetti S, Mora D, Gschwender M, Popp K. Randomized clinical trial: Bifidobacterium bifidum MIMBb75 significantly alleviates irritable bowel syndrome and improve quality of life–a double-blind, placebo-controlled study. Alliment Pharmacol Ther. 2011;33:1123–32.
15. Guyonnet D, Chassany O, Ducrotte P, Picard C, Mouret M, Mercier CH, Matuchansky C. Effect of a fermented milk containing *Bifidobacterium animalis* DN-173 010 on the health-related quality of life and symptoms in irritable bowel syndrome in adults in primary care: a multicenter, randomized, double-blind, controlled trial. Aliment Pharmacol Ther. 2007;26:475–86.
16. Whorwell PJ, Altringer L, Morel J, Bond Y, Charbonneau D, O'Mahony L, Kiely B, Shanahan F, Quigley EM. Efficacy of an encapsulated probiotic Bifidobacterium infantis 35624 in women with irritable bowel syndrome. Am J Gastroenterol. 2006;101:1581–90.
17. O'Mahony L, McCathy J, Kelly P, Hurley G, Luo F, Chen K, O'Sullivan GC, Kiely B, Collins JK, Shanahan F, Quigley EM. Lactobacillus and Bifidobacterium in irritable bowel syndrome: symptom responses and relationship to cytokine profiles. Gastroenterology. 2005;128:541–51.
18. Charbonneau D, Gibb RD, Quigley EM. Fecal excretion of Bifidobacterium infantis 35624 and changes in fecal microbiota after eight weeks of oral supplementation with encapsulated probiotic. Gut Microbes. 2013;4:201–11.
19. Agrawal A, Houghton LA, Morris J, Reilly B, Guyonnet D, Goupil Feuillerat N, Schlumberger A, Jakob S, Whowell PJ. Clinical trial: the effects of a fermented milk product containing Bifidobacterium lactis DN-173010 on abdominal distension and gastrointestinal transit in irritable bowel syndrome with constipation. Aliment Pharmacol Ther. 2009;29:104–14.
20. Nobaek S, Johansson ML, Molin G, Ahrne S, Jeppsson B. Alteration of intestinal microflora is associated with reduction in abdominal bloating and pain in patients with irritable bowel syndrome. Am J Gastroenterol. 2000;95:1231–8.
21. Niedzielin K, Kordecki H, Birkenfeld B. A controlled, double-blind randomized study on the efficacy of Lactobacillus plantarum 299V in patients with irritable bowel syndrome. Eur J Gastroenterol Hepatol. 2001;13:1143–7.
22. Ligaarden SC, Axelsson L, Naterstad K, Lyderson S, Farup PG. A candidate probiotic with unfavourable effects in subjects with irritable bowel syndrome: a randomized controlled trial. BMC Gastroenterol. 2010;10:16.
23. Thijssen AY, Clemens CH, Vankerckhoven V, Goossens H, Jonkers DM, Masclee AA. Efficacy of Lactobacillus casei Shirota for patients with irritable bowel syndrome. Eur J Gastroenterol Hepatol. 2016;28:8–14.
24. Kamiya T, Wang L, Forsythe P, Goettsche G, Mao Y, Wang Y, Tougas G, Bienenstock J. Inhibitory effects of Lactobacillus reuteri on visceral pain induced by colorectal distension in Sprague-Dawley rats. Gut. 2006;55:191–6.
25. Tiequn B, Guanqun C, Shuo Z. Therapeutic effects of Lactobacillus in treating irritable bowel syndrome: a meta-analysis. Intern Med. 2015;54:243–9.
26. Pineton de Chambrun G, Neut C, Chau A, Cazaubiel M, Pelerin F, Justen P, Desreumaux P. A randomized clinical trial of Saccharomyces cerevisiae versus placebo in the irritable bowel syndrome. Dig Liver Dis. 2015;47:119–24.
27. Spiller R, Pelerin F, Cayzeele Decherf A, Maudet C, Housez B, Cazaubiel M, Justen P. a double blind placebo-controlled trial of Saccharomyces cerevisiae CNCMI-3856 in irritable bowel syndrome: improvement in abdominal pain and bloating in those with predominant constipation. United European Gastroenterol J. 2016;4:353–62.

28. Cayzeele-Decherf A, Pelerin F, Leuillet S, Douillad B, Housez B, Cazaubiel M, Jacobson GK, Justen P, Desreumaux P. Saccharomyces cerevisiae CNCMI-3856 in irritable bowel syndrome: an individual subject meta-analysis. World J Gastroenterol. 2017;23:336–44.
29. Bafutto M, Almeida JR, Leite NV, Costa MB, Oliveira EC, Resende-Filho J. Treatment of diarrhea-predominant irritable bowel syndrome with mesalazine and/or Saccharomyces boulardii. Arq Gastroenterol. 2013;50:304–9.
30. Kim HJ, Vazquez Roque MI, Camilleri M, Stephens D, Burton DD, Baxer K, Thomforde G, Zinsmeister AR. A randomized controlled trial of a probiotic combination VSL#3 and placebo in irritable bowel syndrome with bloating. Neurogastroenterol Motil. 2005;17:687–96.
31. Tsuchiya J, Barreto R, Okura R, Kawakita S, Fesce E, Marotta F. Single-blind follow-up study on the effectiveness of a symbiotic preparation in irritable bowel syndrome. Chin J Dig Dis. 2004;5:169–74.
32. Lorenzo-Zuniga V, Llop E, Suarez C, Alvarez B, Abreu L, Espadaler J, Serra J. I.31, a new combination of probiotics, improves irritable bowel syndrome-related quality of life. World J Gastroenterol. 2014;20:8709–16.
33. Plaza-Diaz J, Ruiz-Ojeda FJ, Gill-Campos M, Gill A. Mechanisms of action of probiotics. Adv Nutr. 2019;10(suppl 1):S49–66.
34. Gibson GR, Hutkins R, Sanders ME, Prescott SL, Reimer RA, Salminen SJ, Scott K, Stanton C, Swanson KS, Cani PD, Verbeke K, Reid G. The international scientific association for probiotics and prebiotics (ISAPP) consensus statement on the definition and scope of prebiotics. Nat Rev Gastroenterol Hepatol. 2017;14:491–502.
35. Silk DB, Davis A, Vulevic J, Tzortzis G, Gibson GR. Clinical trial: the effects of a trans-galactooligosaccharide prebiotic on faecal microbiota and symptoms in irritable bowel syndrome. Aliment Pharmacol Ther. 2009;29:508–18.
36. Vulevic J, Tzortzis G, Juric A, Gibson GR. Effect of a prebiotic galactooligosaccharide mixture (B-GOS) on gastrointestinal symptoms in adults selected from a general population who suffer with bloating, abdominal pain, or flatulence. Neurogastroenterol Motil. 2018;30:e13440.
37. Olesen M, Gudmand-Hoyer E. Efficacy, safety and tolerability of fructooligosaccharides in the treatment of irritable bowel syndrome. Am J Clin Nutr. 2000;72:1570–5.
38. Azpiroz F, Dubray C, Bernailer-Donadille A, Cardot JM, Accarino A, Serra J, Wagner A, Respondek F, Dapoigny M. Effects of scFOS on the composition of fecal microbiota and anxiety in patients with irritable bowel syndrome: a randomized, double blind, placebo controlled study. Neurogastroenterol Motil. 2017;29:12911.
39. Min YW, Park SU, Jang YS, Kim YH, Rhee PL, Ko SH, Joo N, Kim SI, Kim CH, Chang DK. Effect of composite yogurt enriched with acacia fiber and Bifidobacterium lactis. World J Gastroenterol. 2012;18:4563–9.
40. Bahrudin MF, Abdul Rani R, Tamil AM, Mokhtar NM, Raja Ali RA. Effectiveness of sterilized symbiotic drink containing Lactobacillus helveticus comparable to probiotic alone in patients with constipation-predominant irritable bowel syndrome. Dig Dis Sci. 2020;65:541–9.
41. Lacy BE, Pimentel M, Brenner DM, Chey WD, Keefer LA, Long MD, Moshiree B. ACG clinical guideline: management of irritable bowel syndrome. Am J Gastroenterol. 2021;116:17–44.
42. Pimentel M, Lembo A, Chey WD, Zakko S, Ringel Y, Yu J, Mareya SM, Shaw AL, Bortey E, Forbes WP, TARGET Study Group. Rifaximin therapy for patients with irritable bowel syndrome without constipation. N Engl J Med. 2011;364:22–32.
43. Lembo A, Rao SSC, Heimanson Z, Pimentel M. Abdominal pain response to rifaximin in patients with irritable bowel syndrome with diarrhea. Clin Transl Gastroenterol. 2020;11:e00144.
44. Rezale A, Heimanson Z, McCallum R, Pimentel M. Lactulose breath testing as a predictor of response to rifaximin in patients with irritable bowel syndrome with diarrhea. Am J Gastroenterol. 2019;114:1886–93.

45. Pimentel M, Chow EJ, Lin HC. Normalization of lactulose breath testing correlates with symptom improvement in irritable bowel syndrome. A double-blind, randomized, placebo-controlled study. Am J Gastroenterol. 2003;98:412–9.
46. Pimentel M, Chow EJ, Lin HC. Eradication of small intestinal bacterial overgrowth reduces symptoms of irritable bowel syndrome. Am J Gastroenterol. 2000;95:3503–6.

Part V
Recent Special

Chapter 17
Fecal Microbiota Transplantation for Treatment of Irritable Bowel Syndrome

Tsuyoshi Yamane, Tatsuhiro Masaoka, and Takanori Kanai

Abstract Fecal microbiota transplantation (FMT) as a treatment option for irritable bowel syndrome (IBS) is emerging, but early studies have led to high expectations. Essential to the success of FMT is the extraction and preservation of gut bacterial flora. Protocols are still in the examination stage and being standardized; however, it has been shown that freeze storage of bacterial extracts is possible. Progress is also being made in recognizing and optimizing factors that may influence the success of FMT as a treatment for IBS including the selection process of identifying the recipient and the donor, the setup criteria of the control group in experimental studies, and the method of administering the transplant. These and other factors are currently being studied to improve the efficacy of FMT in the future.

Keywords Capsule · *Clostridium difficile* infection (CDI) · Dysbiosis · Fecal microbiota transplantation (FMT) · Irritable bowel syndrome (IBS) · Stool extract

17.1 Fecal Microbiota Transplantation (FMT)

The human gastrointestinal tract contains about 1000 bacterial species and about 100 trillion bacteria per person. Bacterial numbers range from 10^1 to 10^4 cfu/g in the stomach and jejunum, but as bile acid decreases, the numbers increase to 10^8 cfu/g

T. Yamane · T. Kanai
Division of Gastroenterology and Hepatology, Department of Internal Medicine, Keio University School of Medicine, Tokyo, Japan
e-mail: takagast@z2.keio.jp

T. Masaoka (✉)
Division of Gastroenterology and Hepatology, Department of Internal Medicine, Keio University School of Medicine, Tokyo, Japan

Center for Endoscopy, Kwasaki Municipal Hospital, Kawasaki, Japan
e-mail: masaoka@keio.jp

© The Editor(s) (if applicable) and The Author(s), under exclusive license to Springer Nature Singapore Pte Ltd. 2024

T. Kamiya, S. Fukudo (eds.), *Irritable Bowel Syndrome*,
https://doi.org/10.1007/978-981-97-8410-3_17

in the ileum and further increase to 10^{11} to 10^{12} cfu/g in the large intestine [1]. The microbiota metabolize undigested food to short-chain fatty acids, and other metabolites, and these metabolites help differentiate and mature immune cells [2]. More than 99% of gut microbiota are bacteria belonging to four phyla: *Firmicutes*, *Actinobacteria*, *Bacteroidetes*, and *Proteobacteria* [3]. Although the stable condition of the human gut microbiota has been maintained for a long time, there are individual differences. Moreover, the human gut microbiota is affected by various factors such as eating behavior and lifestyle [3]. The abnormal constitution of the gut microbiota is termed as dysbiosis, and dysbiosis may be caused by various factors such as inflammation, environment, infection, diet, and the use of antibiotics [4]. Gut microbiota are associated with various diseases such as inflammatory bowel disease, allergic disease, functional gastrointestinal disease, and autism, as well as lifestyle-related diseases such as obesity and diabetes [5].

Currently, various medical treatment strategies are used to improve dysbiosis of the gut microbiota. Although most of them have not shown satisfactory clinical efficacy, FMT is a novel method to improve dysbiosis since FMT can administer larger amounts and types of bacteria compared to probiotics treatment. FMT is a treatment that uses stool extract containing bacterial flora obtained from healthy donors and delivered to the intestinal tract of the recipient. Therefore, FMT is expected to directly change the intestinal flora. Currently, FMT is the accepted treatment option for recurring and intractable *Clostridium difficile* infection (CDI) [6–8], and its effectiveness in treating CDI and other diseases has been examined [9]. Although irritable bowel syndromes (IBS) is strongly related to dysbiosis [10, 11], treatment options are limited; therefore, the expectation for FMT as a successful treatment for IBS is high. The first use of FMT in the treatment of patients with IBS was reported in 2014 [12]; since then, several reports have emerged helping to clarify the efficacy of this treatment approach and the focus of future studies.

17.2 Selection of Donor for FMT

To perform FMT, it is first necessary to select a donor. At present, since the optimal microbiota for FMT is not clear, selection of an effective donor is difficult. A small retrospective study of 13 patients who underwent FMT for the treatment of refractory IBS reported that 38% of the donors were spouses; 31% were other family members such as parents, brothers, or sisters; and the remaining 31% were nonfamily members. However, improvement in IBS symptoms was not affected by recipient-donor relationships [13]. On the other hand, safety must be considered in the selection of donors, not just for IBS patients but all recipients. Specifically, screening for infectious diseases such as human immunodeficiency virus, hepatitis B virus, and hepatitis C virus, syphilis and other bacterial infections, and parasites are needed. The use of illegal drugs, tattooing, or body piercing within 6 months of the transplant date may also exclude a donor. Patients with autoimmune diseases, metabolic diseases, malignancies, and defecation disorders should also be excluded.

The case of a woman successfully treated with FMT who developed new-onset obesity after receiving stool from a healthy but overweight donor was reported [14]. Therefore, appropriate blood tests and thorough evaluations are needed before approving a donor.

17.3 Preparation of Stool Extract for FMT

The methods for extracting stool and obtaining bacterial flora from a donor is outlined in Table 17.1. Whether the extract is administered as is or encapsulated depends on the dosing regimen, but in any case, it is necessary to prepare the bacterial extract relatively quickly with minimal exposure to air, considering the survival of anaerobic bacteria and suppression of the growth of aerobic bacteria [16]. Cui et al. [15] have standardized extraction protocols (Table 17.1). The composition of the bacterial flora in the original stool is not significantly changed in the final extract obtained by suspending the stool and repeated filtration, centrifugation, and concentration [17]. Johnsen et al. [18] reported that the efficacy of FMT for the treatment of IBS did not depend on whether the extract was transplanted immediately or after cryopreservation and thawing. Therefore, it was concluded that stool extract stored at -80°C was preserved. In the case of encapsulation, the extract can be encapsulated directly [19], and, after freeze-drying, the encapsulated stool extract can be stored for long periods [20].

Table 17.1 Fecal microbiota extraction protocol (modified from Cui et al. [15])

1. Feces collection: collect fresh feces in a sterile container and transfer into a sterile blender container
2. Fecal suspension preparation: add 500–1000 mL of a 0.9% saline solution to the blender container, mix feces solution thoroughly to make a suspension, and filter to collect the suspension
3. Filter: filter four times using a micro-strainer and collect the suspension
4. Centrifuge: transfer the suspension to 50-mL centrifuge tubes and centrifuge at 1200 g for 3 min
5. Wash: discard the supernatant and add sterile saline to 50 mL; gently mix by inverting multiple times, and centrifuge again
6. Repeat the centrifugation and wash steps 3–5 times
7. Discard most of supernatant; the desired product is the crudely purified fecal microbiota pellet
8. Fecal microbiota suspension: dilute the flora 1.5-fold with 0.9% saline, and mix gently by inverting the tube several times. The freshly concentrated fecal microbiota suspension should be administered to the patient's intestine immediately
9. Bacteria storage: if the suspension is not going to be used immediately, it can be stored in 10% sterile pharmaceutical-grade glycerol at −80 °C

17.4 Administrative Methods of Stool Extract for FMT

Methods of administrating the stool extract into the intestinal tract include nasogastric, nasojejunal, upper gastrointestinal endoscopy, lower gastrointestinal endoscopy, and enemas. Although lower gastrointestinal endoscopy allows direct observation of lesions, the invasiveness and cost of this optional procedure must be considered [16]. The use of enemas is less invasive and less costly than the lower gastrointestinal endoscopy approach, but the range of reach of the extract by enema is limited, so the effect may be limited [16]. A simpler approach is from the upper gastrointestinal tract, which has been shown to be effective in the case of small intestine bacterial overgrowth (SIBO). However, the development of aspiration pneumonia following the upper gastrointestinal approach has been reported [21]. Studies investigating the impact of the administrative method of FMT on the therapeutic efficacy of IBS are limited, and additional studies are needed [19]. There is also no consensus on how long the changes in the microbiota introduced by FMT are maintained; this is discussed in the following section.

17.5 Efficacy of FMT for IBS

FMT for patients with IBS was firstly reported in 2014, with symptomatic improvements observed in 9 of 13 patients (70%); only 1 adverse event, increased flatus, was noted [12]. The results of this initial study led to increased attention and use of FMT as a new method to improve dysbiosis of patients with IBS. In Japan, FMT using lower gastrointestinal endoscopy was performed in ten IBS patients (eight of whom had diarrhea-type based on Rome III criteria) who were resistant to medical treatment for more than 1 year. In six of ten patients, fecal properties (assessed by the Bristol Stool Scale) and abdominal symptoms were improved, and no severe adverse events were observed [22]. A 16S rRNA gene-based metagenomic analysis of donor and recipient stool samples showed improved bacterial diversity in the FMT-effective recipient group, and abundant *Actinobacteria*, particularly *Bifidobacterium*, were found in the stools of effective donors. Johnsen et al. [23] conducted a randomized controlled trial in which the control group was administered their own stool and the treatment group received donor stool. A significantly higher rate of improvement in symptoms at 3 months after FMT was reported in the treatment group (65%; 36 of 55 patients) compared to the control group (43%; 12 of 28). Mazzawi et al. [24] reported that 13 patients with IBS, based on Rome III criteria, underwent FMT with upper gastrointestinal endoscopy. The observation periods were 28 weeks for nine participants and 20 weeks for four participants. Eight patients showed improved symptoms and remained in the same stable condition during the observation period. A 16S rRNA gene-based metagenomic analysis of donor and recipient stools also showed that stools from effective donors had a significantly smaller signal for *Bacteroides* and *Desulfitispora* than stools from noneffective donors. In a recent report, Johnsen et al. [23] conducted a randomized controlled trial of 90 patients with constipation-type and mixed-type IBS based on Rome III criteria, refractory to medical treatment, and evaluated them 6 and 12 months after FMT. Quality of life and fatigue were both reported to be highly improved in the treatment group compared with the control group. Thus, while some reports have shown the effectiveness of FMT in patients with IBS, others have shown no apparent efficacy. Halkjaer et al. [25] performed a randomized double-blind, placebo-controlled study of IBS patients receiving stool capsules or placebo capsules for 12 days and compared the treatment group (26 cases) and the placebo group (26 cases) at 6 months after administration. In the treatment group, the diversity of intestinal bacteria was improved, but the superior improvement in symptoms was also recognized in the placebo group. A double-blind, randomized, crossover trial of fecal capsule administration followed by placebo capsule administration versus placebo capsule administration followed by fecal capsule administration reported no significant differences in IBS-symptom severity scale (IBS-SSS) scores between the two groups at 12 weeks, after adjustment for baseline scores [26]. In a meta-analysis of randomized controlled trials of FMT for IBS, symptom improvement 3 months after FMT was similar to that of the placebo. A sub-analysis suggested a superiority of donor FMT over autologous fecal transplantation with a single dose of endoscopy as the method of administration ($n = 5$, relative risk [RR] = 1.59; 95% CI 1.06–2.39). However, as a conclusion of the analysis, current evidence from randomized controlled trials does not support a benefit of FMT for global IBS symptoms [27]. Holster et al. [28] conducted a randomized controlled trial of 16 patients with IBS based on Rome III criteria using autologous stool transplantation as a control group. No significant differences were found between the allogenic and the autologous FMT treatment regarding symptom scores. However, symptom scores of patients receiving allogenic fecal material significantly decreased after FMT compared with the baseline, which was not the case in the autologous group. The authors discussed that colonoscopy and routine bowel irrigation prior to FMT may alter the composition of the intestinal flora and contribute to the improvement of IBS symptoms. These reports about the efficacy of FMT for IBS are summarized in Table 17.2.

As mentioned above, a specific view on the use of FMT as a therapy for IBS has not been obtained, and at present, the effectiveness is also not clear and requires further investigation. Therefore, in the evidence-based clinical practice guidelines for irritable bowel syndrome 2020 published by the Japanese Society of Gastroenterology (JSGE), FMT is commented as "Further studies are needed to evaluate the efficacy of FMT" [30]. Although not limited to FMT for IBS treatment, many factors have been implicated in the study design of FMT including the use of endoscopy, enema, and fecal capsules as routes of administration for FMT, study designs of control groups, the origin of donor stool, and the number of doses. There are many unresolved questions at present, such as which bacteria produce IBS symptoms, which are effective in improving the symptoms, whether the changes in intestinal bacteria after FMT are permanent, if not, how long are they stable, and whether repeated dosing is required. In addition, many of the mentioned studies

Table 17.2 Summary of fecal microbiota transplantation (FMT) trials

References	Country Year	Sample size	Route of FMT	Follow-up period	Results
Pinn et al. [12]	USA 2014	13 patients (single-arm study)	Upper gastrointestinal endoscopy	11 months	70% of patients experienced resolution of IBS symptoms after FMT
Mizuno et al. [22]	Japan 2017	10 patients (single-arm study)	Lower gastrointestinal endoscopy	4 weeks	FMT improved stool form and depressed mood; *Bifidobacterium*-rich donor feces was related to successful FMT
Holvoet et al. [29]	Belgium 2017	12 patients (single-arm study)	–	12 months	75% of patients experienced resolution of IBS symptoms after FMT
Johnsen et al. [23]	Norway 2018	55 patients 28 controls (RCT)	Lower gastrointestinal endoscopy	3 months	65% of patients experienced resolution of IBS symptoms after FMT (control 43%)
Mazzawi et al. [24]	Norway 2018	13 patients (single-arm study)	Upper gastrointestinal endoscopy	28 weeks	62% of patients experienced resolution of IBS symptoms after FMT *Bacteroides*- and *Desulfitispora*-poor donor feces were related to unsuccessful FMT
Halkjær et al. [25]	Denmark 2018	26 patients 26 controls (RCT)	Capsules (p.o.)	6 months	Placebo group experienced greater symptom relief Gut microbiota in patients was changed by FMT
Aroniadis et al. [26]	USA 2019	48 patients (crossover study)	Capsules (p.o.)	12 weeks	No significant difference in IBS-SSS score
Xu et al. [27]	USA 2019	4 studies Meta-analysis (RCT)	Nasojejunal tube Lower gastrointestinal endoscopy Capsules (p.o.)	12 weeks	No significant difference between the FMT and control group
Holster et al. [28]	Sweden 2019	8 patients 8 controls (RCT)	Lower gastrointestinal endoscopy	6 months	All participants experienced resolution of IBS symptoms No significant difference between the FMT and control group
Johnsen et al. [18]	Norway 2020	60 patients 30 controls (RCT)	Lower gastrointestinal endoscopy	12 months	Significant improvement of QoL and fatigue were found

IBS irritable bowel syndrome; *p.o.* per os, *QoL* quality of life, *RCT* randomized controlled trial, *SSS* symptom severity scale used Rome III criteria to define IBS symptoms. Although abdominal pain and abdominal discomfort were included as symptoms of IBS, newly defined Rome VI criteria only include abdominal pain [31]. If studies are conducted on the basis of Rome IV criteria, the research results and their interpretation may change. All of these factors need to be investigated.

17.6 Conclusions

FMT is an emerging therapy for IBS; however, its effectiveness is not clear at present and the technique remains under investigation. The bacterial flora extraction protocol is becoming standardized, and the extract is able to withstand cryopreservation. However, there are many issues which remain unanswered and without a unified view among researchers in the field. Some of these issues are the screening and selection of the donor, the criteria used to set the control group, and the method of administration of the bacterial extract. Further large-scale and Rome IV-based patient studies of FMT and continued development of this exciting technology are needed in the future.

References

1. Simrén M, Barbara G, Flint HJ, Spiegel BMR, Spiller RC, Vanner S, et al. Intestinal microbiota in functional bowel disorders: a Rome foundation report. Gut. 2013;62(1):159–76.
2. Nicholson JK, Holmes E, Kinross J, Burcelin R, Gibson G, Jia W, et al. Host-gut microbiota metabolic interactions. Science. 2012;336(6086):1262–7.
3. Mayer EA, Savidge T, Shulman RJ. Brain-gut microbiome interactions and functional bowel disorders. Gastroenterology. 2014;146(6):1500–12.
4. Honda K, Littman DR. The microbiome in infectious disease and inflammation. Annu Rev Immunol. 2012;30:759–95.
5. Collado MC, Rautava S, Isolauri E, Salminen S. Gut microbiota: a source of novel tools to reduce the risk of human disease? Pediatr Res. 2015;77(1-2, 182):–188.
6. Kelly CR, Ihunnah C, Fischer M, Khoruts A, Surawicz C, Afzali A, et al. Fecal microbiota transplant for treatment of *Clostridium difficile* infection in immunocompromised patients. Am J Gastroenterol. 2014;109(7):1065–71.
7. Agrawal M, Aroniadis OC, Brandt LJ, Kelly C, Freeman S, Surawicz C, et al. The long-term efficacy and safety of fecal microbiota transplant for recurrent, severe, and complicated *Clostridium difficile* infection in 146 elderly individuals. J Clin Gastroenterol. 2016;50(5):403–7.
8. Khoruts A, Rank KM, Newman KM, Viskocil K, Vaughn BP, Hamilton MJ, et al. Inflammatory bowel disease affects the outcome of fecal microbiota transplantation for recurrent *Clostridium difficile* infection. Clin Gastroenterol Hepatol. 2016;14(10):1433–8.
9. Smith MB, Kelly C, Alm EJ. Policy: how to regulate faecal transplants. Nature. 2014;506(7488):290–1.
10. Kassinen A, Krogius-Kurikka L, Mäkivuokko H, Rinttilä T, Paulin L, Corander J, et al. The fecal microbiota of irritable bowel syndrome patients differs significantly from that of healthy subjects. Gastroenterology. 2007;133(1):24–33.

11. Wang L, Alammar N, Singh R, Nanavati J, Song Y, Chaudhary R, et al. Gut microbial dysbiosis in the irritable bowel syndrome: a systematic review and meta-analysis of case-control studies. J Acad Nutr Diet. 2019;120(4):565–86.
12. Pinn DM, Aroniadis OC, Brandt LJ. Is fecal microbiota transplantation the answer for irritable bowel syndrome? A single-center experience. Am J Gastroenterol. 2014;109(11):1831–2.
13. Pinn D, Aroniadis O, Brandt L. Follow-up study of fecal microbiota transplantation (FMT) for the treatment of refractory irritable bowel syndrome (IBS). Am J Gastroenterol. 2013;108:563. https://doi.org/10.14309/00000434-201310001-01862.
14. Alang N, Kelly CR. Weight gain after fecal microbiota transplantation. Open Forum Infect Dis. 2015;2(1):4.
15. Cui B, Feng Q, Wang H, Wang M, Peng Z, Li P, et al. Fecal microbiota transplantation through mid-gut for refractory Crohn's disease: safety, feasibility, and efficacy trial results. J Gastroenterol Hepatol. 2015;30(1):51–8.
16. König J, Siebenhaar A, Högenauer C, Arkkila P, Nieuwdorp M, Norén T, et al. Consensus report: faecal microbiota transfer - clinical applications and procedures. Aliment Pharmacol Ther. 2017;45(2):222–39.
17. Cui B, Li P, Xu L, Zhao Y, Wang H, Peng Z, et al. Step-up fecal microbiota transplantation strategy: a pilot study for steroid-dependent ulcerative colitis. J Transl Med. 2015;12(13):298.
18. Johnsen PH, Hilpüsch F, Valle PC, Goll R. The effect of fecal microbiota transplantation on IBS related quality of life and fatigue in moderate to severe non-constipated irritable bowel: secondary endpoints of a double blind, randomized, placebo-controlled trial. EBioMedicine. 2020;51:102562.
19. Kelly CR, Kahn S, Kashyap P, Laine L, Rubin D, Atreja A, et al. Update on fecal microbiota transplantation 2015: indications, methodologies, mechanisms, and outlook. Gastroenterology. 2015;149(1):223–37.
20. Jiang ZD, Ajami NJ, Petrosino JF, Jun G, Hanis CL, Shah M, et al. Randomised clinical trial: faecal microbiota transplantation for recurrent *Clostridium difficile* infection - fresh, or frozen, or lyophilised microbiota from a small pool of healthy donors delivered by colonoscopy. Aliment Pharmacol Ther. 2017;45(7):899–908.
21. Baxter M, Ahmad T, Colville A, Sheridan R. Fatal aspiration pneumonia as a complication of fecal microbiota transplant. Clin Infect Dis. 2015;61(1):136–7.
22. Mizuno S, Masaoka T, Naganuma M, Kishimoto T, Kitazawa M, Kurokawa S, et al. *Bifidobacterium*-rich fecal donor may be a positive predictor for successful fecal microbiota transplantation in patients with irritable bowel syndrome. Digestion. 2017;96(1):29–38.
23. Johnsen PH, Hilpüsch F, Cavanagh JP, Leikanger IS, Kolstad C, Valle PC, et al. Faecal microbiota transplantation versus placebo for moderate-to-severe irritable bowel syndrome: a double-blind, randomised, placebo-controlled, parallel-group, single-centre trial. Lancet Gastroenterol Hepatol. 2018;3(1):17–24.
24. Mazzawi T, Lied GA, Sangnes DA, El-Salhy M, Hov JR, Gilja OH, et al. The kinetics of gut microbial community composition in patients with irritable bowel syndrome following fecal microbiota transplantation. PLoS One. 2018;13(11):e0194904.
25. Halkjær SI, Christensen AH, Lo BZS, Browne PD, Günther S, Hansen LH, et al. Faecal microbiota transplantation alters gut microbiota in patients with irritable bowel syndrome: results from a randomised, double-blind placebo-controlled study. Gut. 2018;67(12):2107–15.
26. Aroniadis OC, Brandt LJ, Oneto C, Feuerstadt P, Sherman A, Wolkoff AW, et al. Faecal microbiota transplantation for diarrhoea-predominant irritable bowel syndrome: a double-blind, randomised, placebo-controlled trial. Lancet Gastroenterol Hepatol. 2019;4(9):675–85.
27. Xu D, Chen VL, Steiner CA, Berinstein JA, Eswaran S, Waljee AK, et al. Efficacy of fecal microbiota transplantation in irritable bowel syndrome: a systematic review and meta-analysis. Am J Gastroenterol. 2019;114(7):1043–50.
28. Holster S, Lindqvist CM, Repsilber D, Salonen A, de Vos WM, König J, et al. The Effect of allogenic versus autologous fecal microbiota transfer on symptoms, visceral perception and

fecal and mucosal microbiota in irritable bowel syndrome: a randomized controlled study. Clin Transl Gastroenterol. 2019;10(4):e00034.

29. Holvoet T, Joossens M, Wang J, Boelens J, Verhasselt B, Laukens D, et al. Assessment of faecal microbial transfer in irritable bowel syndrome with severe bloating. Gut. 2017;66(5):980–2.
30. Fukudo S, Okumura T, Inamori M, Okuyama Y, Kanazawa M, Kamiya T, et al. Evidence-based clinical practice guidelines for irritable bowel syndrome 2020. J Gastroenterol. 2021;56(3):193–217.
31. Mearin F, Lacy BE, Chang L, Chey WD, Lembo AJ, Simren M, et al. Bowel disorders. Gastroenterology. 2016;150(6):1393–407.

Chapter 18
Clinical Study Design and Evaluation of the Efficacy in the Treatment

Takeshi Kamiya, Hiromi Hagiwara, and Hidekatsu Fukuta

Abstract Irritable bowel syndrome (IBS) is diagnosed based on subjective symptoms, and the aim of treatment is to improve the symptoms of IBS. Patients' symptom reporting is essential to evaluate the severity of symptoms. Furthermore, study design and endpoint are very important in IBS clinical trials. Both the Food and Drug Administration (FDA) and the European Medicines Agency (EMA) released a general guidance on the evaluation of medical products for the treatment of IBS based on patient-reported outcome (PRO) measures. The primary endpoint should be clinically meaningful and demonstrate the efficacy of therapeutic agents, and the best endpoint for IBS clinical trials need to be determined.

Keywords Irritable bowel syndrome · Clinical study design · Treatment efficacy · Endpoint

18.1 Introduction

Irritable bowel syndrome (IBS) is a highly prevalent bowel disorder [1–5] but not an organic disease, which might explain its symptoms. It has a heterogeneous pathophysiology, with various factors contributing to the causation of symptoms. However, the underlying mechanisms are still unclear. Although IBS can be diagnosed using subjective valuables, no biomarkers are available. A wide range of management strategies, such as diet, pharmaceutical therapy, psychological therapy, and alternative medicine, have been proposed according to the possible underlying etiology; however, these remain mostly unsatisfactory. Further treatment strategies such as new drugs for IBS are currently being anticipated. With regard to the

T. Kamiya (✉) · H. Hagiwara · H. Fukuta
Department of Medical Innovation, Nagoya City University Graduate School of Medical Sciences, Nagoya, Japan
e-mail: kamitake@med.nagoya-cu.ac.jp; crhiroha@med.nagoya-cu.ac.jp; fukuta-h@med.nagoya-cu.ac.jp

© The Editor(s) (if applicable) and The Author(s), under exclusive license to Springer Nature Singapore Pte Ltd. 2024

T. Kamiya, S. Fukudo (eds.), *Irritable Bowel Syndrome*,
https://doi.org/10.1007/978-981-97-8410-3_18

development of new drugs, it is necessary to demonstrate their efficacy and safety in clinical trials. In general, the design and endpoint of a clinical trial are extremely important for evaluating the effectiveness of new therapies. This article summarizes the design of clinical trials including their primary endpoint for IBS.

18.2 Evaluation of Symptoms

IBS is diagnosed based on subjective symptoms and by excluding structural diseases, and the treatment is aimed at improving the symptoms of IBS. More than 10 years earlier, the symptoms of patients were primarily evaluated by physicians. However, patients' symptom reporting had been believed to be very important to evaluate the severity of symptoms. It has been reported [6] that there were significant differences between physician and patient assessment of health-related quality of life (HR-QOL) among patients with prostate cancer. Patients' symptom reporting is essential to evaluate the severity of symptoms, and it is highly important to assess the effectiveness of IBS therapies. The visual analogue scale (VAS) or Likert scale is used to rate the severity of IBS symptoms such as abdominal pain and abdominal distension. Moreover, there are several questionnaires for evaluating functional gastrointestinal disorders (FGIDs), including IBS, to assess their subjective symptoms (Table 18.1). The Gastrointestinal Symptom Rating Scale [7], which is designed to evaluate common gastrointestinal symptoms, consists of 15 items that generate the 5 subscales of gastroesophageal reflux, abdominal pain, indigestion, diarrhea, and constipation. It was originally developed to evaluate dyspeptic symptoms but was later validated in patients with IBS. The IBS severity scoring system (IBS-SSS) [8], a digestive symptom frequency questionnaire (DSFQ) [9], and the IBS quality of life (IBS-QOL) [10, 11] are generally used for patients with IBS to evaluate IBS-specific symptoms and HR-QOL, respectively. The IBS-SSS consists of five items: severity of abdominal pain, frequency of abdominal pain, severity of abdominal distension, dissatisfaction with bowel habits, and interference with quality of life over the past 10 days. Each item is rated according to severity on a 100-point VAS ranging from 0 to 500. Patients with IBS are categorized as having mild (75–175), moderate (175–300), or severe (>300) disease. The IBS-QOL is a 34-question survey that evaluates the degree to which IBS interferes with the quality of life of a

Table 18.1 Questionnaires for IBS patients

Gastrointestinal symptoms rating scale (GSRS)	IBS severity index (IBS-SI)
Functional bowel disease severity index (FBDSI)	IBS severity scoring system (IBS-SSS)
Digestive symptom frequency questionnaire (DSFQ)	IBS quality of life (IBS-QOL)
Izumo scale for abdominal symptom related QOL	Social functioning-36 (SF-36)
Hospital anxiety and depression scale (HADS)	State-trait anxiety inventory (STAI)
Psychological general well-being index (PGWB)	
Hamilton depression rating Scale (HDRS)	

subject over the past 30 days. Each item is rated on a 1–5 Likert scale, with higher scores indicating a lower QOL. In addition, questionnaires on anxiety/depression in psychometry such as the Hospital Anxiety and Depression Scale (HADS) [12], State-Trait Anxiety Inventory (STAI) [13], the Social Functioning-36 (SF-36) [14], and the Psychological General Well-Being Index (PGWB) [15] are useful for evaluating the degree of psychological disturbance related to the pathophysiology in patients with IBS.

The Food and Drug Administration (FDA) released a general guidance [16] for the evaluation of symptom benefit in clinical trials based on patient-reported outcome (PRO) measures in 2006. A PRO is the measurement of any aspect of a patient's health status that is derived directly from the patient's response outcome (i.e., without the interpretation of the patients' responses by a physician or anyone else). The process for developing new or for modifying existing instruments for clinical trials is as follows [17, 18]. The starting point in developing a valid and meaningful outcome measure is to identify concepts and to construct a conceptual framework. This is followed by the creation of the instrument in closing the generation of items, choice of the administration method and response scales, formatting the instrument, pilot testing of the draft instrument, and refinement of the instrument and procedure. The next step is the evaluation of the measurement of properties, such as score reliability, validity, and ability to detect change. After finalizing the instrument formats, scoring, procedures, and training materials, the process of modifying the instrument is completed. The European Medical Agency (EMA) also said that any outcome directly evaluated by the patients themselves and based on patients' perception of a disease and its treatment(s) is known as a PRO. The SPIRIT (Standard Protocol Items: Recommendations for Interventional Trials) PRO-specific guidelines [19], which were published in 2018, provide recommendations for items that should be addressed in clinical trials in which PROs are primary or key secondary outcomes. Improving the design of clinical trials, including PROs, could help ensure high-quality data. The FDA emphasizes that PROs must be embedded in a conceptual framework. However, there are few PROs in IBS development based on an explicit conceptual framework, and an uncertainty exists on how best to measure PROs in IBS. Spiegel et al. [20] applied the FDA guidance to develop a conceptual framework for measuring the physical symptom experience in IBS. Symptom experience may be determined by 35-item categories within the 5 domains of pain, gas/bloating, diarrhea, constipation, and extraintestinal symptoms. They concluded that the framework can be applied to develop and initially validate a novel PRO for use in future IBS clinical trials. These PRO measures had a major influence on trial designs in IBS.

18.3 Clinical Study Design

Clinical treatment trials on IBS have not yet been established sufficiently, although there have been substantial advances in several aspects of clinical trial design after the publication of Rome III criteria. IBS is a symptom-based disease without specific biomarkers, and there are still several uncertain factors regarding how to conduct the best clinical trials incorporating symptom variability. As there are no "gold standard" treatments for IBS, candidate drugs are generally compared with placebo. Today, the double-masked, placebo-controlled, parallel group design remains the accepted standard for evaluating treatment efficacy. Other designs have also been generally implemented. For instance, crossover designs are sometimes used in IBS clinical trials. Patients receive both treatments during a distinct time period, separated by a washout phase, in a randomized order to compare the treatments. The trial of equivalence or noninferiority is sometimes performed whenever a new therapy is more convenient or less expensive.

Placebo effects [21] can be defined as "the beneficial effects that are attributable to the responses of the patient to the context in which the treatment is delivered, rather than to specific actions of the treatment." Placebo effect is a common phenomenon in clinical research, and there are several possible associated factors, such as the quality of the relationship between patients and physicians and the frequency of visit. Using placebo as a control is the gold standard in randomized controlled trials (RCTs). In general, treatment is considered to be effective when it is proven to be superior to placebo in clinical trials. However, FGIDs, including IBS, are known to have high placebo response rates [22–24] than those of organic diseases such as gastrointestinal cancers with objective markers. Patients-physicians interaction plays a vital role in the pathophysiology of FGIDs. Ford et al. [25] reported that the pooled placebo response rate in 73 RCTs of IBS was 37.5% (95% confidence internal 34.4–40.6%). Estimates of placebo response rates in randomized controlled IBS pharmacological trials are approximately 40%. Several factors may be associated with placebo effects, and several reviews have attempted to identify them in IBS. Ballou et al. [26] identified variations in baseline pain symptom, severity of baseline symptoms, and early improvement of abdominal pain as the baseline factors associated with placebo response in female patients with IBS with constipation (IBS-C). In terms of study duration, the results have been a controversial issue. Some reviews found that longer study duration is associated with higher placebo response rates, whereas others suggest that shorter study duration predicts higher response rates. Spiller et al. [22] demonstrated that placebo response rates increased from trial entry and then decreased with time peaking at 8–12 weeks and that the optimum duration of a trial was probably >3 months. Hence, IBS clinical trials of <7 weeks are not recommended. Moreover, it is believed that the placebo effect of psychological interventions [27], such as cognitive behavioral therapy and hypnotherapy, is larger than that of pharmacological interventions. We must carefully consider the psychological impact of being entered into a placebo-controlled trial. Several approaches such as using a run-in period and a longer study period with less frequent follow-up visits should be attempted to investigate how to minimize placebo response across RCTs of therapies in IBS. A placebo run-in period implies that all patients receive placebo for a specified time period, and their responses are evaluated using study outcome measures to evaluate patient eligibility. Patients who show significant improvement during this period are excluded before treatment. It is very important to ensure that RCTs are designed to reduce placebo response.

18.4 Endpoints

There are several novel treatment approaches for IBS according to the different mechanisms of action. In particular, several new drugs in development are being investigated in ongoing or planned clinical trials for IBS. These new drugs would be approved by regulatory agencies based on achieving the primary endpoint in phase III trials. Secondary endpoints support or explain the results of the primary outcome in clinical trials. The primary endpoints for evaluating drug efficacy in IBS trials have changed over the past two decades. A systematic review conducted before the publication of Rome IV [1] and Rome III [2] criteria supported the use of binary endpoints as a standard primary outcome for IBS clinical trials. The binary endpoint incorporating overall assessment of adequate, satisfactory, or considerable relief provides a dichotomous responder status of yes/no. Several high-quality RCTs on IBS have used a binary endpoint that evaluated the global effects of medications or a global improvement scale. An overall assessment of adequate relief has been used as a primary endpoint in treatment trials with alosetron, cilansetron, and tegaserod. However, the FDA presented the guidance [28] with a focus on providing interim endpoints and recommendations for IBS clinical trials in 2012. According to the FDA guidance on PRO, the effects of treatment on the severity of a specific sign or symptom are not completely captured by overall measures. The FDA recommended evaluating a co-primary endpoint that focuses on the two major IBS symptoms of abdominal pain and abnormal defecation for assessing the efficacy of pharmacological treatments in IBS. The standard 11-point numeric rating scale should be used to measure abdominal pain in IBS. For abnormal defecation, the FDA recommended measuring stool frequency for trials on IBS-C and measuring stool form using the Bristol Stool Form Scale (BSFS) [29, 30] for trials on IBS with diarrhea (IBS-D). The most recent updated the European Medicines Agency (EMA) guideline [31] primarily follows the same principles as the co-primary endpoint (Table 18.2). It was reported [32] that the FDA-recommended co-primary endpoints yielded similar responder rates as those by the EMA-recommended co-primary endpoints, whereas the binary endpoint of adequate relief generated higher response rates. In Japan, the Evidence-based Clinical Practice Guidelines for IBS, based on the Rome III criteria and the increasing knowledge on the differences between Japan and Western countries, were published in Japanese in 2014 and English in 2015 [4], updated in 2020 [5]. IBS therapy aims to improve IBS symptoms according to these Japanese clinical practice guidelines for IBS (Table 18.3). Assessment of PROs is recommended although no worldwide consensus has been reached.

We investigated the primary endpoint of 20 high-quality RCTs on IBS in 5 high-citation journals of *Gastroenterology*, *Clinical Journal of Gastroenterology*, *Gut*, *American Journal of Gastroenterology* (AJG), and *Alimentary Pharmaceutical and Therapeutics* (APT) from 2015 to 2017 (Table 18.4). The co-primary endpoints of abdominal pain and abnormal defecation according to the FDA guideline were used in 4 of 20 studies. Three studies were published in USA journals (*Gastroenterology*, CGH, and AJG), and one study was published in a European journal (APT). Other

Table 18.2 Primary endpoints of IBS clinical trials in both FDA and EMA guideline

FDA
Co-primary endpoints
IBS-C
• Abdominal pain intensity (0–10 11-point scale, at least 30% compared with baseline)
• Stool frequency (increase of one or more CSBM per week compared with baseline)
IBS-D
• Abdominal pain intensity (0–10 11-point scale, at least 30% compared with baseline)
• Stool frequency (using BSFS, decrease at least 50% in the number of days per week with at least one stool that has a consistency of type 6 or 7 compared with baseline)
EMA
Co-primary endpoint
IBS-C
• Abdominal pain intensity (11-point scale, improved at least 30% compared with baseline)
• Stool frequency (increase of at least 1 CSBM per week compared to baseline)
IBS-D
• Abdominal pain intensity (11-point scale, improved at least 30% compared with baseline)
• Stool frequency (using BSFS, at least 50% reduction in the number of days with at least one stool that has a consistency of 6 or 7 compared to baseline)
IBS-M, IBS-unsubtyped, mixed IBS-C and IBS-D populations
• Global assessment of efficacy scale of the highest improvement
• Abdominal pain score (Improved at least 30% compared to baseline)

FDA Food and Drug Administration, *EMA* European Medicines Agency, *IBS-C* IBS with predominant constipation, *IBS-D* IBS with predominant diarrhea, *IBS-M* mixed IBS, *BSFS* Bristol Stool Form Scale

Table 18.3 The aim of IBS therapy in Japanese clinical guidelines for IBS [4]

CQ. Is the aim of IBS therapy improvement of IBS symptoms?
• The aim of IBS therapy is improvement of IBS symptoms
• Strong recommendation, evidence level A, grade 1, 100% agreed

studies used overall IBS symptoms, global symptom improvement, satisfactory relief, or adequate relief of IBS symptoms as the primary endpoint. Three studies used the co-primary endpoints of overall IBS symptoms and abdominal pain/discomfort, overall IBS symptoms and increased stool consistency, and adequate symptom relief and stool *Bifidobacterium* species concentration. Recently, two new drugs, ramosetron and linaclotide, were approved for treating IBS in Japan. Ramosetron, a potent and selective 5-hydroxytriptamine 3 (5-HT_3) receptor antagonist, was approved in 2008 for male patients with IBS-D and in 2015 for female patients with IBS-D. The primary endpoint of the first Japanese phase III study of ramosetron was overall improvement rating in IBS symptoms, whereas the global assessment of relief of overall IBS symptoms and improvement in stool consistency measured by BSFS were used as co-primary endpoints [33] for female patients. Linaclotide, which acts as a novel activator of guanylate cyclase C, was approved for treating IBS-C in 2017. The co-primary endpoints of the Japanese phase III [34]

Table 18.4 The primary endpoint of 20 high-quality RCTs on IBS in 5 high-citation journals

	Gastro	Gut	AJG	CGH	APT
Overall IBS symptoms	2	2	1	1	3
Satisfactory relief of IBS symptoms Change in overall GI symptoms Adequate relief of IBS symptoms Global symptoms improvement					
Satisfactory relief of abdominal pain/discomfort		1			
Total score on GSRS-IBS			1		
Abdominal pain frequency					1
CSBMs			1		
Co-primary					
FDA guidance	1		1	1	1
Overall IBS symptoms and abdominal pain/discomfort	1				
Adequate symptom relief and stool bifidobacterium conc.	1				
Overall IBS symptoms and increased stool consistency	1				

RCT randomized controlled trial, *Gastro* gastroenterology, *AJG* American Journal of Gastroenterology, *CGH* clinical gastroenterology and hepatology, *APT* aliment pharmacology and therapy

study of linaclotide were global improvement of IBS symptoms and complete spontaneous bowel movement. These co-primary endpoints were approved by the Japanese pharmaceutical medical device agency. The primary endpoint should be clinically meaningful and demonstrate the efficacy of therapeutic agents. Further studies are required to determine the best endpoint in IBS clinical trials.

References

1. Lacy BE, Mearin F, Chang L, Chey WD, Lembo AJ, Simren M, Spiller R. Bowel disorder. Gastroenterology. 2016;150:1393–407.
2. Longstreth GF, Thompson WG, Chey WD, Houghton LA, Mearin F, Spiller RC. Functional bowel disorders. Gastroenterology. 2006;130:1480–91.
3. Thompson WG, Longstreth GF, Drossman DA, Heaton KW, Irvine EJ, Müller-Lissner SA. Functional bowel disorders and functional abdominal pain. Gut. 1999;45(Suppl2):1143–7.
4. Fukudo S, Kaneko H, Akiho H, Inamori M, Endo Y, Okumura T, Kanazawa M, Kamiya T, Sato K, Chiba T, Furuta K, Yamato S, Arakawa T, Fujiyama Y, Azuma T, Fujimoto K, Mine T, Miura S, Kinoshita Y, Sugano K, Shimosegawa T. Evidence-based clinical practice guidelines for irritable bowel syndrome. J Gastroenterol. 2015;50:11–50.
5. Fukudo S, Okumura T, Inamori M, Okuyama Y, Kanazawa M, Kamiya T, Sato K, Shiotani A, Naito Y, Fujikawa Y, Hokari R, Masaoka T, Fujimoto K, Kaneko H, Torii A, Matsueda K, Miwa H, Enomoto N, Shimosegawa T, Koike K. Evidence-based clinical practice guidelines for irritable bowel syndrome 2020. J Gastroenterol. 2021;56:193–217.
6. Litwin MS, Lubeck DP, Henning JM, Carroll PR. Differences in urologist and patient assessments of health related quality of life in men with prostate cancer: results of the CaPSURE database. J Urol. 1998;159:1988–92.
7. Svedlund J, Sjodin I, Dotevall G. GSRS-a clinical rating scale for gastrointestinal symptoms in patients with irritable bowel syndrome and peptic ulcer disease. Dig Dis Sci. 1998;33:129–34.

8. Francis CY, Moris J, Whorwell PJ. The irritable bowel severity scoring system: a simple method of monitoring irritable bowel syndrome and its progress. Aliment Pharmacol Ther. 1997;11:395–402.
9. Azpiroz F, Guyonnet D, Donazzolo Y, Gendre D, Tanguy J, Guarner F. Digestive symptoms in healthy people and subjects with irritable bowel syndrome: validation of symptom frequency questionnaire. J Clin Gastroenterol. 2015;49:64–70.
10. Patrick DL, Drossman DA, Frederick IO, DiCesare J, Puder KL. Quality of life in persons with irritable bowel syndrome: development and validation of a new measure. Dig Dis Sci. 1998;43:400–11.
11. Drossman DA, Patrick DL, Whitehead WE, Toner BB, Diamant NE, Hu Y, Jia H, Bangdiwala SI. Further validation of the IBS-QOL: a disease-specific quality-of-life questionnaire. Am J Gastroenterol. 2000;95:999–1007.
12. Zigmond AS, Snaith RP. The hospital anxiety and depression scale. Acta Psychiatr Scand. 1983;67:361–70.
13. Marteau TM, Bekker H. The development of a six-item short-form of the state scale of the Spielberger State-Trait Anxiety Inventory (STAI). Br J Clin Psychol. 1992;31:3010306.
14. Brazier JE, Harper R, Jones NM, Cathain A, Thomas KJ, Usherwood T, Westlake L. Validating the SF-36 health survey questionnaire: new outcome measure for primary care. BMJ. 1992;305:160–4.
15. Hunt SM, McKenna S. A British adaptation of the general well-being index: a new tool for clinical research. Br J Med Econ. 1992;2:49–60.
16. US Food and Drug Administration (FDA). Guidance for industry: patient-reported outcome measures-use in medical product development to support labeling claims. Health Qual Life Outcomes. 2006;4:79.
17. Camilleri M, Chang L. Challenges to the therapeutic pipeline for irritable bowel syndrome: endpoints and regulatory hurdles. Gastroenterology. 2008;135:1877–91.
18. Burke LB, Kennedy DL, Miskala PH, Papadopoulos EJ, Trentacosti AM. The use of patient-reported outcome measures in the evaluation of medical products for regulatory approval. Clin Pharmacol Ther. 2008;84:281–3.
19. Calvert M, Kyte D, Mercieca-Bebber R, Shade A, Chan AW, King MT, SPIRIT-PRO Group. Guidelines for inclusion of patient-reported outcomes in clinical protocols. The SPIRIT-PRO extension. JAMA. 2018;319:483–93.
20. Spiegel BM, Bolus R, Agarwal N, Sayuk G, Haris LA, Lucak S, Esrallian E, Chey WD, Lembo A, Karsan H, Tillsch K, Talley J, Chang L. Measuring symptoms in the irritable bowel syndrome: development of a framework for clinical trials. Aliment Pharmacol Ther. 2010;32:1275–91.
21. Kaptchuk TJ. Powerful placebo: the dark side of the randomized controlled trial. Lancet. 1998;351:1722–5.
22. Spiller RC. Problems and challenges in the design of irritable bowel syndrome clinical trials: experience from published trials. Am J Med. 1999;107:91S–7S.
23. Dorn SD, Kaptchuk TJ, Park JB, Nguyen LT, Canenguez K, Nam BH, Woods KB, Conboy LA, Stason WB, Lembo AJ. A meta-analysis of the placebo response in complementary and alternative medicine trials of irritable bowel syndrome. Neurogastroenterol Motil. 2007;19:630–7.
24. Miller LE. Study design considerations for irritable bowel syndrome clinical trials. Ann Gastroenterol. 2014;27:338–45.
25. Ford AC, Moayyedi P. Meta-analysis: factors affecting placebo response rate in the irritable bowel syndrome. Aliment Pharmacol Ther. 2010;32:144–58.
26. Ballou S, Beath A, Kaptchuk TJ, Hirsch W, Sommers T, Nee J, Iturrino J, Rangan V, Singh P, Jones M, Lembo A. Factors associated with response to placebo in patients with irritable bowel syndrome and constipation. Clin Gastroenterol Hepatol. 2018;16:1738–44.
27. Filk CE, Bakker L, Laan W, Rood YR, Smout AJ, de Wit NJ. Systematic review: the placebo effect of psychological interventions in the treatment of irritable bowel syndrome. World J Gastroenterol. 2017;23:2223–33.

28. US Department of Health and Human services Food and Drug Administration Center for Drug Evaluation and research (CDER). Guidance for industry. irritable bowel syndrome–clinical evaluation of drugs for treatment. 2012.
29. Levis SJ, Heaton KW. Stool form scale as a useful guide to intestinal transit time. Scand J Gastroenterol. 1997;32:920–4.
30. O'Donnell LJ, Virjee J, Heaton KW. Detection of pseudodiarrhoea by simple clinical assessment of intestinal transit rate. BMJ. 1990;300:439–40.
31. European Medicines Agency. Points to consider on the evaluation of medicinal product for the treatment of irritable bowel syndrome. Adopted guideline. 2012.
32. Corsetti M, Tack J. FDA and EMA end points: which outcome end points should we use in clinical trials in patients with irritable bowel syndrome? Neurogastroenterol Motil. 2013;25:453–7.
33. Fukudo S, Kinoshita Y, Okumura T, Ida M, Akiho H, Nakashima Y, Nishida A, Haruma K. Ramosetron reduces symptoms of irritable bowel syndrome with diarrhea and improves quality of life in women. Gastroenterology. 2016;150:358–66.
34. Fukudo S, Miwa H, Nakajima A, Haruma K, Kosako M, Nakagawa A, Akiho H, Yamaguchi Y, Johnston JM, Currie M, Kinoshita Y. A randomized controlled and long-term linaclotide study of irritable bowel syndrome with constipation patients in Japan. Neurogastroenterol Motil. 2018;30:e13444.

Chapter 19
Future Direction of Research and Treatment Possibility for Irritable Bowel Syndrome

Shin Fukudo, Yuhei Yamaguchi, Yuka Endo, Tomotaka Shoji, Shunya Moue, Kan Goto, Yasuhiro Sato, Tomohiko Muratsubaki, Michiko Kano, and Motoyori Kanazawa

Abstract There are many unsolved problems in the field of irritable bowel syndrome (IBS). Actually considerable patients with IBS do not respond to the standard treatments. This fact implies that we do not fully understand the pathogenesis and pathophysiology of IBS. Besides, treatment for IBS has not been completed systematically. Therefore, it is necessary to investigate unsolved aspects of pathogenesis and pathophysiology of IBS and develop new treatments for IBS in the very near future. The first point is whether Rome IV IBS patients are more homogenous in pathophysiology than Rome III IBS patients. The second point is whether there is more clinical merit

S. Fukudo (✉)
Department of Behavioral Medicine, Tohoku University Graduate School of Medicine, Sendai, Japan

Department of Psychosomatic Medicine, Tohoku University Hospital, Sendai, Japan

Research Center for Accelerator and Radioisotope Science, Tohoku University, Sendai, Japan

Department of Psychosomatic Medicine, Japanese Red Cross Ishinomaki Hospital, Ishinomaki, Japan
e-mail: shin.fukudo.c6@tohoku.ac.jp

Y. Yamaguchi · Y. Endo · T. Shoji · S. Moue · K. Goto · Y. Sato
Department of Psychosomatic Medicine, Tohoku University Hospital, Sendai, Japan
e-mail: yendo@hosp.tohoku.ac.jp; tshoji@hosp.tohoku.ac.jp; shunya.moue.e6@tohoku.ac.jp; kan.goto.a2@tohoku.ac.jp; yassat@hosp.tohoku.ac.jp

T. Muratsubaki · M. Kano
Department of Behavioral Medicine, Tohoku University Graduate School of Medicine, Sendai, Japan
e-mail: t-mura@med.tohoku.ac.jp

M. Kanazawa
Department of Behavioral Medicine, Tohoku University Graduate School of Medicine, Sendai, Japan

Department of Psychosomatic Medicine, Tohoku University Hospital, Sendai, Japan
e-mail: m-kanazawa@med.tohoku.ac.jp

© The Editor(s) (if applicable) and The Author(s), under exclusive license to Springer Nature Singapore Pte Ltd. 2024

T. Kamiya, S. Fukudo (eds.), *Irritable Bowel Syndrome*,
https://doi.org/10.1007/978-981-97-8410-3_19

to diagnose IBS with Rome IV criteria than that to do with Rome III criteria. The most important things are to increase studies measuring pathophysiology of IBS including difference among IBS subtypes. Future direction of pathogenesis will be a combination of following factors: gut microbiota, stress, and susceptible genes. Future direction of treatment will be 5-HT3 antagonist, 5-HT4 agonist, intestinal secretagogues, ileal bile acid transporter inhibitor, sodium-glucose cotransporter 1 inhibitors, and many other novel agents and treatments. Research interest in IBS is largely expanding in the world. Further research including pathophysiology, pathogenesis, and treatment will improve the quality of life of IBS patients.

Keywords Irritable bowel syndrome · Pathophysiology · Pathogenesis · Treatment Rome IV criteria · Microbiota · Stress · Gene

Abbreviations

5-HT	5-hydroxytryptamine
CDH1	E-cadherin-1
CI	Confidence interval
COVID-19	Coronavirus disease 2019
CRH	Corticotropin-releasing hormone
CRH-BP	Corticotropin-releasing hormone binding protein
CRH-R1	Corticotropin-releasing hormone receptor 1
CRH-R2	Corticotropin-releasing hormone receptor 2
FBD	Functional bowel disorder
FGF	Fibroblast growth factor
FXR	Farnesoid X receptor
GLUL	Glutamine synthetase
GPER	G protein-coupled estrogen receptor
GRID2IP	Glutamate receptor, ionotropic, delta 2-interacting protein
IBAT	Ileal bile acid transporter
IBS	Irritable bowel syndrome
IBS-C	Irritable bowel syndrome with predominant constipation
IBS-D	Irritable bowel syndrome with predominant diarrhea
IBS-M	Irritable bowel syndrome with mixed bowel habits
IBS-U	Irritable bowel syndrome unclassified
IL	Interleukin
JSGE	Japanese Society of Gastroenterology
KDELR2	KDEL endoplasmic reticulum protein retention receptor 2

NK2	Neurokinin-2
PAR	Protease-activated receptor
QOL	Quality of life
SARS-CoV-2	Severe acute respiratory syndrome coronavirus-2
SGLT-1	Sodium-glucose cotransporter 1
TLR	Toll-like receptor
TNFSF15	Tumor necrosis factor superfamily member 15
TRPM8	Transient receptor potential melastatin 8
TSPO	Translocator protein 18 kDa

19.1 Introduction: Future Direction

There are many unsolved problems in the field of irritable bowel syndrome (IBS). Actually considerable patients with IBS do not respond to the standard treatments [1]. This fact implies that we do not fully understand the pathogenesis and pathophysiology of IBS. Besides, treatment for IBS has not been completed systematically. Therefore, it is necessary to investigate unsolved aspects of pathogenesis and pathophysiology of IBS and develop new treatments for IBS in the very near future.

19.2 Future Direction of Pathophysiology

Research on IBS was substantially developed after the publication of Rome I criteria [2]. The most recent definition and diagnostic criteria for IBS is Rome IV [3]. Internationally unified diagnostic criteria have been useful to erase the heterogeneity of the study population of IBS. Simultaneous epidemiological survey in the world indicated that prevalence of IBS is 4.1% [4]. This prevalence is lower than that (10.1%) of IBS diagnosed with Rome III criteria [5]. Thus, Rome IV criteria are apparently stringent criteria to diagnose IBS. Two things must be considered in the future direction of pathophysiology of IBS after using the stringent criteria.

The first point is whether Rome IV IBS patients [4] are more homogenous in pathophysiology than Rome III IBS patients [5]. Unfortunately, biological studies which compare Rome IV IBS patients with Rome III IBS patients are lacking. However, there are several studies on clinical features of Rome III IBS patients comparing between Rome IV-positive subjects and Rome IV-negative subjects [6, 7]. In the Dutch study with 404 IBS patients, Rome IV positive subjects were more often female, younger, more recruited from secondary/tertiary care, higher abdominal pain scores and gastrointestinal symptom severity, higher psychological symptom scores, and lower quality of life (QOL) [6]. We performed large populational internet survey with 30,000 subjects in Japan which identified 428 Rome III IBS with constipation (IBS-C) subjects with abdominal pain or discomfort more than once per week [7]. Among them, 126 (29.4%) surrogate Rome IV-positive IBS-C subjects and 302 (70.6%) surrogate Rome IV-negative IBS-C (unspecified functional bowel disorder, FBD) subjects were identified [7]. Surrogate Rome IV-positive IBS-C subjects had more anxiety than surrogate Rome IV-negative IBS-C subjects (FBD) especially in women and 20–49 ages [7]. These studies suggest that Rome IV IBS patients are severer especially on the psychological aspects than Rome III IBS patients.

The second point is whether there is more clinical merit to diagnose IBS with Rome IV criteria than that to do with Rome III criteria. The original idea of Rome I criteria was that unified diagnostic criteria for IBS would facilitate IBS research [2]. The concept was realized in general [1, 3–5, 8]. However, diagnostic criteria must be scientifically concordant with understanding of objective measure of the disease. One distinct disease will have the essential cause and pathophysiology of a disease. By the time of Rome III criteria, subtyping of IBS as IBS-C, IBS with diarrhea (IBS-D), IBS with mixed bowel habits (IBS-M), and unclassified IBS (IBS-U) was useful to develop therapeutic agents depending on the dominant bowel habits [9, 10]. By contrast, Rome IV criteria for IBS and its related disorders were conceptualized as the spectrum disorders [3, 8]. This conceptualization allows us to treat IBS-C patients and patients with functional constipation with the same agents that are effective on the phenomena to cause constipation. The same things are true in IBS-D patients and patients with functional diarrhea. Because the stringent diagnostic criteria of IBS reduced prevalence of IBS [4, 9], it is reasonable to have chance to diagnose Rome III IBS patients as either functional constipation, functional diarrhea, or unspecified FBD instead of diagnosing IBS with Rome IV criteria. From the first point above and the point of view on spectrum disorders, one practical merits of diagnosing IBS with Rome IV may be earlier application of neurological and/or psychobehavioral treatments.

The most important things are to increase studies measuring pathophysiology of IBS. Even though diagnostic criteria were internationally unified, IBS remains “syndrome.” It is still unknown whether IBS is a cruster of several diseases or not. Subtyping of IBS into IBS-C, IBS-D, IBS-M, and IBS-U seems to be successful to develop new agents [10, 11]. However, it is only partially true. There is no approved agents which target to patients with IBS-M or IBS-U. Moreover, a study that followed the phenotypic changes in dominant bowel patterns for 15 months revealed only 25% patients with IBS-C and those with IBS-C remaining the same subtypes [12]. Remaining 75% patients with IBS changed the dominant bowel patterns during the follow-up time [12]. Patients with IBS-C, IBS-M/U, and IBS-D showed statistically delayed, intermediate, and rapid whole gut transit time [13]. Besides, only 15% of IBS-C patients have abnormally delayed gut transit time, and 36% of IBS-D patients have abnormally rapid gut transit time [13]. Biological markers of IBS subtypes are explored, and some candidates of them are toll-like receptor 2 (TLR2) and toll-like receptor 4 (TLR4) [14]. IBS-M patients show increased expression of TLR2 and TLR4 in the colonic mucosa resulting immune activation via increase in interleukin-1β and interleukin 8 [14]. From these studies, at least in part on the dominant bowel habits, IBS subtypes may have different pathophysiology.

There are also several studies that express IBS patients have common pathophysiology regardless of subtypes. In a study using colonic barostat and manometry, IBS patients had visceral hypersensitivity compared with healthy controls [15]. IBS patients also showed increased colonic motility in response to colonic distention or meal ingestion compared with healthy controls [15]. However, there was no difference in visceral hypersensitivity or reflex colonic motility response to distention or meal loading among IBS subtypes [15]. IBS patients showed increased mucosal permeability regardless of IBS subtypes [16]. Lower expression of zonula occludens-1 (ZO-1) and α-catenin was also detected in IBS and quiescent inflammatory bowel diseases (IBD) with IBS-like symptoms [16]. Further studies are necessary to identify the pathognomonic findings of IBS per se.

19.3 Future Direction of Pathogenesis

At least on IBS, probably no further development of science would be expected from the repetition of revision of symptoms-based diagnosis. The realistic way of research is fixation or, if we have any necessity to do so, minor arrangement with limited degree, of Rome IV criteria for a while. Because Rome IV-defined IBS patients are more concentrated population than Rome III-defined IBS patients [4, 6, 7, 9], objective biomarkers should be accumulated extensively for a longer time. This approach will enable us to identify the etiological or pathogenic factors of IBS. From the knowledge accumulated by the present time [1], pathogenesis of IBS would be combination of following factors: gut microbiota, stress, and susceptible genes.

The role of gut microbiota as well as the other microorganisms in the pathogenesis of IBS has been proven by the existence of postinfectious IBS [17, 18]. The great mystery exists in the cause of postinfectious IBS. Although infectious acute gastroenteritis is reported to trigger the newly generated IBS [18], specificity of pathogens for developing postinfectious IBS is still unknown. Recent systematic review and meta-analyses examined the pooled prevalence and odds ratios of representative pathogens, i.e., *Campylobacter* spp., *Salmonella* spp., *Shigella* spp., *Escherichia coli*, *Clostridium difficile*, norovirus, rotavirus, *Cryptosporidium* spp., or *Giardia intestinalis* [19]. Pooled prevalence of IBS after the infection of the specific pathogen was as follows: *Campylobacter* spp.: 12% (confidence interval 95% [CI]: 10–15%), *Salmonella* spp.: 12% (CI: 9–15%), *Shigella* spp.: 11% (CI: 8–15%), *Clostridium difficile*: 14% (CI: 4–29%), and *Escherichia coli* spp.: 12% (CI: 5–20%) [19]. Odds ratio of IBS after *Salmonella* infection was 5.5 (CI: 2.3–12.8) and that after *Shigella* infection was 13.8 (CI: 4.2–45.4). Odds ratio of IBS after overall bacterial acute gastroenteritis showed 5.8 (CI: 4.0–8.3) and that after acute gastroenteritis caused by any pathogen revealed 4.9 (CI: 3.9–6.1) [19]. Thus, at this moment, there is no obvious evidence that proves the high-risk pathogens at the timing of acute gastroenteritis for IBS.

IBS patients as a group or as some subtypes show altered gut microbiota [20, 21]. The previous study from our group disclosed that IBS patients have increased abundance of *Lactobacillus* spp. and *Veillonella* spp. in the feces [21]. Combination of these two microbiota resulted in increased fecal concentration of acetic acid and propionic acid [21]. Moreover, IBS symptoms worsened depending on the fecal acetic/propionic acid concentration [21]. There is no study to bridge between the insult by the acute gastroenteritis and commensal bacteria in the gut lumen in IBS patients. However, microbial differences appear to underlie between IBS-D and IBS-C [22]. Mechanistically, the pathogens that cause gastroenteritis and trigger subsequent IBS development produce a common toxin, cytolethal distending toxin B, and antibodies raised against this toxin cross-react with the cytoskeletal protein vinculin and impair gut motility, facilitating bacterial overgrowth in IBS-D patients [22]. Methane gas produced by methanogenic archaea slows intestinal contractility, which may facilitate the development of constipation in IBS-C patients [22]. Detailed analyses are necessary to clarify the biological mechanism from the bacterial infection to development of IBS.

The role of stress in pathogenesis of IBS has been repeatedly reported. Regression coefficient between psychosocial stress and abdominal symptoms in IBS patients is steeper than that in healthy controls or in patients with other functional bowel disorders [23]. A history of sexual and physical abuse is a frequent experience in women seen in referral-based gastroenterology practice and is particularly common in those with functional gastrointestinal disorders including IBS [24]. Systematic reviews and meta-analyses revealed that early psychosocial stress is surely a risk factors of IBS [25, 26]. However, the mechanism of stress-induced onset and/or exacerbation of IBS is only partially explored. One of the candidates to contribute to the development of IBS is serotonin (5-hydroxytryptamine: 5-HT) and allied molecules including serotonin transporter, 5-HT_3 receptors, 5-HT_4 receptors, and so on [27]. The other candidate is corticotropin-releasing hormone (CRH) and relating substances including CRH receptor 1 (CRH-R1), CRH receptor 2 (CRH-R2), CRH binding protein (CRH-BP), glucocorticoid receptors, and so on [27, 28]. Brain imaging studies clarified the certain role of these substances [29, 30]. Structural changes of the neurons with relation to these molecules are suggested in IBS [31]. The next step is proving etiological roles of these substances.

There are some candidate genes in IBS. A relatively large number study comparing monozygotic twins with dizygotic twins clarified the existence of heredity in IBS [31]. To date, representative studies reported the following genes to be associated with IBS: α_{2A} (C-1291G), α_{2C} (Del 332-325), GNβ_3 (C825T)[32], serotonin transporter [32–35], 5-HT_3 receptor [36], mitochondrial DNA 7028C [37], CRH, CRH-BP [38], CRH-R1 [39, 40], CRH-R2 [41], TLR-9, interleukin-6 (IL-6), E-cadherin-1 (CDH1) [42], excessive expression of micro-RNA-29a for glutamine synthetase (GLUL) [43], G298S mutation of SCN5A for sodium channel Nav1.5 [44], tumor necrosis factor superfamily member 15 (TNFSF15) [45], KDEL endoplasmic reticulum protein retention receptor 2 (KDELR2), and glutamate receptor, ionotropic, delta 2 (Grid2) interacting protein (GRID2IP) [46]. Among them, KDELR2 and GRID2IP were identified from the genome-wide association study with a relatively large number of patients in the Europe and the United States [46]. Although the function of these genes are still unknown, KDELR2 and GRID2IP are suggested to be related to signal transduction of the bacterial toxin and neurotoxin which activates cholinergic neurons [46]. Adrenergic α_{2A} receptor (C-1291G), α_{2CA} receptor (Del 332-325), GNβ_3 (C825T) [32], serotonin transporter [32–35], 5-HT3 receptor [36], CRH, CRH-BP [38], CRH-R1 [39, 40], and CRH-R2 [41] are regulating molecules of the neurons. Therefore, these genes may play a role in stress physiology at the onset of IBS. TLR-9, IL-6, and CDH1 are identified molecule from patients with postinfectious IBS [42]. Apparently this is phenomenon of gene-environment interaction [47]. There also is another combination of pathogenic factors. Anxiety and

Table 19.1 Treatment options for irritable bowel syndrome

Q	Step	Subtype	Contents	Recommendation	Level
BQ1-1			Prevalence		
BQ1-2			Postinfectious IBS		
BQ1-3			Stress		
BQ1-4			Microbiota, mucosal permeability, low-grade inflammation		
BQ1-5			Neurotransmitters, endocrine substances		
BQ1-6			Psychological disturbance		
BQ1-7			Genetics		
BQ1-8			Pathophysiology among C, D, M, and U subtypes		
BQ2-1			Diagnosis based on Rome IV criteria		
CQ2-1			Colonoscopy	Weak	B
CQ2-2			Laboratory tests for differential diagnosis	Strong	B
CQ2-3			Some clinical tests for identifying IBS	Weak	B
CQ2-4			Laboratory tests for follow-up	Strong	A
CQ3-1	1		Diet therapy	Weak	B
CQ3-2	1		Behavioral modification: exercise	Weak	B
CQ3-3	1		Bulking polymer/dietary fiber	Strong	A
CQ3-4	1		Gastrointestinal motility modifiers	Weak	B
CQ3-5	1		Anticholinergics	Weak	B
CQ3-6	1		Probiotics	Strong	A
CQ3-7	1	D	5-HT3 receptor antagonists	Strong	A
CQ3-8	1	D	Antidiarrheal agents	Weak	C
CQ3-9	1	C	Intestinal secretagogues	Strong	A
CQ3-10	1	C	Bile acids/ileal bile acid transporter inhibitor	Weak	B
CQ3-11	1	C	5-HT4 agonists	Weak	B
CQ3-12	1	C	Non-stimulant (osmotic) laxatives	Weak	C

(continued)

Table 19.1 (continued)

Q	Step	Subtype	Contents	Recommendation	Level
CQ3-13	1	C	Stimulant laxatives, on-demand use	Weak	D
CQ3-14	2		Antidepressants	Weak	A
CQ3-15	2		Anxiolytics for a short period	Weak	B
CQ3-16	3		Psychotherapy	Strong	B
CQ3-17	1/2		*Kampo*	Weak	C
CQ3-18	1/2		Anti-allergic agents	Strong	A
CQ3-19	1/2		Antibiotics	Weak	A
CQ3-20	2		Comprehensive alternative medicine: peppermint oil	Weak	A
CQ3-21	2		Narcotics	Weak no	C
CQ3-22	1-3		Preventing patients from leaving without treatment	Weak	C
FRQ3-1	2/3		Anti-psychotics, mood stabilizers		
FRQ3-2	2/3		Fecal microbiota transplantation		
FRQ3-3	1-3		Severity-dependent treatment		
BQ4-1			Quality of life, healthcare-seeking behavior		
BQ4-2			Comorbidity with FD, GERD, or IBD		
BQ4-3			Comorbidity with extraintestinal disorders		

BQ background question, *CQ* clinical question, *FRQ* future research question, *5-HT* 5-hydroxytryptamine, *FD* functional dyspepsia, *GERD* gastroesophageal reflux disease, *IBD* inflammatory bowel disease, *Level A* high evidence, *Level B* moderate evidence, *Level C* low evidence, *Level D* very low evidence, *Step 1* first step in the therapeutic algorithm, *Step 2* second step in the therapeutic algorithm, *Step 3* third step int therapeutic algorithm, *Subtype C* constipation-predominant IBS, *Subtype D* diarrhea-predominant IBS

Summarized from the [55], JSGE clinical practice guidelines 2020

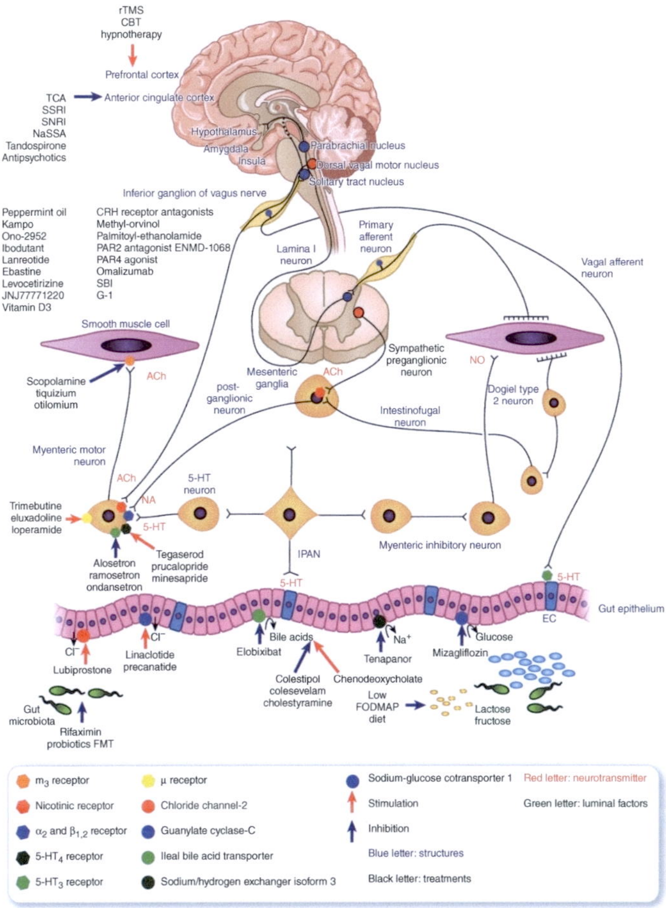

Fig. 19.1 Mechanistic schema of present and possible treatments for irritable bowel syndrome. The figure illustrated site of actions of therapeutic agents with special reference to the brain-gut interactions. The gut epithelium is the boundary the inside (shown upper 4/5) and the outside (shown lower 1/5) of the human body. Foods pass from oral (left) to aboral (right) site. Mechanical and/or chemical stimulation to enterochromaffin cells (EC) releases 5-hydroxytryptamine (5-HT) which stimulates intrinsic primary afferent neurons (IPAN). The signal which is conducted to the aboral side releases nitric oxide (NO), resulting relaxation of the smooth muscle cells. The signal which is conducted to the oral side releases 5-HT, stimulating 5-HT_4 and 5-HT_3 receptors in the surface of excitatory motor neurons in the myenteric plexus. The motor neurons releases acetylcholine (ACh) which makes smooth muscle cells contract. Exaggerated contractions and/or impaired accommodations cause gut dysmotility and raise the gut intraluminal pressure which cause excitation of the primary afferent neurons. There are the other pathways to stimulate afferent neurons: increased mucosal permeability, low-grade inflammation, and gut dysbiosis. The visceral pain signal ascends lamina I neurons in the dorsal horn and via the parabrachial nucleus it spreads to the specific regions of the brain. *rTMS* repetitive transcranial magnetic stimulation, *CBT* cognitive behavioral therapy, *TCA* tricyclic antidepressants, *SSRI* selective serotonin reuptake inhibitor, *SNRI* serotonin noradrenaline reuptake inhibitor, *NaSSA* noradrenergic and specific serotonergic antidepressant, *CRH or CRF* corticotropin-releasing hormone, *PAR* protease-activated receptor, *SBI* serum-derived bovine immunoglobulin/protein isolate, *NA* noradrenaline, *FMT* fecal microbiota transplantation, *FODMAP* fermentable oligosaccharides, disaccharides, monosaccharides, and polyols

depression presumably based on stress physiology are risk factors for postinfectious IBS [48]. Further research of additive or modifiable effects among gut microbiota, stress, and susceptible genes is warranted.

19.4 Future Direction of Treatment

There are many guidelines or consensus for the treatment of IBS [11, 49–53]. Among them, guidelines by the Japanese Society of Gastroenterology (JSGE) in 2014/2015 [11] were evaluated as the top 2 rank [54]. The Japanese version of clinical practice guidelines for IBS by JSGE was revised in 2020, and its English version was published in 2021 [55]. Apparently JSGE guidelines showed the most clinical questions and answers with grading system (Table 19.1) [55]. Future treatments for IBS patients will be in line with revising evidence and adding the new data of new therapies (Fig. 19.1).

19.5 5-HT$_3$ Antagonist

Alosetron was the first drug introduced for IBS-D women in the United States, but it was soon withdrawn due to severe constipation and ischemic colitis [50]. Now it was reintroduced under a risk evaluation and mitigation strategy for women suffering with severe IBS-D that is disabling. Some studies showed efficacy of ondansetron or cilansetron in IBS-D patients, but it has not been approved yet [49]. By contrast, ramosetron has high specificity to 5-HT$_3$ receptors, effective in IBS-D men [56] and IBS-D women [57, 58], and less serious side effects [59]. Ramosetron has been approved in Japan and several Asian countries [11, 51]. Because ramosetron is the only 5-HT$_3$ receptor antagonist that can be administered to men and women with IBS-D, it had better get available in the worldwide.

19.6 5-HT$_4$ Agonist

Tegaserod was the first drug introduced for IBS-C women in the United States, but it was withdrawn due to ischemic heart disease [50]. Now it was reintroduced for IBS-C women under 65 years old [60]. Prucalopride is indicated for chronic constipation but can be used for constipating symptoms in IBS-C patients [51]. Mosapride facilitates human gastric accommodation [61] and colonic motility [62] measured with gastric and colonic barostat. Mosapride is only indicated for patients with chronic gastritis or patients needed colon cleansing in Japan and several Asian countries. Although efficacy has not been proven with phase III trial, a novel 5-HT$_4$ receptor agonist minesapride showed improvement of symptoms in IBS-C patients in Japan [63, 64].

19.7 Intestinal Secretagogues

Lubiprostone is a chloride channel-2 activator which enhances fluid secretion from the intestinal epithelium and improves constipating symptoms [65]. It is also effective in IBS-C patients [66]. In Western countries, lower dose for IBS-C patients is indicated than the usual dose for chronic idiopathic constipation [49, 50, 52]. Linaclotide is a guanylate cyclase C receptor agonist resulting increased fluid secretion in the lower gastrointestinal tract [67]. In Western countries, optimal dose of linaclotide is higher for IBS-C patients than for patients with chronic idiopathic constipation [49, 50, 52]. By contrast in Japan, there were no difference in an optimal dose of linaclotide between IBS-C patients [67, 68] and patients with chronic idiopathic constipation [69, 70]. Plecanatide is the similar drug to linaclotide with different amino acid sequence [71]. Tenapanor is a sodium/hydrogen exchanger 3 inhibitor for IBS-C in the United States [71]. Based on the risk of severe dehydration, it is contraindicated for pediatric patients below 6 years of age.

19.8 IBAT Inhibitor and Related Substances

Elobixibat is an ileal bile acid transporter (IBAT) inhibitor which blocks ileal absorption of bile acids by interrupting the enterohepatic circulation of bile acids and increasing the flow of bile acids into the colon [72]. Increasing colonic bile acids causes mucosal fluid secretion and enhances colonic motor activity. A Japanese study in patients with chronic constipation including IBS-C disclosed that elobixibat is effective to increase spontaneous bowel movement [72]. It is necessary to make sure whether abdominal pain is relieved by the administration of elobixibat. The relating treatment is oral administration of chenodeoxycholic acid to accelerate colonic transit time in IBS-C patients [73]. There are some trials using bile acid sequestrants including cholestyramine, colestipol, and colesevelam for IBS-D patients [71]. Farnesoid X receptor (FXR) agonist obeticholic acid is also expected to reduce bile acid synthesis via fibroblast growth factor (FGF)-19 [71].

19.9 SGLT-1 Inhibitor

Mizagliflozin is a sodium-glucose cotransporter 1 inhibitor [74]. The intestinal absorption of glucose is inhibited by the administration of mizagliflozin [75]. As a result, patients with chronic constipation including IBS-C showed relief of symptoms [74]. Therefore, SGLT-1 inhibition is a novel strategy to improve bowel movement.

19.10 Other Novel Agents and Treatments

International trials were performed to develop novel agents for IBS as follows [71]: opioid μ-receptor agonist and δ-receptor antagonist eluxadoline for IBS-D; opioid μ-and κ-receptor agonist and δ-receptor antagonist methyl-orvinol for IBS; cannabinoid 2 and peroxisome proliferator-activated receptor-α (PPAR-α) receptors agonist palmitoylethanolamide for IBS; neurokinin-2 (NK2) receptor antagonist ibodutant for IBS-D; translocator protein 18 kDa (TSPO) antagonist ONO-2952 for IBS; somatostatin analogs lanreotide for idiopathic refractory diarrhea; histamine H1 receptor antagonists pyrilamine or ebastine for IBS; histamine H4 receptor antagonist levocetirizine or JNJ7777120 for IBS; transient receptor potential melastatin 8 (TRPM8) agonist peppermint oil for IBS; protease-activated receptor (PAR)-targeting molecules and serine protease inhibitors PAR2 antagonist (ENMD-1068), PAR-4 agonist (PAR-4-AP, Cat-G, AYPGKF-NH2), aprotinin, cathepsin-G inhibitor, and soybean trypsin inhibitor for IBS; vitamin D3 for IBS; immunoglobulin E blocker omalizumab for IBS; serum-derived bovine immunoglobulin/protein isolate therapy for IBS-D; G protein-coupled estrogen receptor (GPER) agonist G-1 for IBS; and estradiol, a nonselective ER agonist for IBS.

There are some attempts to develop CRH receptors antagonist, to find more efficacious probiotics, to produce evidence of fecal microbiota transplantation, to extend approval of rifaximin to IBS, and Kampo medicine for IBS [76]. A little evidence was reported in serotonin noradrenaline reuptake inhibitors (SNRI), noradrenergic and specific serotonergic antidepressant (NaSSA), atypical antipsychotics, or mood stabilizers [11, 55]. More effective programs of psychotherapy including cognitive behavioral therapy (CBT) are being developed [77, 78]. Based on neurological understanding of brain-gut interactions in IBS [79], neuromodulation like repetitive transcranial magnetic stimulation (rTMS) will be applied in the near future [80, 81].

19.11 Further Future Research

As described above, progression of pathophysiology or pathogenesis and that in treatment is not always harmonized in IBS research. Probably that is because IBS development is multifactorial [1], because IBS consists of many different diseases, or because present treatments modify only pathophysiology without diminishing pathogenetic factors. In the near future, concordant placebo-controlled randomized clinical trials with a large number of patients including pathophysiological and pathogenetic factors will solve this problem.

The last topic is coronavirus disease 2019 (COVID-19) which is a life-threatening infectious disease caused by severe acute respiratory syndrome coronavirus-2 (SARS-CoV-2) all over the world [82]. Considerable rate (17.6%) of patients with COVID-19 showed positive gastrointestinal symptoms including diarrhea, abdominal pain, and constipation [82]. Fecal specimen revealed positive viral RNA in 25.4% of 59 patients. Meta-analysis from 138 patients indicated 48.1% positive viral RNA from the stool. Pediatric COVID-19 patients showed 80% positive viral RNA in their fecal samples [83]. A life-threatening condition and social isolation by SARS-CoV-2 infection cause definitely stressful situation. Whether epithelial damage and inflammation due to SARS-CoV-2 together with psychosocial stress also cause more postinfectious IBS than other viruses or not should be examined.

19.12 Conclusion: Future Direction

Research interest in IBS is largely expanding in the world. Further research including pathophysiology, pathogenesis, and treatment will improve QOL of IBS patients.

Grant Support This research was supported by Grant-in-Aid for Scientific Research from the Ministry of Education, Science, and Culture of Japan, Grant-in-Aid for Scientific Research from the Ministry of Health, Welfare, and Labor of Japan, SRF, and AMED-Moon Shot 20356688.

Employment No conflict of interests.

Personal Financial Interests All authors declares no conflict of interest with any companies on this article. SF declares the potential conflict of interest but no direct relationship to this article with the following companies; Astellas, Biofermin, EA pharma, Mylan EPD, Tsumura, and Zespri.

References

1. Enck P, Aziz Q, Barbara G, Farmer A, Fukudo S, Mayer E, Niesler B, Quigley E, Rajilic-Stojanović M, Schemann M, Schwille-Kiuntke J, Simren M, Zipfel S, Spiller R. Irritable bowel syndrome (IBS). Nat Rev Dis Prim. 2016;2:16014.
2. Thompson WG, Creed F, Drossman DA, Heaton KW, Mazzacca G. Functional bowel disorders and functional abdominal pain. Gastroenterol Int. 1992;5:75–91.
3. Lacy BE, Mearin F, Chang L, Chey WD, Lembo AJ, Simren M, Spiller R. Bowel disorders. Gastroenterology. 2016;150:1393–407.
4. Sperber AD, Bangdiwala SI, Drossman DA, Ghoshal UC, Simren M, Tack J, Whitehead WE, Dumitrascu DL, Fang X, Fukudo S, Kellow J, Okeke E, Quigley EM, Schmulson M, Whorwell P, Archampong T, Adibi P, Andresen V, Benninga MA, Bonaz B, Bor S, Fernandez LB, Choi SC, Corazziari ES, Francisconi C, Hani A, Lazebnik L, Lee YY, Mulak A, Rahman MM, Santos J, Setshedi M, Syam AF, Vanner S, Wong RK, Lopez-Colombo A, Costa V, Dickman R, Kanazawa M, Keshteli AH, Khatun R, Maleki I, Poitras P, Pratap N, Stefanyuk O, Thomson S, Zeevenhooven J, Palsson OS. Worldwide prevalence and burden of functional gastrointestinal disorders, results of Rome Foundation global study. Gastroenterology. 2021;160:99–114.
5. Longstreth GF, Thompson WG, Chey WD, Houghton LA, Mearin F, Spiller RC. Functional bowel disorders. Gastroenterology. 2006;130:1480–91.
6. Vork L, Weerts ZZRM, Mujagic Z, Kruimel JW, Hesselink MAM, Muris JWM, Keszthelyi D, Jonkers DMAE, Masclee AAM. Rome III vs Rome IV criteria for irritable bowel syndrome:

a comparison of clinical characteristics in a large cohort study. Neurogastroenterol Motil. 2018;30:13189. https://doi.org/10.1111/nmo.13189.
7. Kosako M, Akiho H, Miwa H, Kanazawa M, Fukudo S. Influence of the requirement for abdominal pain in the diagnosis of irritable bowel syndrome with constipation (IBS-C) under the Rome IV criteria using data from a large Japanese population-based internet survey. BioPsychoSoc Med. 2018;12:18.
8. Drossman DA, Hasler WL. Rome IV - functional GI disorders: disorders of gut-brain interaction. Gastroenterology. 2016;150:1257–61.
9. Palsson OS, Whitehead W, Törnblom H, Sperber AD, Simren M. Prevalence of Rome IV functional bowel disorders among adults in the United States, Canada, and the United Kingdom. Gastroenterology. 2020;158:1262–73.
10. Kux L. Department of Health and Human Services, Food and Drug Administration [docket no. FDA–2012–D–0146]: guidance for industry on irritable bowel syndrome—clinical evaluation of drugs for treatment: availability. Fed Regist. 2012;77:32124–5.
11. Fukudo S, Kaneko H, Akiho H, Inamori M, Endo Y, Okumura T, Kanazawa M, Kamiya T, Sato K, Chiba T, Furuta K, Yamato S, Arakawa T, Fujiyama Y, Azuma T, Fujimoto K, Mine T, Miura S, Kinoshita Y, Sugano K, Shimosegawa T. Evidence-based clinical practice guidelines for irritable bowel syndrome. J Gastroenterol. 2015;50:11–30.
12. Drossman DA, Morris CB, Hu Y, et al. A prospective assessment of bowel habit in irritable bowel syndrome in women: defining an alternator. Gastroenterology. 2005;128:580–9.
13. Törnblom H, Van Oudenhove L, Sadik R, et al. Colonic transit time and IBS symptoms: what's the link? Am J Gastroenterol. 2012;107:754–60.
14. Belmonte L, Beutheu Youmba S, Bertiaux-Vandaële N, et al. Role of toll like receptors in irritable bowel syndrome: differential mucosal immune activation according to the disease subtype. PLoS One. 2012;7:e42777.
15. Kanazawa M, Palsson OS, Thiwan SI, et al. Contributions of pain sensitivity and colonic motility to IBS symptom severity and predominant bowel habits. Am J Gastroenterol. 2008;103:2550–61.
16. Vivinus-Nébot M, Frin-Mathy G, Bzioueche H, Dainese R, Bernard G, Anty R, Filippi J, Saint-Paul MC, Tulic MK, Verhasselt V, Hébuterne X, Piche T. Functional bowel symptoms in quiescent inflammatory bowel diseases: role of epithelial barrier disruption and low-grade inflammation. Gut. 2014;63:744–52.
17. Gwee KA, Graham JC, McKendrick MW, Collins SM, Marshall JS, Walters SJ, Read NW. Psychometric scores and persistence of irritable bowel after infectious diarrhoea. Lancet. 1996;347:150–3.
18. Spiller R, Garsed K. Postinfectious irritable bowel syndrome. Gastroenterology. 2009;136:1979–88.
19. Svendsen AT, Bytzer P, Engsbro AL. Systematic review with meta-analyses: does the pathogen matter in post-infectious irritable bowel syndrome? Scand J Gastroenterol. 2019;54:546–62.
20. Tana C, Umesaki Y, Imaoka A, et al. Altered profiles of intestinal microbiota and organic acids may be the origin of symptoms in irritable bowel syndrome. Neurogastroenterol Motil. 2010;22:512–9.
21. Pimentel M, Lembo A. Microbiome and its role in irritable bowel syndrome. Dig Dis Sci. 2020;65:829–39.
22. Kassinen A, Krogius-Kurikka L, Mäkivuokko H, et al. The fecal microbiota of irritable bowel syndrome patients differs significantly from that of healthy subjects. Gastroenterology. 2007;133:24–33.
23. Whitehead WE, Crowell MD, Robinson JC, et al. Effects of stressful life events on bowel symptoms: subjects with irritable bowel syndrome compared with subjects without bowel dysfunction. Gut. 1992;33:825–30.
24. Drossman DA, Leserman J, Nachman G, Li ZM, Gluck H, Toomey TC, Mitchell CM. Sexual and physical abuse in women with functional or organic gastrointestinal disorders. Ann Intern Med. 1990;113:828–33.

25. Chitkara DK, van Tilburg MA, Blois-Martin N, Whitehead WE. Early life risk factors that contribute to irritable bowel syndrome in adults: a systematic review. Am J Gastroenterol. 2008;103:765–74.
26. Afari N, Ahumada SM, Wright LJ, Mostoufi S, Golnari G, Reis V, Cuneo JG. Psychological trauma and functional somatic syndromes: a systematic review and meta-analysis. Psychosom Med. 2014;76:2–11.
27. Fukudo S. Stress and visceral pain: focusing on irritable bowel syndrome. Pain. 2013;154(Suppl 1):S63–70.
28. Fukudo S. Hypothalamic-pituitary-adrenal axis in gastrointestinal physiology. In: Johnson L, editor. Physiology of the gastrointestinal tract. 5th ed. Oxford: Elsevier; 2012. p. 795–815.
29. Tanaka Y, Kanazawa M, Kano M, Morishita J, Hamaguchi T, Van Oudenhove L, Ly HG, Dupont P, Tack J, Yamaguchi T, Yanai K, Tashiro M, Fukudo S. Differential activation in amygdala and plasma noradrenaline during colorectal distention by administration of corticotropin-releasing hormone between healthy individuals and patients with irritable bowel syndrome. PLoS One. 2016;11:e0157347.
30. Kano M, Muratsubaki T, Van Oudenhove L, Morishita J, Yoshizawa M, Kono K, Yagihashi M, Tanaka Y, Mugikura S, Dupont P, Ly HG, Takase K, Kanazawa M, Fukudo S. Altered brain and gut responses to corticotropin-releasing hormone (CRH) in patients with irritable bowel syndrome. Sci Rep. 2017;7:12425.
31. Fukudo S. A neurological approach to biopsychosocial medicine: lessons from irritable bowel syndrome. BioPsychoSoc Med. 2011;5:1.
32. Camilleri M, Busciglio I, Carlson P, et al. Candidate genes and sensory functions in health and irritable bowel syndrome. Am J Physiol Gastrointest Liver Physiol. 2008;295:G219–25.
33. Fukudo S, Kanazawa M, Mizuno T, et al. Impact of serotonin transporter gene polymorphism on brain activation by colorectal distention. NeuroImage. 2009;47:946–51.
34. Kilpatrick LA, Mayer EA, Labus JS, Gupta A, Hamaguchi T, Mizuno T, Komuro H, Kano M, Kanazawa M, Aoki M, Fukudo S. Serotonin transporter gene polymorphism modulates activity and connectivity within an emotional arousal network of healthy men during an aversive visceral stimulus. PLoS One. 2015;10:e0123183.
35. Zhu Y, Zheng G, Hu Z. Association between SERT insertion/deletion polymorphism and the risk of irritable bowel syndrome: a meta-analysis based on 7039 subjects. Gene. 2018;679:133–7.
36. Kilpatrick LA, Labus JS, Coveleskie K, et al. The HTR3A polymorphism c. -42C>T is associated with amygdala responsiveness in patients with irritable bowel syndrome. Gastroenterology. 2011;140:1943–51.
37. Camilleri M, Carlson P, Zinsmeister AR, et al. Mitochondrial DNA and gastrointestinal motor and sensory functions in health and functional gastrointestinal disorders. Am J Physiol Gastrointest Liver Physiol. 2009;296:G510–6.
38. Sasaki A, Sato N, Suzuki N, Kano M, Tanaka Y, Kanazawa M, Aoki M, Fukudo S. Associations between single-nucleotide polymorphisms in corticotropin-releasing hormone-related genes and irritable bowel syndrome. PLoS One. 2016;11(2):e0149322.
39. Sato N, Suzuki N, Sasaki A, Aizawa E, Obayashi T, Kanazawa M, Mizuno T, Kano M, Aoki M, Fukudo S. Corticotropin-releasing hormone receptor 1 gene variants in irritable bowel syndrome. PLoS ONE. 2012;7:e42450.
40. Orand A, Naliboff B, Gadd M, Shih W, Ju T, Presson AP, Mayer EA, Chang L. Corticotropin-releasing hormone receptor 1 (CRH-R1) polymorphisms are associated with irritable bowel syndrome and acoustic startle response. Psychoneuroendocrinology. 2016;73:133–41.
41. Komuro H, Sato N, Sasaki A, Suzuki N, Kano M, Tanaka Y, Yamaguchi-Kabata Y, Kanazawa M, Warita H, Aoki M, Fukudo S. Corticotropin-releasing hormone receptor 2 gene variants in irritable bowel syndrome. PLoS One. 2016;11:e0147817.
42. Villani AC, Lemire M, Thabane M, et al. Genetic risk factors for post-infectious irritable bowel syndrome following a waterborne outbreak of gastroenteritis. Gastroenterology. 2010;138:1502–13.
43. Zhou Q, Souba WW, Croce CM, et al. MicroRNA-29a regulates intestinal membrane permeability in patients with irritable bowel syndrome. Gut. 2010;59:775–84.

44. Saito YA, Strege PR, Tester DJ, et al. Sodium channel mutation in irritable bowel syndrome: evidence for an ion channelopathy. Am J Physiol Gastrointest Liver Physiol. 2009;296:G211–8.
45. Czogalla B, Schmitteckert S, Houghton LA, Sayuk GS, Camilleri M, Olivo-Diaz A, Spiller R, Wouters MM, Boeckxstaens G, Bermejo JL, Niesler B. A meta-analysis of immunogenetic case-control association studies in irritable bowel syndrome. Neurogastroenterol Motil. 2015;27:717–27.
46. Ek WE, Reznichenko A, Ripke S, Niesler B, Zucchelli M, Rivera NV, Schmidt PT, Pedersen NL, Magnusson P, Talley NJ, Holliday EG, Houghton L, Gazouli M, Karamanolis G, Rappold G, Burwinkel B, Surowy H, Rafter J, Assadi G, Li L, Papadaki E, Gambaccini D, Marchi S, Colucci R, Blandizzi C, Barbaro R, Karling P, Walter S, Ohlsson B, Tornblom H, Bresso F, Andreasson A, Dlugosz A, Simren M, Agreus L, Lindberg G, Boeckxstaens G, Bellini M, Stanghellini V, Barbara G, Daly MJ, Camilleri M, Wouters MM, D'Amato M. Exploring the genetics of irritable bowel syndrome: a GWA study in the general population and replication in multinational case-control cohorts. Gut. 2015;64:1774–82.
47. Fukudo S, Kanazawa M. Gene, environment, and brain-gut interactions in irritable bowel syndrome. J Gastroenterol Hepatol. 2011;26(3):110–5.
48. Thabane M, Kottachchi DT, Marshall JK. Systematic review and meta-analysis: the incidence and prognosis of post-infectious irritable bowel syndrome. Aliment Pharmacol Ther. 2007;26:535–44.
49. Quigley EM, Fried M, Gwee KA, Khalif I, Hungin AP, Lindberg G, Abbas Z, Fernandez LB, Bhatia SJ, Schmulson M, Olano C, Le Mair A, Review Team. World Gastroenterology Organisation global guidelines irritable bowel syndrome: a global perspective update September 2015. J Clin Gastroenterol. 2016;50:704–13.
50. Ford AC, Moayyedi P, Chey WD, Harris LA, Lacy BE, Saito YA, Quigley EMM, ACG Task Force on Management of Irritable Bowel Syndrome. American College of Gastroenterology monograph on management of irritable bowel syndrome. Am J Gastroenterol. 2018;113(2):1–18.
51. Song KH, Jung HK, Kim HJ, Koo HS, Kwon YH, Shin HD, Lim HC, Shin JE, Kim SE, Cho DH, Kim JH, Kim HJ, Clinical Practice Guidelines Group Under the Korean Society of Neurogastroenterology and Motility, Clinical practice guidelines for irritable bowel syndrome in Korea, 2017 Revised Edition. J Neurogastroenterol Motil. 2018;24:197–215.
52. Moayyedi P, Andrews CN, MacQueen G, Korownyk C, Marsiglio M, Graff L, Kvern B, Lazarescu A, Liu L, Paterson WG, Sidani S, Vanner S. Canadian Association of Gastroenterology clinical practice guideline for the management of irritable bowel syndrome (IBS). J Can Assoc Gastroenterol. 2019;2:6–29.
53. Gwee KA, Gonlachanvit S, Ghoshal UC, Chua ASB, Miwa H, Wu J, Bak YT, Lee OY, Lu CL, Park H, Chen M, Syam AF, Abraham P, Sollano J, Chang CS, Suzuki H, Fang X, Fukudo S, Choi MG, Hou X, Hongo M. Second Asian consensus on irritable bowel syndrome. J Neurogastroenterol Motil. 2019;25:343–62.
54. Li H, Xing X, Yao L, Li M, Xun Y, Yan P, Yang X, Yang K. Assessment of the quality and content of clinical practice guidelines on irritable bowel syndrome using the AGREE II instrument. Digestion. 2020;101:355–65.
55. Fukudo S, Okumura T, Inamori M, Okuyama Y, Kanazawa M, Kamiya T, Sato K, Shiotani A, Naito Y, Fujikawa Y, Hokari R, Masaoka T, Fujimoto K, Kaneko H, Torii A, Matsueda K, Miwa H, Enomoto N, Shimosegawa T, Koike K. Evidence-based clinical practice guidelines for irritable bowel syndrome 2020. J Gastroenterol. 2021;56:193–217.
56. Fukudo S, Ida M, Akiho H, Nakashima Y, Matsuada K. Effect of ramosetron on stool consistency in male patients with irritable bowel syndrome with diarrhea. Clin Gastroenterol Hepatol. 2014;12:953–9.
57. Fukudo S, Matsueda K, Haruma K, Ida M, Hayase H, Akiho H, Nakashima Y, Hongo M. Optimal dose of ramosetron in female patients with irritable bowel syndrome with diarrhea: a randomized, placebo-controlled phase II study. Neurogastroenterol Motil. 2017;29:13023. https://doi.org/10.1111/nmo.13023.

58. Fukudo S, Kinoshita Y, Okumura T, Ida M, Akiho H, Nakashima Y, Nishida A, Haruma K. Ramosetron reduces symptoms of irritable bowel syndrome with diarrhea and improves quality of life in women. Gastroenterology. 2016;150:358–66.
59. Fukudo S, Kinoshita Y, Okumura T, Ida M, Hayashi K, Akiho H, Nakashima Y, Haruma K. Effect of ramosetron in female patients with irritable bowel syndrome with diarrhea: phase III, long-term study. J Gastroenterol. 2016;51:874–82.
60. Madia VN, Messore A, Saccoliti F, Tudino V, De Leo A, De Vita D, Bortolami M, Scipione L, Pindinello I, Costi R, Di Santo R. Tegaserod for the treatment of irritable bowel syndrome. Antiinflamm Antiallergy Agents Med Chem. 2020;19:342–69.
61. Amano T, Ariga H, Kurematsu A, Yamato S, Morioka S, Masaka A, Kanazawa M, Fukudo S. Effect of 5-hydroxytryptamine receptor 4 agonist mosapride on human gastric accommodation. Neurogastroenterol Motil. 2015;27:1303–9.
62. Kanazawa M, Watanabe S, Tana C, Komuro H, Aoki M, Fukudo S. Effect of 5-HT(4) receptor agonist mosapride citrate on rectosigmoid sensorimotor function in patients with irritable bowel syndrome. Neurogastroenterol Motil. 2011;23:754.
63. Fukudo S, Nakamura M, Hamatani T, Kazumori K, Miwa H. Efficacy and safety of 5-HT4 receptor agonist minesapride for irritable bowel syndrome with constipation in a randomized controlled trial. Clin Gastroenterol Hepatol. 2021;19:538–46.
64. Hamatani T, Fukudo S, Nakada Y, Inada H, Kazumori K, Miwa H. Randomised clinical trial: minesapride vs placebo for irritable bowel syndrome with predominant constipation. Aliment Pharmacol Ther. 2020;52:430–41.
65. Fukudo S, Hongo M, Kaneko H, Takano M, Ueno R. Lubiprostone increases spontaneous bowel movement frequency and quality of life in patients with chronic idiopathic constipation. Clin Gastroenterol Hepatol. 2015;13:249–301.
66. Fukudo S, Hongo M, Kaneko H, Ueno R. Efficacy and safety of oral lubiprostone in constipated patients with or without irritable bowel syndrome: a randomized, placebo-controlled and dose-finding study. Neurogastroenterol Motil. 2011;23:544.
67. Fukudo S, Nakajima A, Fujiyama Y, Kosako M, Nakagawa A, Akiho H, Nakashima Y, Johnston JM, Miwa H. Determining an optimal dose of linaclotide for use in Japanese patients with irritable bowel syndrome with constipation: a phase II randomized, double-blind, placebo-controlled study. Neurogastroenterol Motil. 2018;30:e13275.
68. Fukudo S, Miwa H, Nakajima A, Haruma K, Kosako M, Nakagawa A, Akiho H, Yamaguchi Y, Johnston JM, Currie M, Kinoshita Y. A randomized-controlled and long-term linaclotide study of irritable bowel syndrome with constipation patients in Japan. Neurogastroenterol Motil. 2018;30:e13444.
69. Fukudo S, Miwa H, Nakajima A, Kinoshita Y, Kosako M, Nakagawa A, Akiho H, Kuroishi K, Johnston JM, Currie M, Ohkusa T. Dose-finding study of linaclotide in Japanese patients with chronic constipation: a phase II randomized, double-blind, and placebo-controlled study. Neurogastroenterol Motil. 2018;30:e13442.
70. Fukudo S, Miwa H, Nakajima A, Kinoshita Y, Kosako M, Hayashi K, Akiho H, Kuroishi K, Johnston JM, Currie M, Ohkusa T. High-dose linaclotide is effective and safe in patients with chronic constipation: a phase III randomized, double-blind, placebo-controlled study with a long-term open-label extension study in Japan. Neurogastroenterol Motil. 2019;31:e13487.
71. Bharucha AE, Wouters MM, Tack J. Existing and emerging therapies for managing constipation and diarrhea. Curr Opin Pharmacol. 2017;37:158–66.
72. Nakajima A, Seki M, Taniguchi S, Ohta A, Gillberg PG, Mattsson JP, Camilleri M. Safety and efficacy of elobixibat for chronic constipation: results from a randomised, double-blind, placebo-controlled, phase 3 trial and an open-label, single-arm, phase 3 trial. Lancet Gastroenterol Hepatol. 2018;3:537–47.
73. Rao AS, Wong BS, Camilleri M, Odunsi-Shiyanbade ST, McKinzie S, Ryks M, Burton D, Carlson P, Lamsam J, Singh R, Zinsmeister AR. Chenodeoxycholate in females with irritable bowel syndrome-constipation: a pharmacodynamic and pharmacogenetic analysis. Gastroenterology. 2010;139:1549–58.

74. Fukudo S, Endo Y, Hongo M, Nakajima A, Abe T, Kobayashi H, Nakata T, Nakajima T, Sameshima K, Kaku K, Mizagliflozin Study Group. Safety and efficacy of the sodium-glucose cotransporter 1 inhibitor mizagliflozin for functional constipation: a randomised, placebo-controlled, double-blind phase 2 trial. Lancet Gastroenterol Hepatol. 2018;3:603–13.
75. Fukudo S, Kaku K. Effect of mizagliflozin on postprandial plasma glucose in patients with functional constipation. J Neurogastroenterol Motil. 2019;25:332–3.
76. Nakaya K, Nagura Y, Hasegawa R, Ito H, Fukudo S. Dai-Kenchu-To, a herbal medicine, attenuates colorectal distention-induced visceromotor responses in rats. J Neurogastroenterol Motil. 2016;22:686–93.
77. Kawanishi H, Sekiguchi A, Funaba M, Fujii Y, Yoshiuchi K, Kikuchi H, Kawai K, Maruo K, Sugawara N, Hatano K, Shoji T, Yamazaki T, Toda K, Murakami M, Shoji M, Ohara C, Tomita Y, Fukudo S, Ando T. Cognitive behavioral therapy with interoceptive exposure and complementary video materials for irritable bowel syndrome (IBS): protocol for a multicenter randomized controlled trial in Japan. BioPsychoSoc Med. 2019;13:14.
78. Funaba M, Kawanishi H, Fujii Y, Higami K, Tomita Y, Maruo K, Sugawara N, Oe Y, Kura S, Horikoshi M, Ohara C, Kikuchi H, Ariga H, Fukudo S, Sekiguchi A, Ando T. Hybrid cognitive behavioral therapy with interoceptive exposure for irritable bowel syndrome: a feasibility study. Front Psychiatry. 2021. https://doi.org/10.3389/fpsyt.2021.673939.
79. Tayama J, Saigo T, Ogawa S, Takeoka A, Hamaguchi T, Inoue K, Okamura H, Yajima J, Matsudaira K, Fukudo S, Shirabe S. Effect of attention bias modification on event-related potentials in patients with irritable bowel syndrome: a preliminary brain function and psycho-behavioral study. Neurogastroenterol Motil. 2018;30:e13402.
80. Aizawa Y, Morishita J, Kano M, Mori T, Izumi SI, Tsutsui K, Iijima T, Kanazawa M, Fukudo S. Effect of repetitive transcranial magnetic stimulation on rectal function and emotion in humans. J Gastroenterol. 2011;46:1071–80.
81. Aizawa Y, Morishita J, Kano M, Kanazawa M, Fukudo S. Modification of rectal function and emotion by repetitive transcranial magnetic stimulation in humans. Neurosci Res. 2021;168:54–63.
82. Cheung KS, Hung IF, Chan PP, Lung KC, Tso E, Liu R, Ng YY, Chu MY, Chung TW, Tam AR, Yip CC, Leung KH, Yim-Fong Fung A, Zhang RR, Lin Y, Cheng HM, Zhang AJ, To KK, Chan KH, Yuen KY, Leung WK. Gastrointestinal manifestations of SARS-CoV-2 infection and virus load in fecal samples from the Hong Kong cohort and systematic review and meta-analysis. Gastroenterology. 2020;159(1):81–95. https://doi.org/10.1053/j.gastro.2020.03.065.
83. Xu Y, Li X, Zhu B, Liang H, Fang C, Gong Y, Guo Q, Sun X, Zhao D, Shen J, Zhang H, Liu H, Xia H, Tang J, Zhang K, Gong S. Characteristics of pediatric SARS-CoV-2 infection and potential evidence for persistent fecal viral shedding. Nat Med. 2020;26:502–5.